THE BRUTAL ART OF RIPPING, POKING, AND PRESSING VITAL TARGETS

To my teachers, friends, and students in the martial arts: thank you for helping me search for simplicity.

THE BRUTAL ART OF RIPPING, POKING, AND PRESSING VITAL TARGETS

LOREN W. CHRISTENSEN

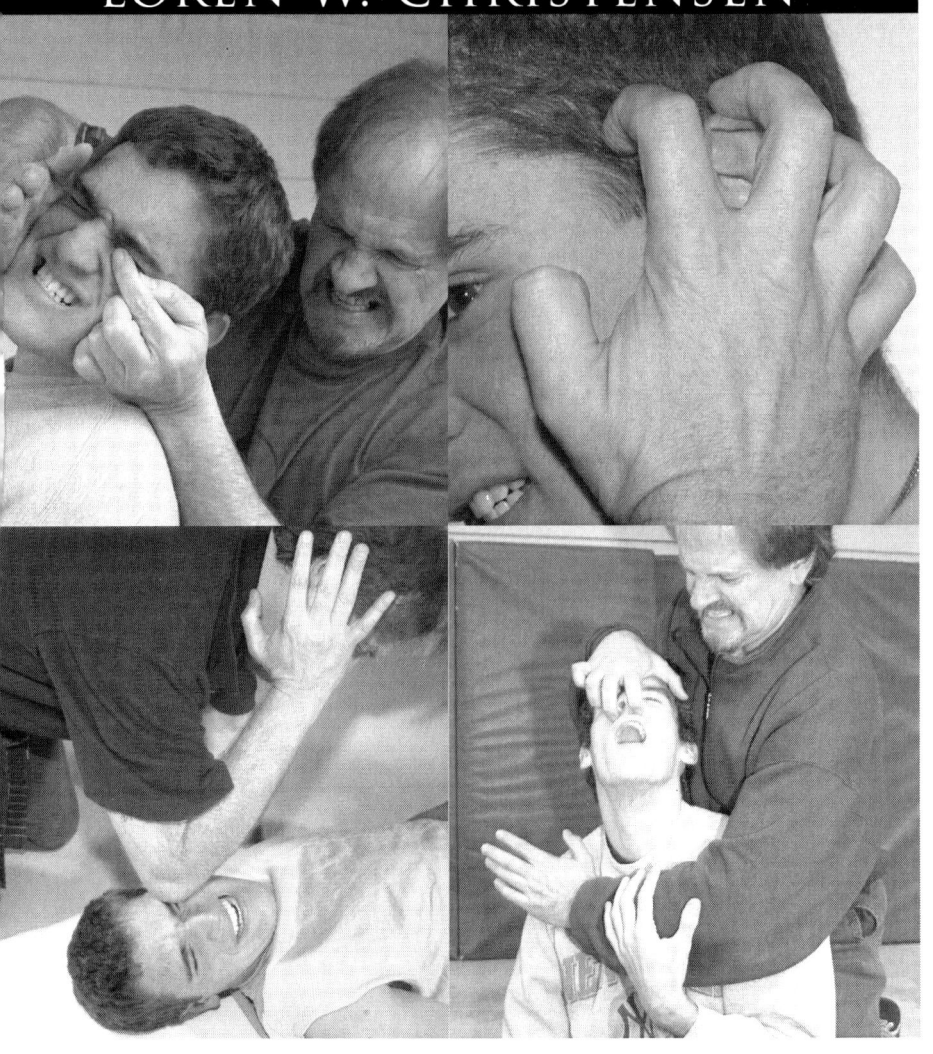

PALADIN PRESS · BOULDER, COLORADO

Also by Loren W. Christensen
Brutal Art of Ripping, Poking, and Pressing Vital Targets: The Video
Deadly Force Encounters
Extreme Joint Locking and Breaking
Fighter's Guide to Hard-Core Heavy Bag Training (with Wim Demeere)
Fighting Dirty (video)
Fighting in the Clinch (with Mark Mireles)
Fighting Power
Hookers, Tricks, and Cops
Restraint and Control Strategies (video)
Riot
Speed Training
Speed Training: The Video
Surviving a School Shooting
Surviving Workplace Violence
Vital Targets (video)

Brutal Art of Ripping, Poking, and Pressing Vital Targets
by Loren W. Christensen

Copyright © 2006 by Loren W. Christensen

ISBN 13: 978-0-87364-525-9
Printed in the United States of America

Published by Paladin Press, a division of Paladin Enterprises, Inc.
Gunbarrel Tech Center, 7077 Winchester Circle
Boulder, Colorado 80301 USA, +1.303.443.7250

Direct inquiries and/or orders to the above address.

PALADIN, PALADIN PRESS, and the "horse head" design are trademarks belonging to Paladin Enterprises and registered in United States Patent and Trademark Office.

All rights reserved. Except for use in a review, no portion of this book may be reproduced, stored in or introduced into a retrieval system, or transmitted in any form without the express written permission of the publisher. The scanning, uploading, and distribution of this book by the Internet or any other means without the permission of the publisher is illegal and punishable by law. Please respect the author's rights and do not participate in any form of electronic piracy of copyrighted material.

Neither the author nor the publisher assumes any responsibility for the use or misuse of information contained in this book.

Visit our website at www.paladin-press.com

Contents

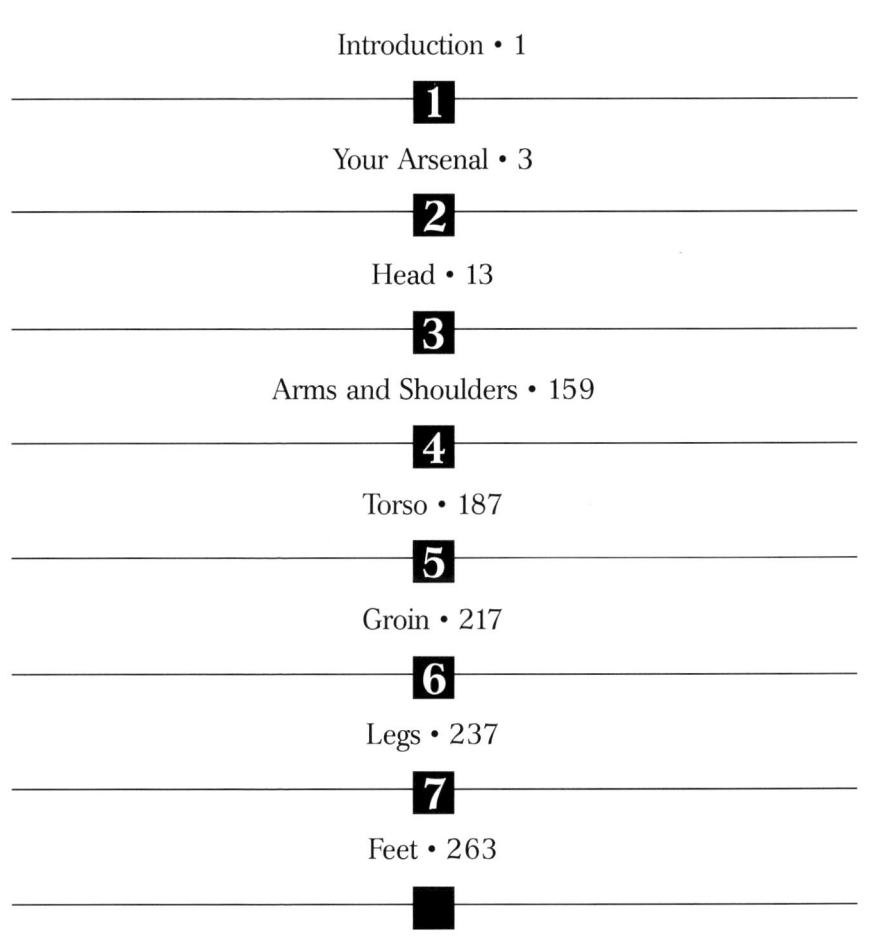

Introduction • 1

1
Your Arsenal • 3

2
Head • 13

3
Arms and Shoulders • 159

4
Torso • 187

5
Groin • 217

6
Legs • 237

7
Feet • 263

A Concluding Comment • 273

Warning

This book presents techniques designed to control and restrain through the application of pain. These techniques also have the potential to cause extreme injury, including damage to tendons, ligaments, and joints. In some cases, permanent injury or even death could result.

It is the reader's responsibility to research and comply with all laws regarding self-defense, justified use of force in defense of one's life, and related areas. The author, publisher, and distributors of this book disclaim any liability from any damage or injuries of any type that a reader or user of information contained in this book may incur or cause from its use or misuse. This book is presented *for academic study only.*

Acknowledgments

I give a respectful bow to all who generously volunteered their help, skill, critiques, and patience during the writing of this book and the long hours behind and in front of the camera. A big hug goes to my love, Lisa Place, for her patience and skill shooting most of the pics. A big thanks to:

Lisa Place
Dr. Dan L. Christensen
Mark Whited
Wim Demeere
Rock Dehon
Alex Larson
Max Brockbank
Oh, and to B.O.B., the dummy

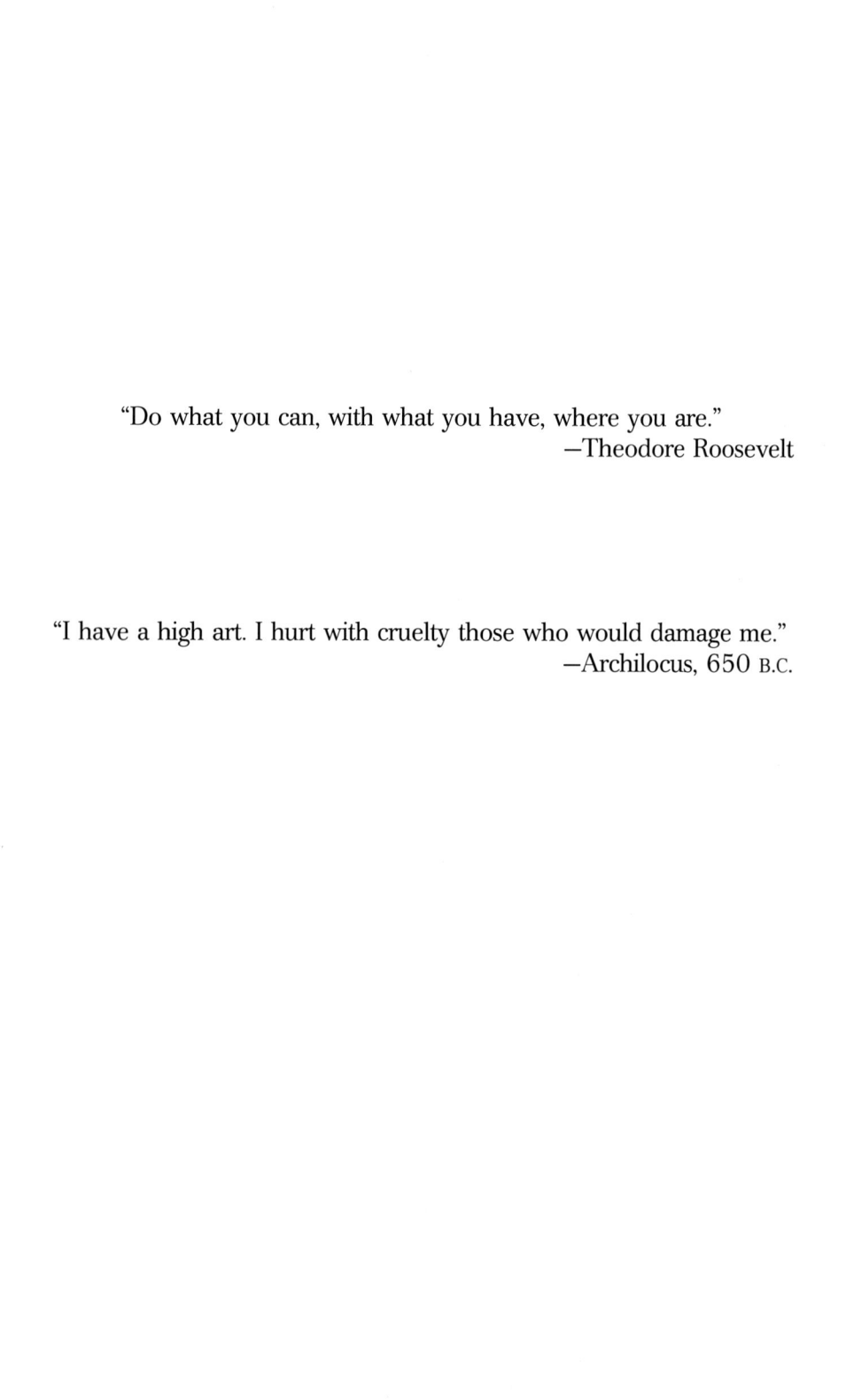

"Do what you can, with what you have, where you are."
—Theodore Roosevelt

"I have a high art. I hurt with cruelty those who would damage me."
—Archilocus, 650 B.C.

Introduction

". . . in every fight there is always the possibility that when one hand goes out it will come back red."

Interviewer to Woody Allen: "Do you think sex is dirty?"
Allen: "If it's done right, yes."

My personal path of martial arts study has evolved from using mostly power techniques (what I call my locomotive style) to one in which I now emphasize quick techniques delivered to the eyes, throat, ears, groin, nerve points, and other acutely vulnerable targets. This has led people not involved in the martial arts to ask me, "Isn't that dirty fighting?" To my amazement I've even been asked this by other martial artists. Now, I can understand it coming from a white-haired, canasta-playing senior citizen. But a martial artist? My answer to both groups is to paraphrase comedian Woody Allen: "If it's done right, yes, it is dirty fighting."

But then, all fighting is dirty. Ram your fist into someone's nose and his facial features momentarily distort as snot, saliva, and blood flies. He staggers back, trips, and falls with a sickening thump as his head meets the sidewalk. That's dirty. So is a powerful kick to the thigh that buckles the leg and sends the receiver down a flight of stairs, and so is an armbar that damages the tendons and ligaments around an elbow. A hard blow to the abdomen can make a guy upchuck his chili dog, and a hard slap to the face can disrupt his vision and send him stumbling over the furniture and into the fireplace.

I think the question of dirty fighting reveals much about the person asking. My guess is that he has had little to no experience fighting for real. If the questioner is a martial artist, no doubt he is a point fighting competitor for whom attacking these vital targets is considered a foul. Or, he practices a style where the students and the teacher are only fooling themselves into thinking that their "clean" techniques are going to help them in the ugliness that is a street fight.

As a military policeman in Saigon, Vietnam, and as a retired 25-year veteran of the Portland (Oregon) Police Bureau, I learned first-hand that there is nothing pretty or clean about brawling. It hurts, it's frightening, it's brutal, and it's ugly. Every fight has the potential for serious injury, even death. A shove or a trip can mean a nasty fall where a limb gets twisted and breaks, a skull hits something hard and cracks, or a torso lands on something sharp and gets punctured. In my nearly three decades working law enforcement, I saw many seemingly no-big-deal fights end tragically and I saw incredibly violent fights end with no one getting seriously hurt.

There is no way to know the outcome when two or more people enter battle. But in every fight there is always the possibility that when one hand goes out it will come back red.

For that reason you must bring to the fight every tool at your disposal and remove from your mind any thought that this technique or that one is dirty fighting. It's all about using the right tool at the right moment to finish the job.

The techniques in this book range from annoying to devastatingly destructive. Annoying techniques are used to distract an attacker and get him to shift in a certain direction so that you can execute other moves. Devastating techniques are used when there are no other options but to apply intense pain and potential injury.

I began studying the martial arts in 1965 and, ever since that first day, I have stolen techniques. If one works for the situation I'm in, I use it, and I couldn't care less if it came from China, Korea, Japan, or Kansas. Such is the case with this book. The techniques within this text have been lifted from a host of fighting styles over the years. Others, through trial and error, I made up, though I'm sure they exist in some fighting system somewhere.

My primary criteria for techniques included in this book are:

- They must be simple.
- They must hurt.
- They must be executable within just a few inches of space.
- They must give direction to the attacker.
- They must have psychological and physical shock value.

It's my hope that you find these techniques as useful as I have. And don't fret over dirty and clean. Just do what you've got to do to survive.

1
Your Arsenal

*". . . when we're talking about defending ourselves,
we ought to be in the right mind-set and use the right words."*

Many martial artists talk about their "fighter's toolbox," meaning their techniques, concepts, and principles. Frankly, I think this term is getting a little worn. When I hear the word toolbox I think of the plumber and the mechanic and that red, metal box they carry with all the unfolding drawers. But when I think of the warrior arts, I don't think of screwdrivers and wrenches. I think of an arsenal, a cache of weapons used to inflict leverage, pain, injury, and even death.

I know it's just semantics and I know I'm probably getting a little cantankerous, but I think that when talking about defending ourselves, we ought to be in the right mind-set and use the right words. I don't want to use a wrench out of my shiny red toolbox to tighten the lug nuts on my attacker's car. I want to choose the right weapons from my arsenal to crush his nuts, period. See the difference? I just think things ought to be straightforward in the fighting arts.

The following pages show some of the weapons you will use in this book . . .

PINCHING
Fingers

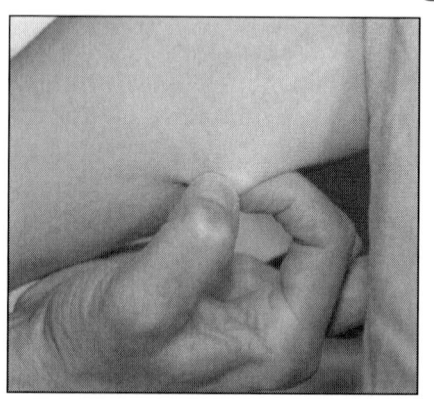

Figure 1

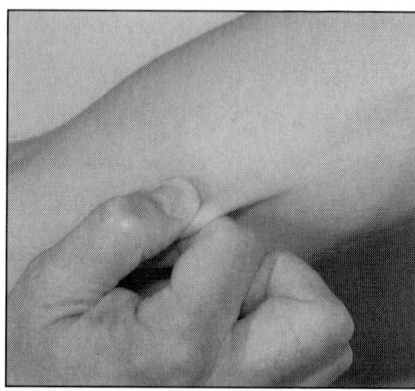

Figure 2

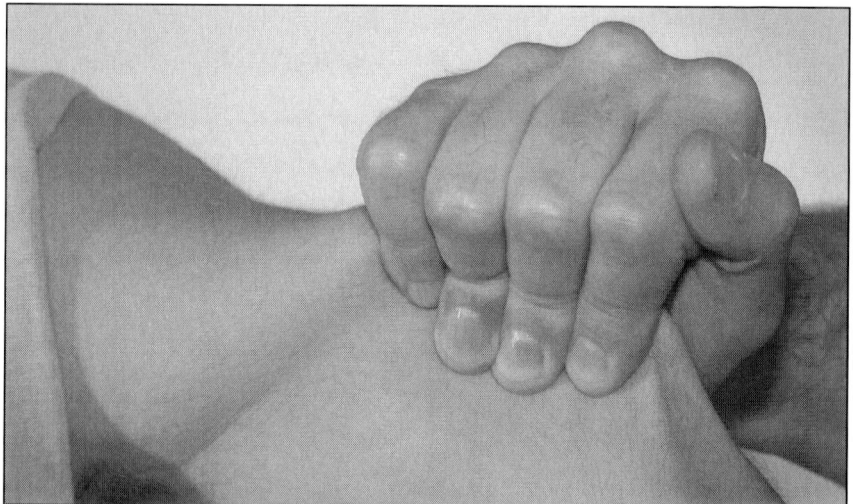

Figure 3

- Crab bite: Trap a tender piece of your attacker's skin between the fingernails of your thumb and index finger, or thumb and middle finger, and then dig in. (Fig. 1)
- Thumb and index finger: Trap a tender piece of your attacker's skin between the pad of your thumb and the middle section of your index finger, and squeeze. (Fig. 2)

Knees

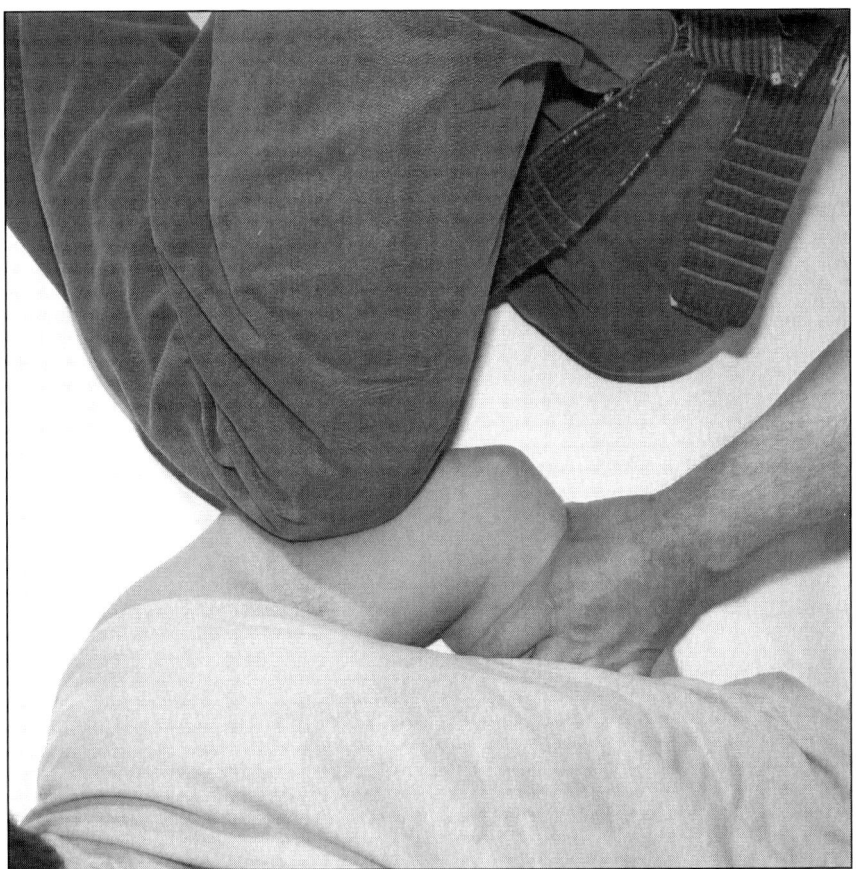

Figure 4

- Four-fingers-to-palm: Trap a large section of your attacker's tender skin or a tender muscle, and squeeze. You can press with the pads of your four fingers or use the nails to slice into the skin. (Fig. 3)
- Use your knee to press skin or muscles into a hard surface, usually the floor. (Fig. 4)

Heel of Foot

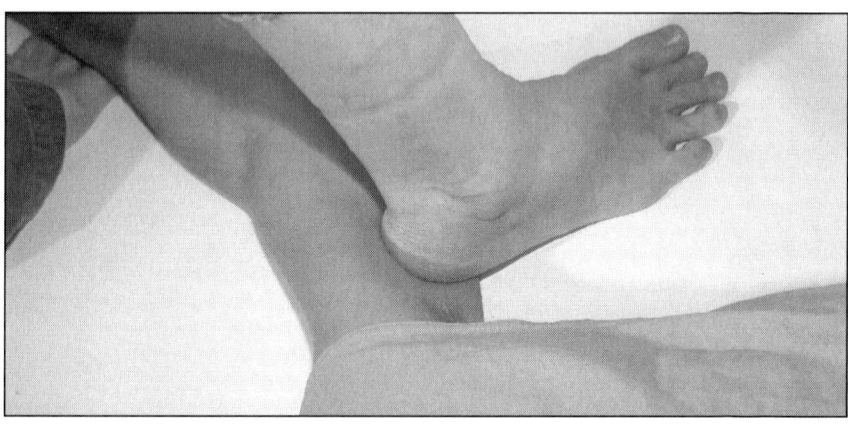

Figure 5

- Use your heel to pinch skin or muscle into a hard surface, usually the floor. (Fig. 5)

TWISTING
Fingers

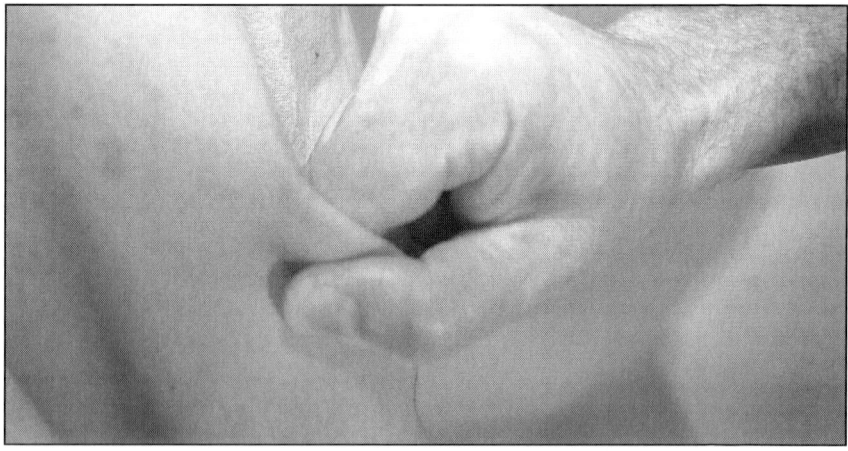

Figure 6

- Use the same grips as in "crab bite," "thumb and index finger," and "four-fingers-to-palm" to grab a section of skin, tendons, and muscles. Forcefully twist the flesh clockwise or counterclockwise. (Fig. 6)

RIPPING
Mantis Finger

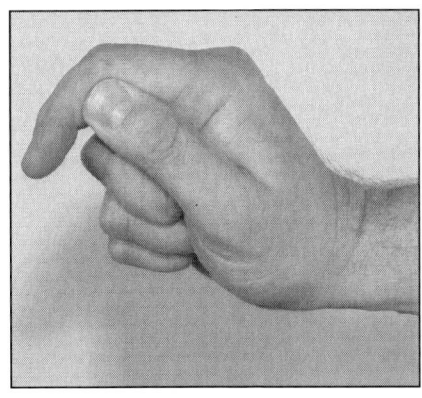
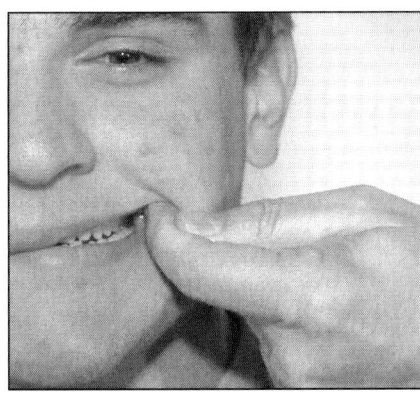

Figure 7   **Figure 8**

- Point your index finger, bend it inward slightly, and stiffen it as hard as you can. (Fig. 7)
- Press your thumb against the middle section of your index finger as you press your index finger back against it. This makes a powerful hooking weapon. (Fig. 8)

Four-Fingers Hook

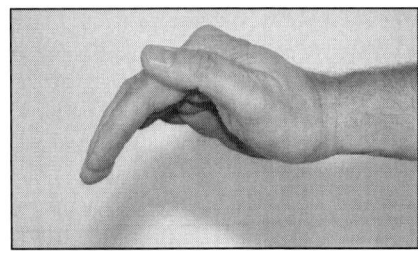
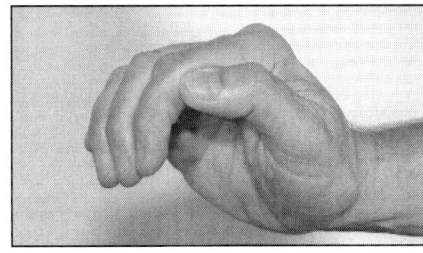

Figure 9   **Figure 10**

- Method 1: Form your hand into a hook with your four fingers bent and pressed together. Hold your bent thumb against your hand. (Fig. 9)
- Method 2: Form your hand into a hook with your four fingers bent slightly more than in Method 1. Push the pad of your thumb against the middle of your index finger and resist the push with your little finger. This stiffens all four fingers into a virtual hook. (Fig. 10)

Five-Fingered Claw

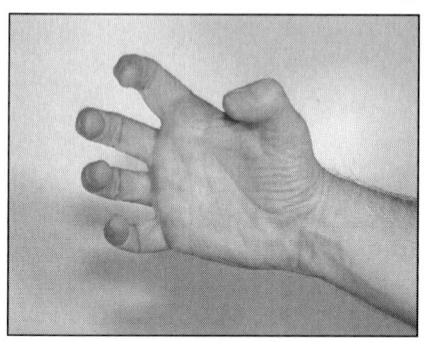

Figure 11

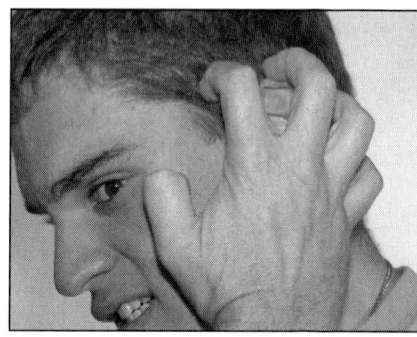

Figure 12

- Form your hand like a jungle cat's claw, all five fingers bent and stiffened, their tips pointing toward the target. (Fig. 11)
- Use it to claw/rip sensitive targets. (Fig. 12)

PRESSING
Forehead

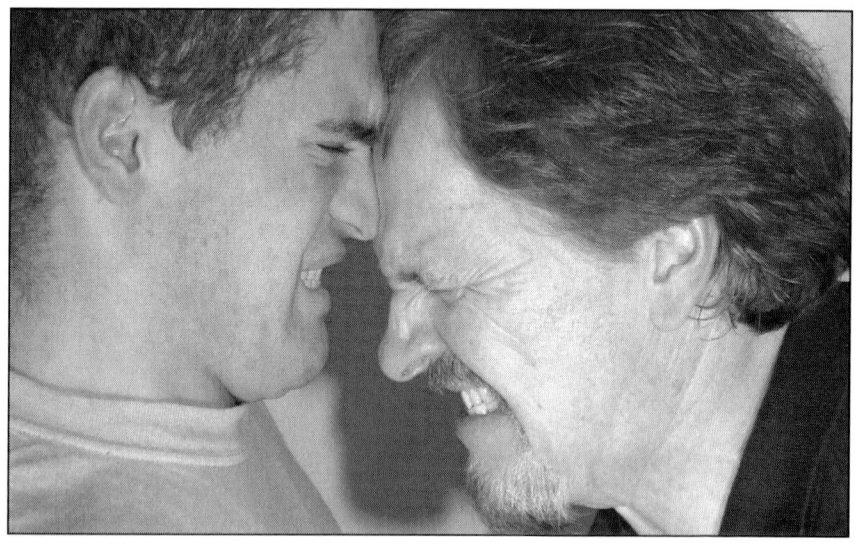

Figure 13

- Use your forehead to press against a vulnerable target. (Fig. 13)

Thumb

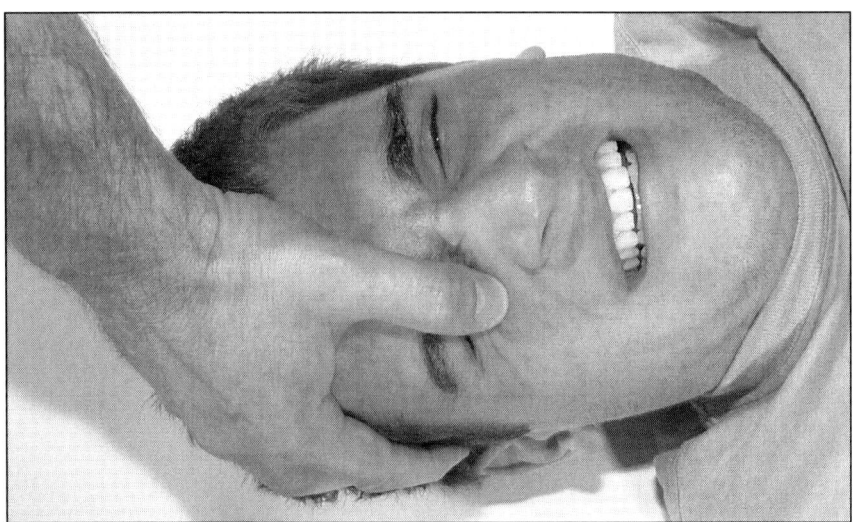

Figure 14

- Use the pad of your thumb to press into a vulnerable area. (Fig. 14)

Knuckles

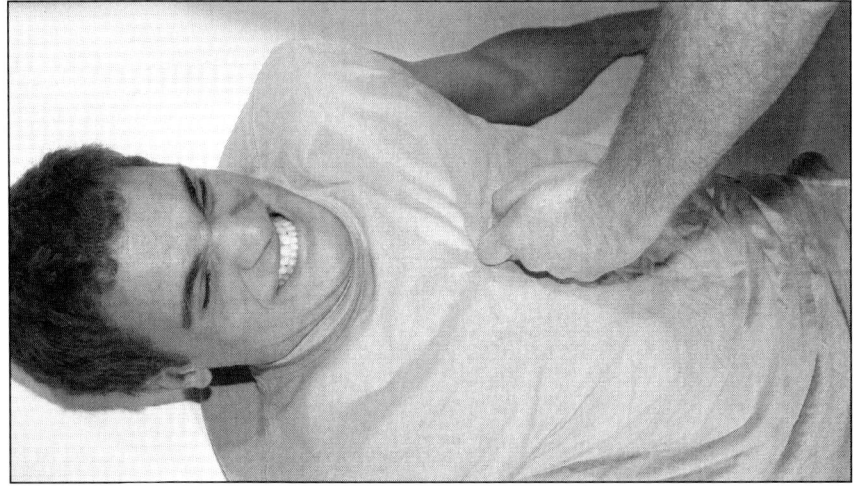

Figure 15

- Use a single knuckle to press into a vulnerable area. (Fig. 15)

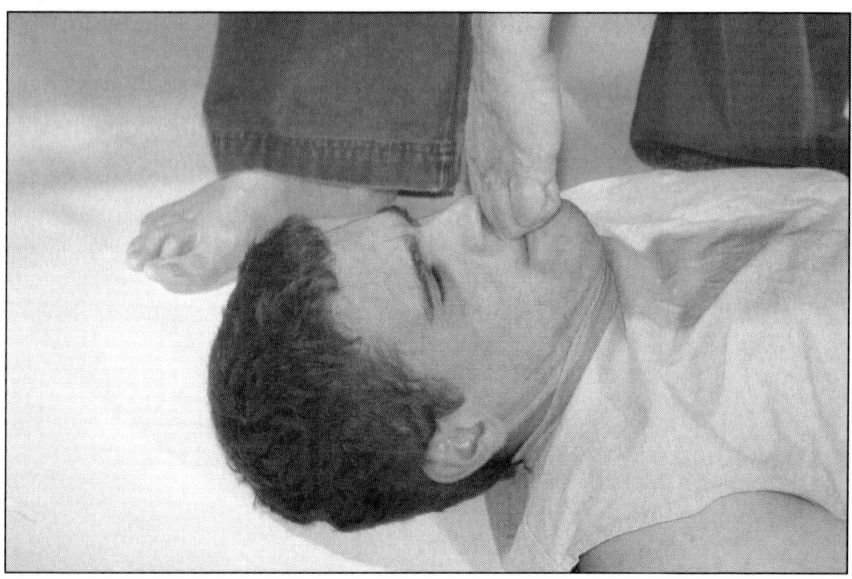

Figure 16

- Use the middle three knuckles to press particularly vulnerable targets. (Fig. 16)

Elbow

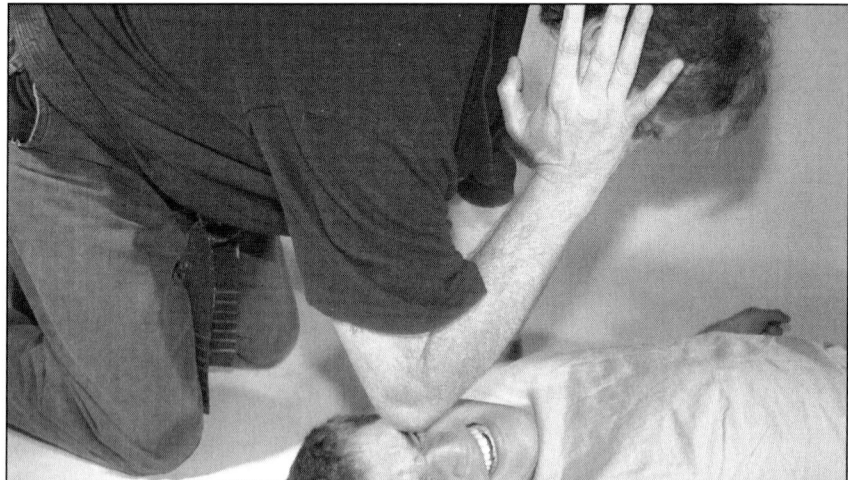

Figure 17

- Use the point of your elbow to press into a vulnerable area. (Fig. 17)

Knee

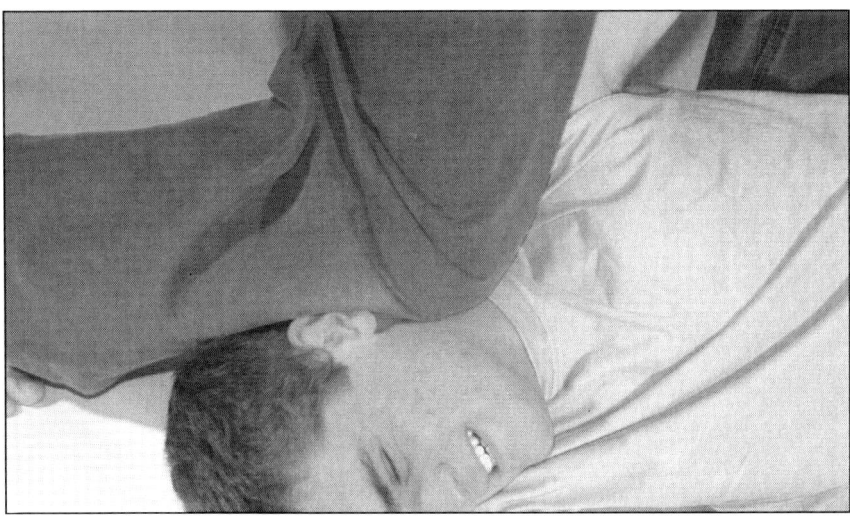

Figure 18

- Use your knee to press into a vulnerable target and to restrain your attacker with your body weight. (Fig. 18)

Shin

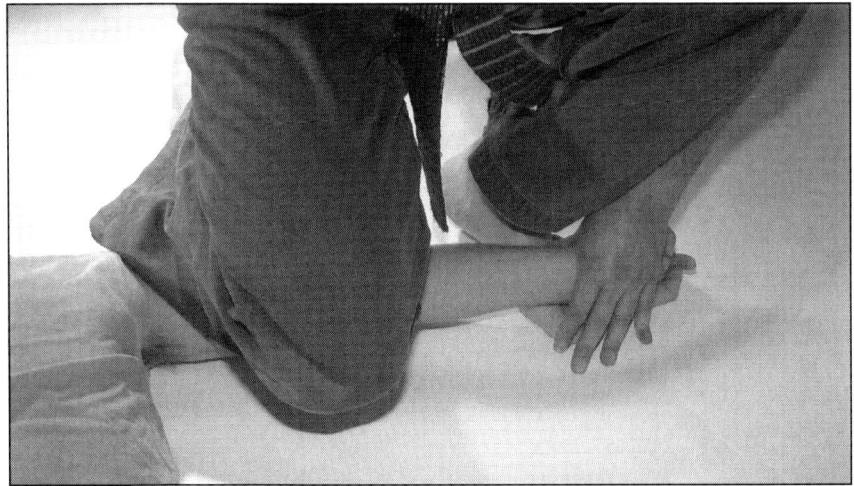

Figure 19

- Use your shin bone to press and "saw" a vulnerable target. (Fig. 19)

FLICKING
Fingers

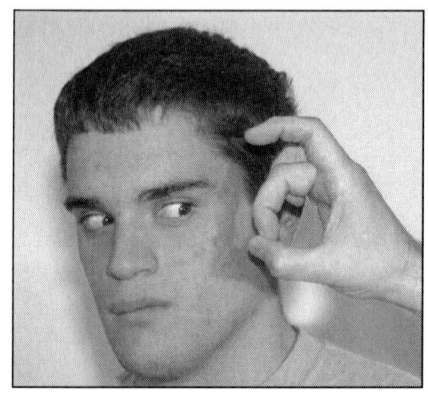 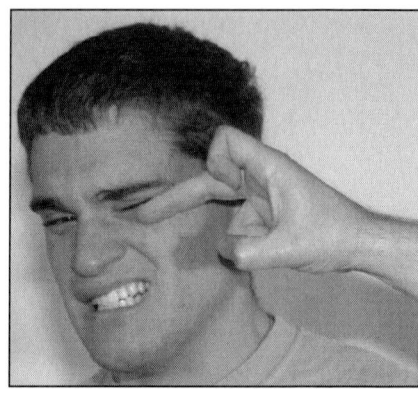

Figure 20 **Figure 21**

- Place your index or middle finger against the pad of your thumb. Your thumb restrains your finger. (Fig. 20)
- Release your finger forcefully. (Fig. 21)

2
Head

"When a person can't see, it's hard for him to shoot, stab, or hit you . . ."

The head—especially the face—is a playground of places to press, pinch, poke, and pull. Nerves there run close to the surface, making that part of the body especially vulnerable. For most people there is an intense psychological effect produced by attacking the head, too, since it is the center of their being. Most of their perception—sight, hearing, balance, and general sense of place—happens there. So when you apply pain to vulnerable targets on the head, it can be disorientating and psychologically overwhelming to your attacker.

Let's begin with the most vulnerable head target, which is perhaps the most vulnerable target in all the body.

EYES

Usually when the conversation turns to universal phobias, people are quick to list snakes, darkness, fire, and debilitating disease. Interestingly, few mention having their eyes gouged, perhaps because they take these wondrous gifts for granted. They shouldn't, though, because without them life would be hard and self-defense nearly impossible. A logical fact missed by too many fighters is this: When a person can't see, it's hard for him to shoot, stab, or punch you. This is what makes the eyes such a good target when you're forced to defend yourself.

This isn't brain surgery. Stick your finger in someone's eyes and it hurts like the dickens. For a few seconds or a few minutes, that person's life is all about the agony in his face and his inability to see and keep fighting. It was an easy-to-do technique, too. It didn't require power, strength and, in some cases, it didn't even require speed to do damage. All it needed was an opportunity to get to the target.

The eyes can be poked, raked, clawed, flicked, pressed, ripped, and pinched. Which technique you use depends on the situation and especially your position in relation to the attacker's. When you're at arm's reach with him, you can use rakes, claws, and pokes. When you're literally on top of him, you can add presses and pinches to the mix.

Good Techniques You Won't Find Here

There are all kinds of gouging, raking, punching, and kicking techniques you can execute to an attacker's eyes, but they are outside the parameters of this book. The interested reader can find these in abundance in my DVD *Vital Targets: A Street Savvy Guide to Targeting the Eyes, Ears, Nose, and Throat* produced by Paladin Press. In this text we are examining only ripping, pressing, pinching, and twisting techniques.

PRESSING

Pressing the eyes is extraordinarily painful and psychologically powerful. A pressing technique lasts longer than a poke, claw, or rake, which gives time for the pain to build and for your attacker's imagination to kick in as he wonders if your fingers are going all the way into his brain. (They probably aren't, but don't tell him that.) Once you start experimenting with eye presses in your training you will find all kinds of places to use them.

There are two kinds: a long press and a short press. A short press lasts a second or less. A long press, with few exceptions, lasts longer than a couple of seconds.

Leg Sweep Takedown with Long Press

Too many fighters act in training as if taking the attacker down is going to end the confrontation. Unless the fall knocked the wind out of him or he broke his arm or neck on the asphalt, you've probably only made him mad. You need to run away or follow with additional techniques.

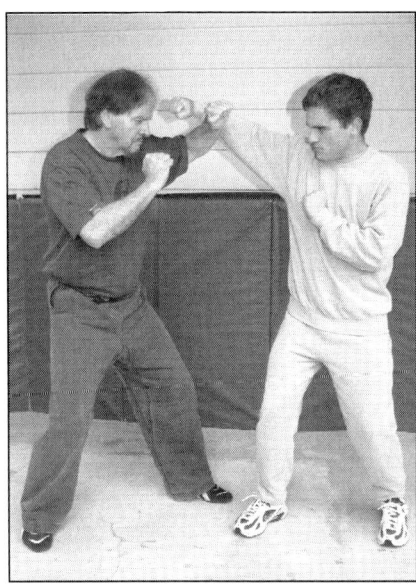

Figure 22

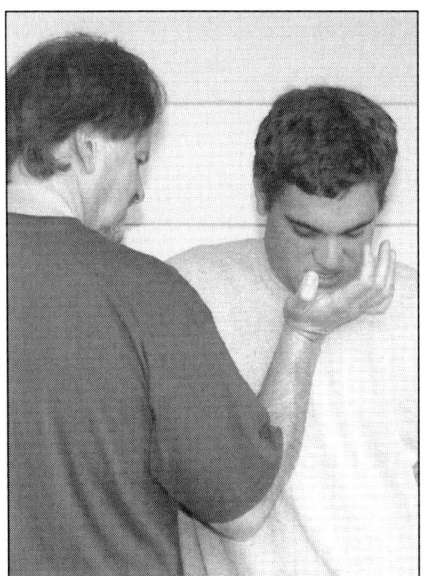

Figure 24

Figure 23

Your attacker throws a sloppy arcing punch at you.

- Block the punch. (Fig. 22)
- Step in and begin to sweep his leg. Your right hand can push his throat, chin, or face. (Fig. 23)
- Say you're pushing his chin but he resists by pushing his head forward and downward. (Fig. 24)

- With your hand still on his chin, press one or two fingers into his eyes to make him snap his head back. This gets his energy moving back and down. (Fig. 25)
- Sweep his leg to take him down. Either run away or keep pressing his eyes until you establish a control hold. (Fig. 26)

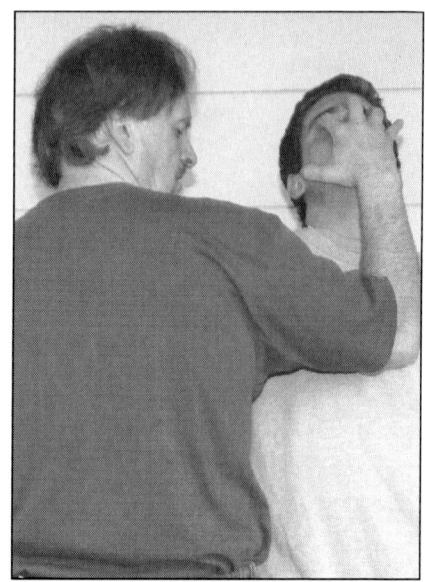

Figure 25

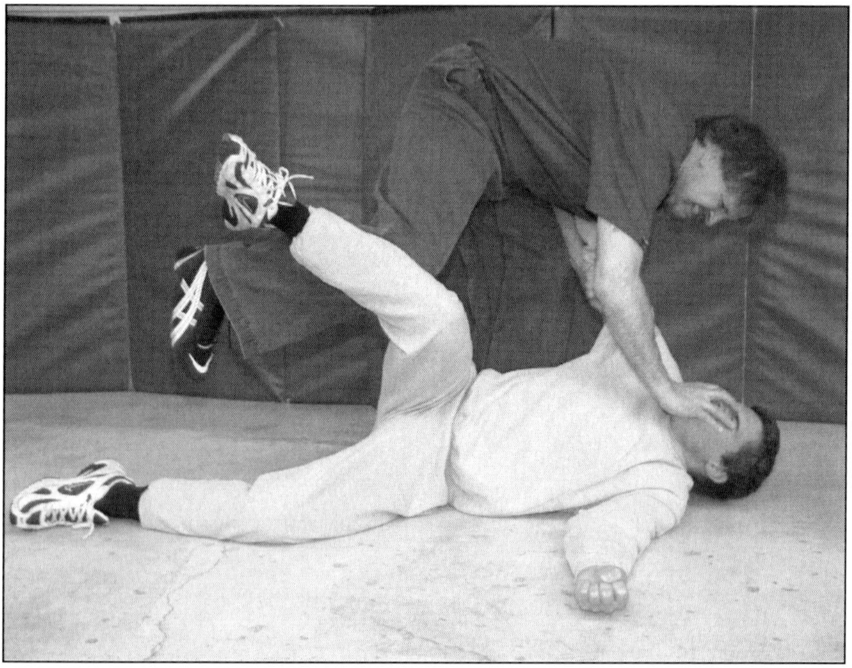

Figure 26

Block a Round Kick and Long Press from Behind

Your attacker throws a roundhouse kick at you.

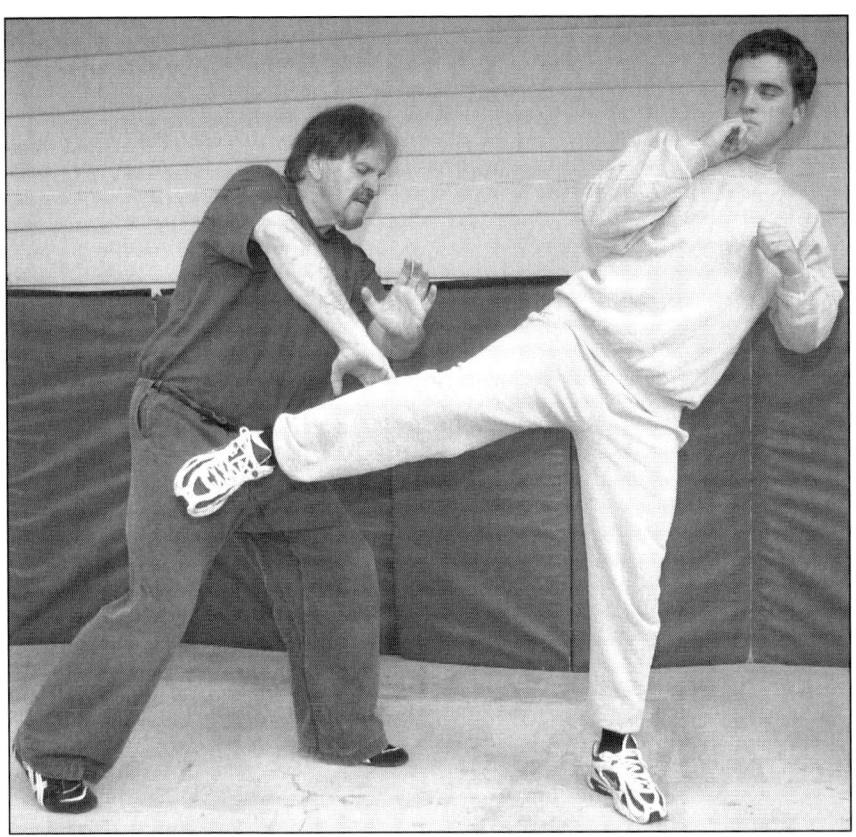

Figure 27

- Sweep it with enough force to spin him around. (Fig. 27)

18 *The Brutal Art of Ripping, Poking, and Pressing Vital Targets*

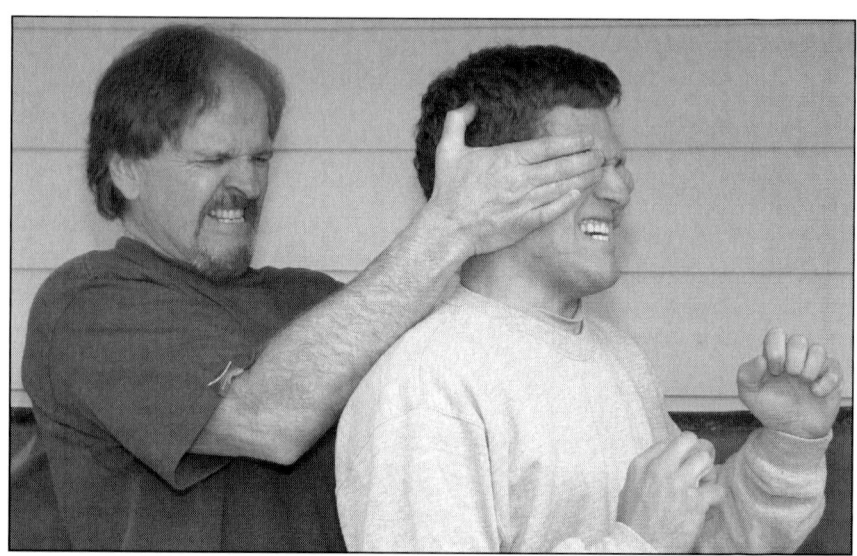

Figure 28

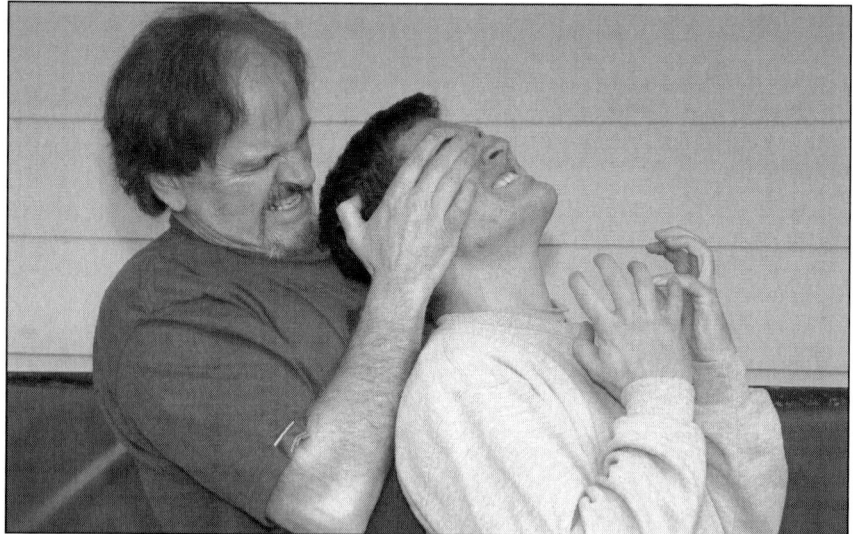

Figure 29

- Slap both hands against his face and ears as you hook your fingers into his eyes. (Fig. 28)
- Dig into his eye sockets as you pull his head against your chest. (Fig. 29)

Long Press to Escape from a Tackle

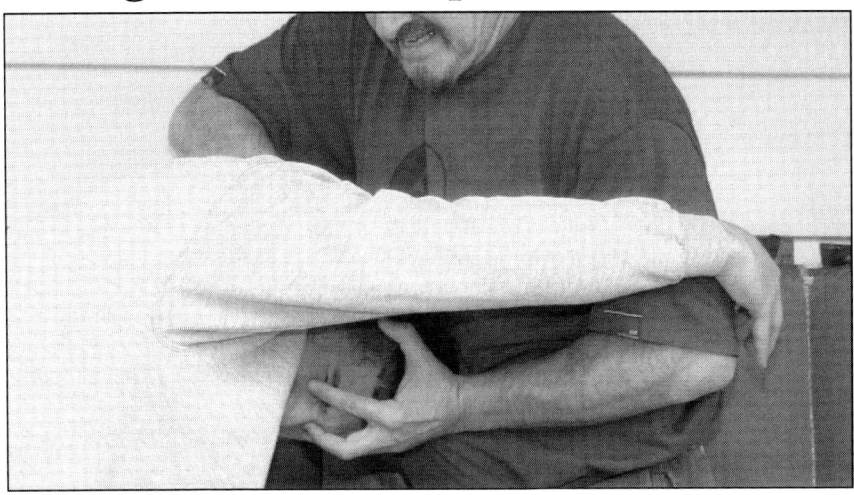

Figure 30

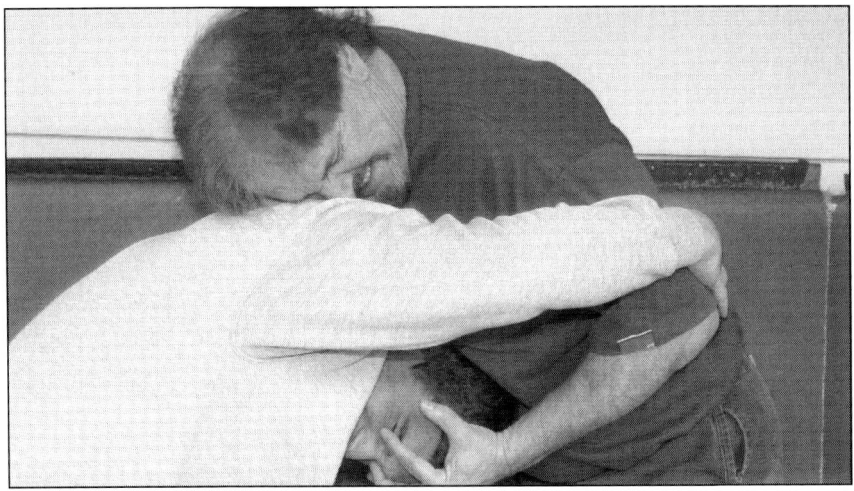

Figure 31

- Your attacker catches you in a tackle and drives you into a wall. Grab his head to hold it in place and shoot your other hand under his face to press your fingers into his eyes. (Fig. 30)
- You can lean your chest on the back of his head for added pressure. (Fig. 31)

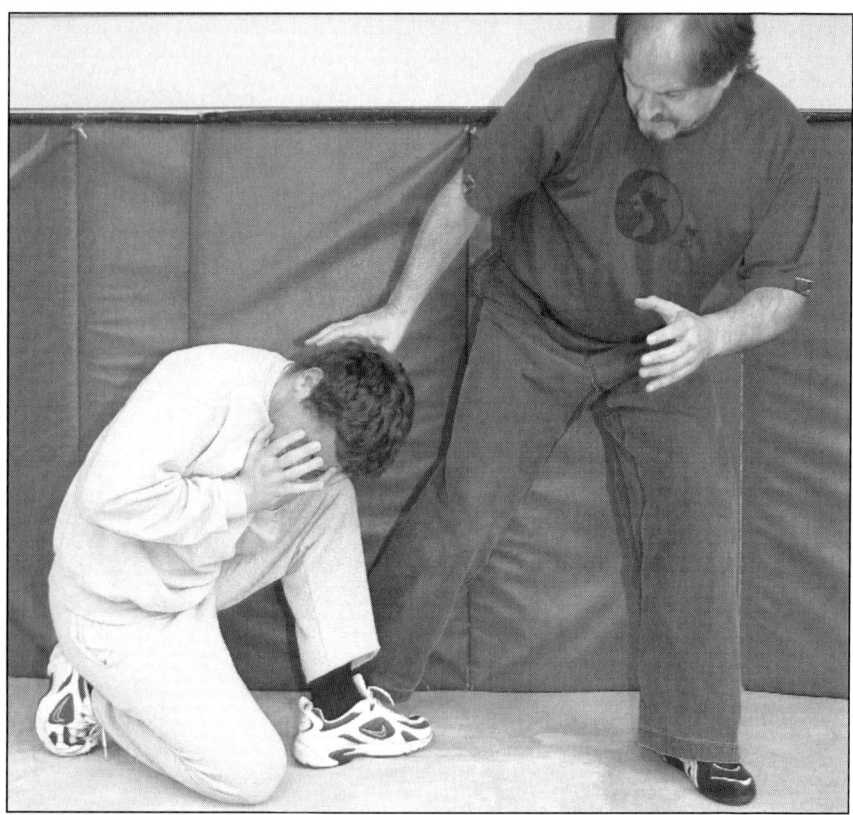

Figure 32

- When he drops in pain, push him away and run. (Fig. 32)

The Power of the Brace

For our purposes here, a "brace" is any movement that solidifies the target and allows the full energy of the technique to penetrate. For example, in the last technique, "Long press to escape from a tackle," you lean your chest on the back of the attacker's head as you press your fingers into his eyes. Since his head can't move, all the energy of the press goes into his eyes.

Whenever possible, brace the target to prevent it from moving.

Long Press When the Attacker Reaches for a Weapon

A bully is verbally threatening you.

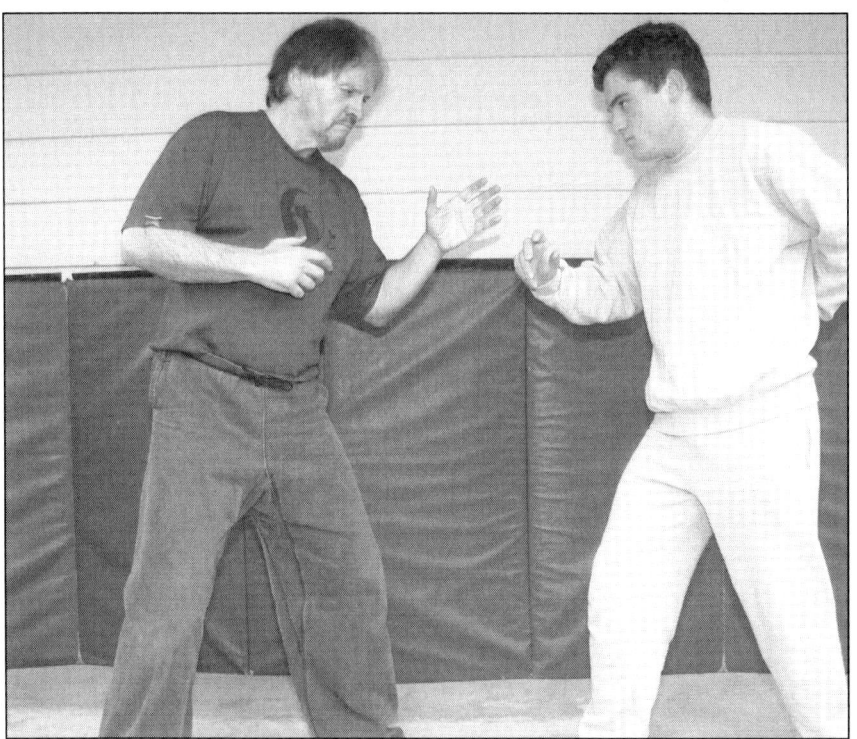

Figure 33

- He says he's going to cut you and he reaches toward his mid-back. (Fig. 33)
- Grab his arm and spin him toward the arm that is reaching. Shoot your other hand toward his face. (Fig. 34)
- Press your fingers into his eyes, lift his arm, and push his head . . . (Fig. 35)
- . . . until he falls over backwards. Don't release the pressure on his eyes as he falls. (Fig. 36)
- Apply pressure to his eyes as you apply an armlock, or run away. (Fig. 37)

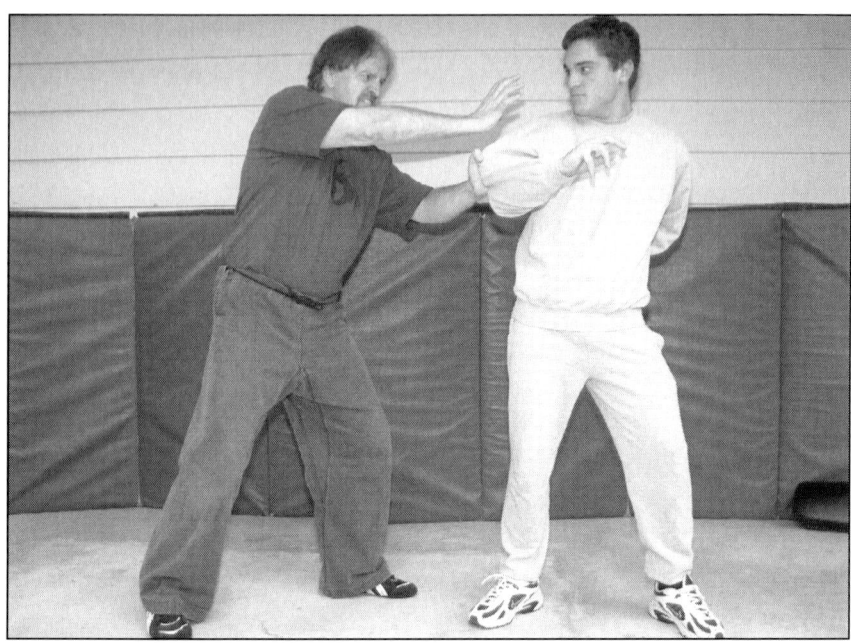

Figure 34

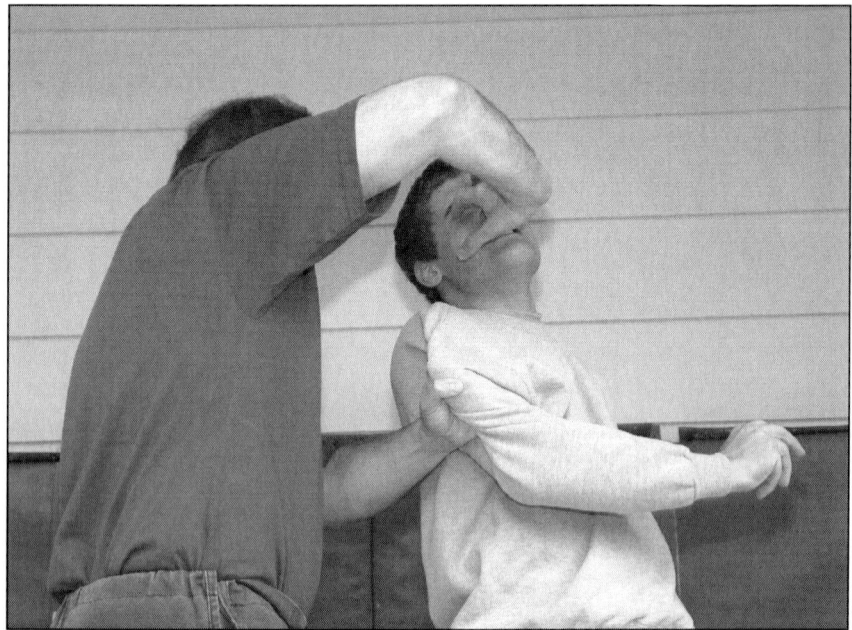

Figure 35

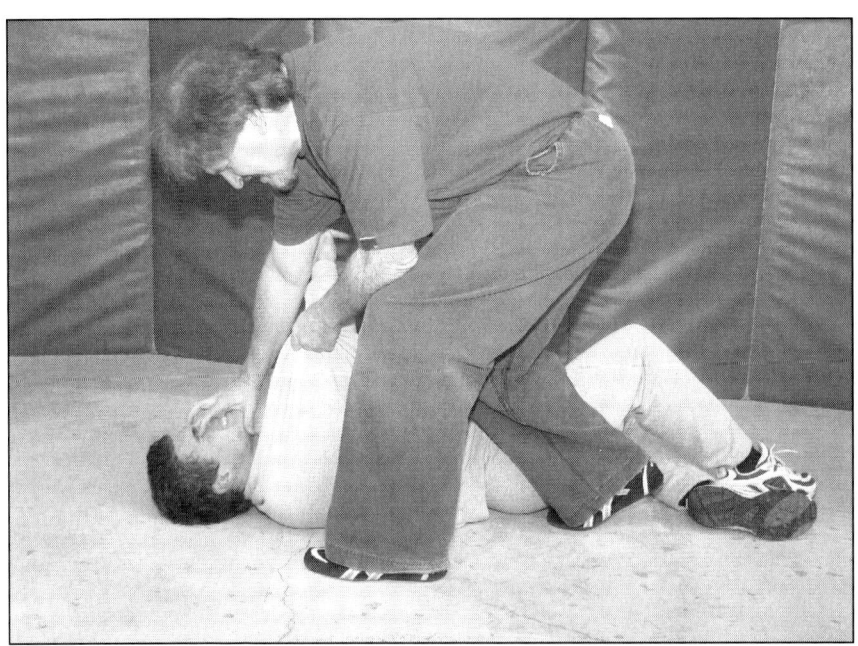

Figure 36

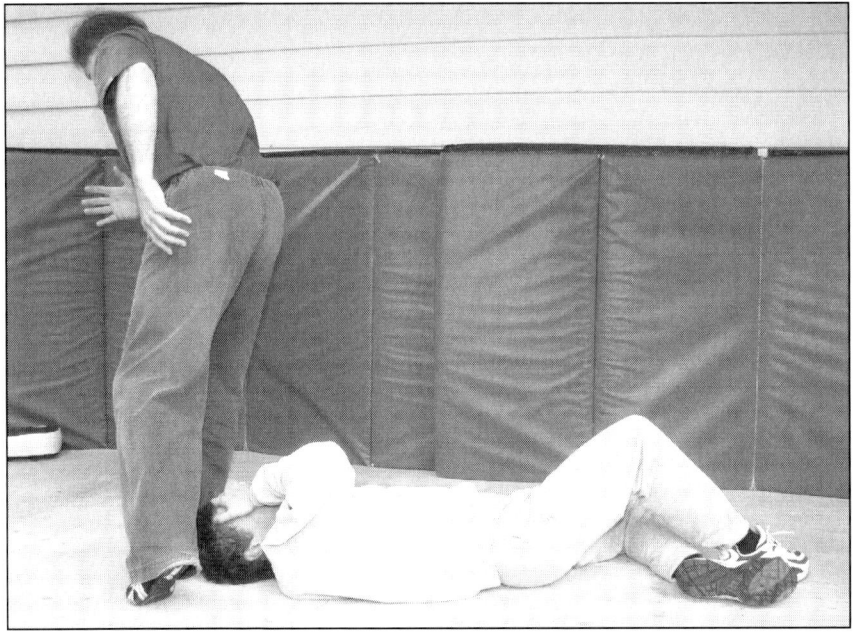

Figure 37

Long Press Into a Wall

The attacker attempts to strangle you.

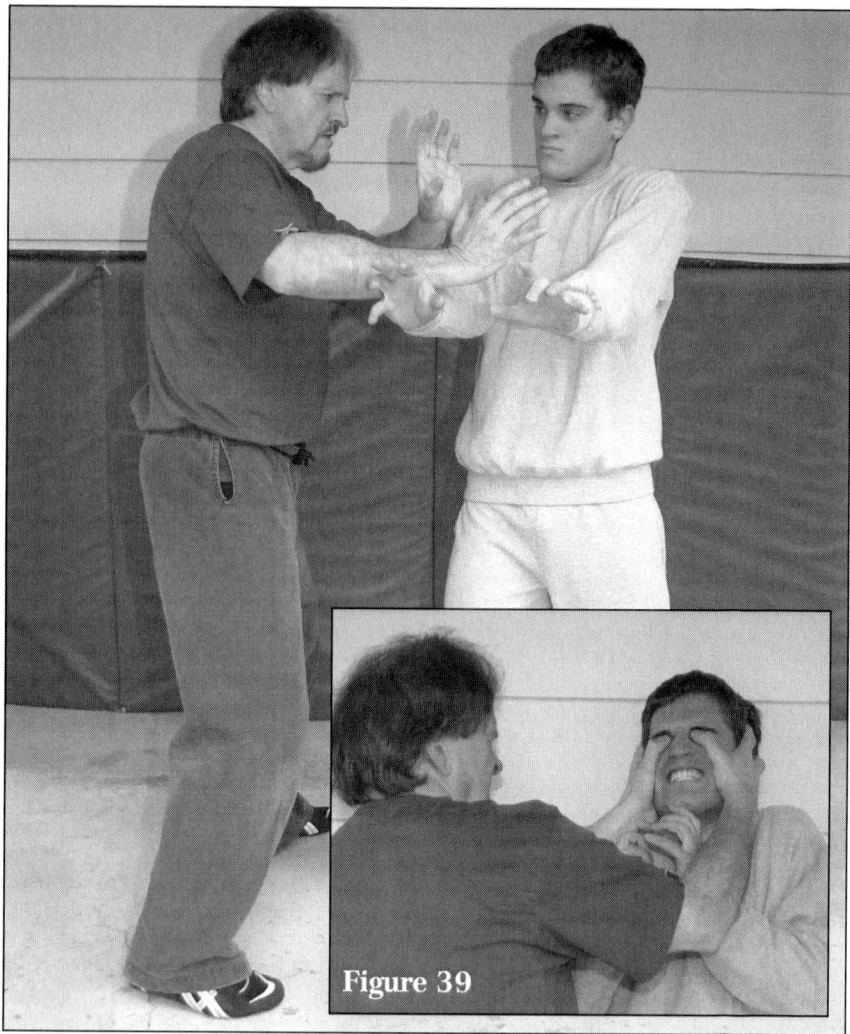

Figure 38

- Swat his arms aside. (Fig. 38)
- Ram your thumbs into his eyes and drive him into a wall. (Fig. 39)
- Kick his feet out from under him and push him by his eyes to the floor. (Fig. 40)

Head

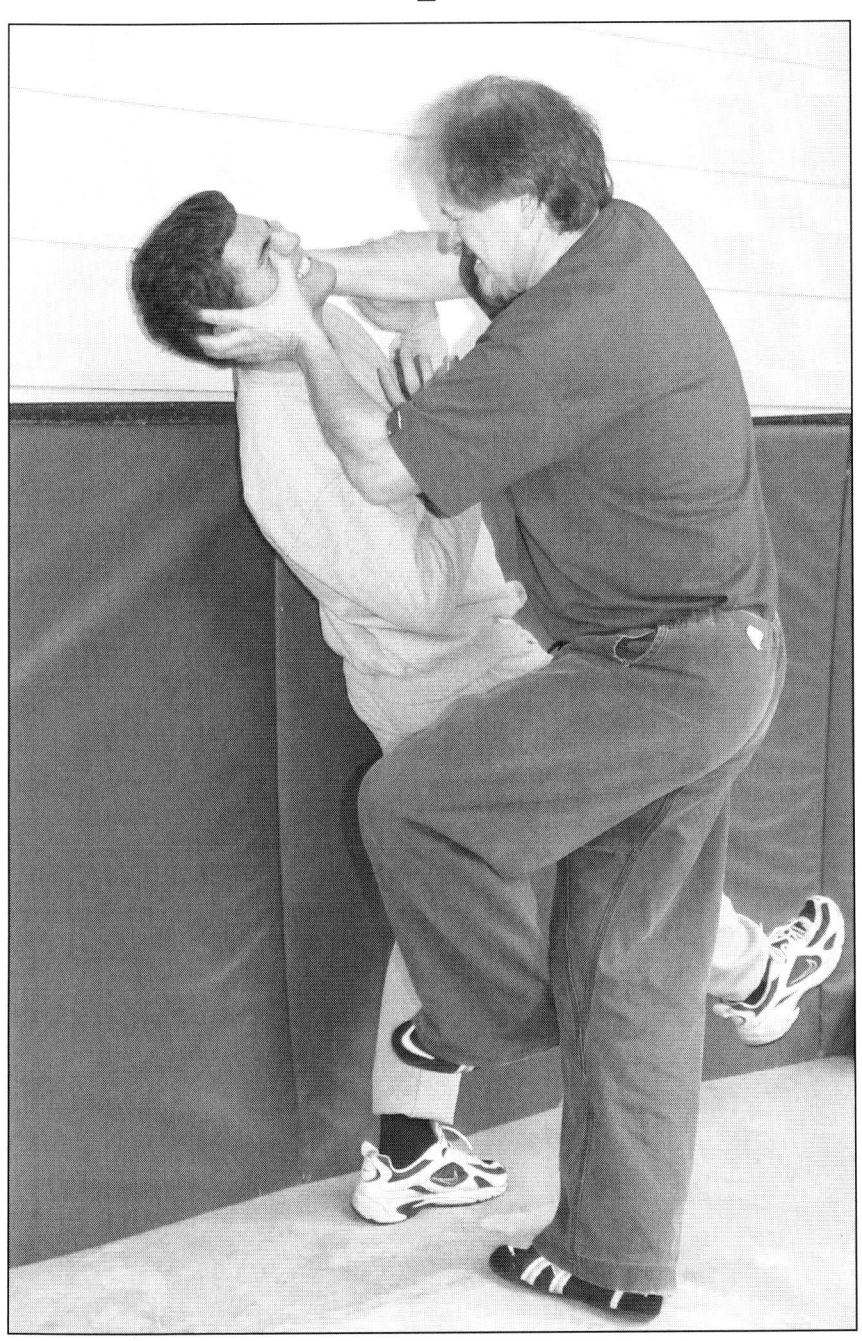

Figure 40

Long Press on the Floor

An attacker says he is going to cut you and reaches behind his back.

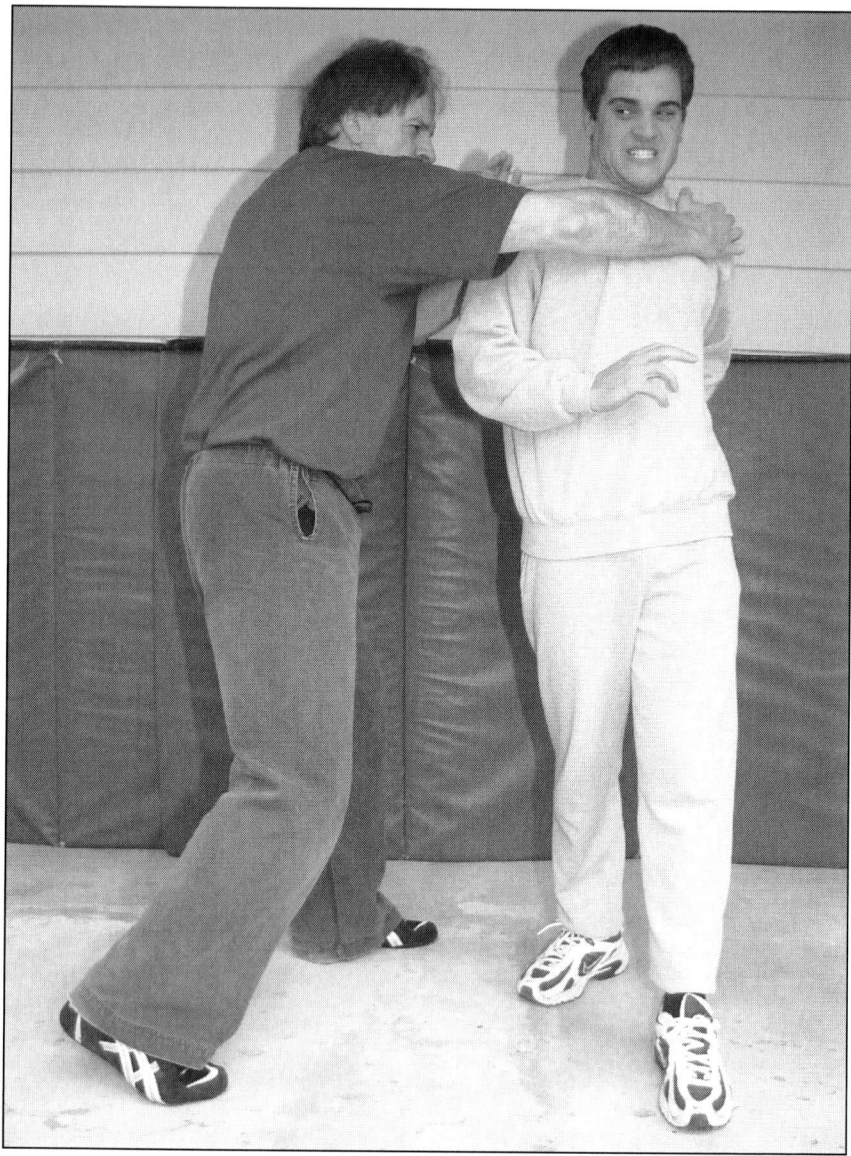

Figure 41

- Before he grabs his knife, spin him around by pushing on one shoulder and pulling on the other. (Fig. 41)
- Jerk his shoulders downward as you point your elbows toward the floor. (Fig. 42)
- Let's say that for some reason you slip and fall, too. You haven't hurt the guy and now you're lying on his face. (Fig. 43)
- To keep him from trying again to get his weapon, distract him by pressing your thumbs into his eyes as you get up. He will scream and flail around, so get up quickly and run. (Fig. 44)

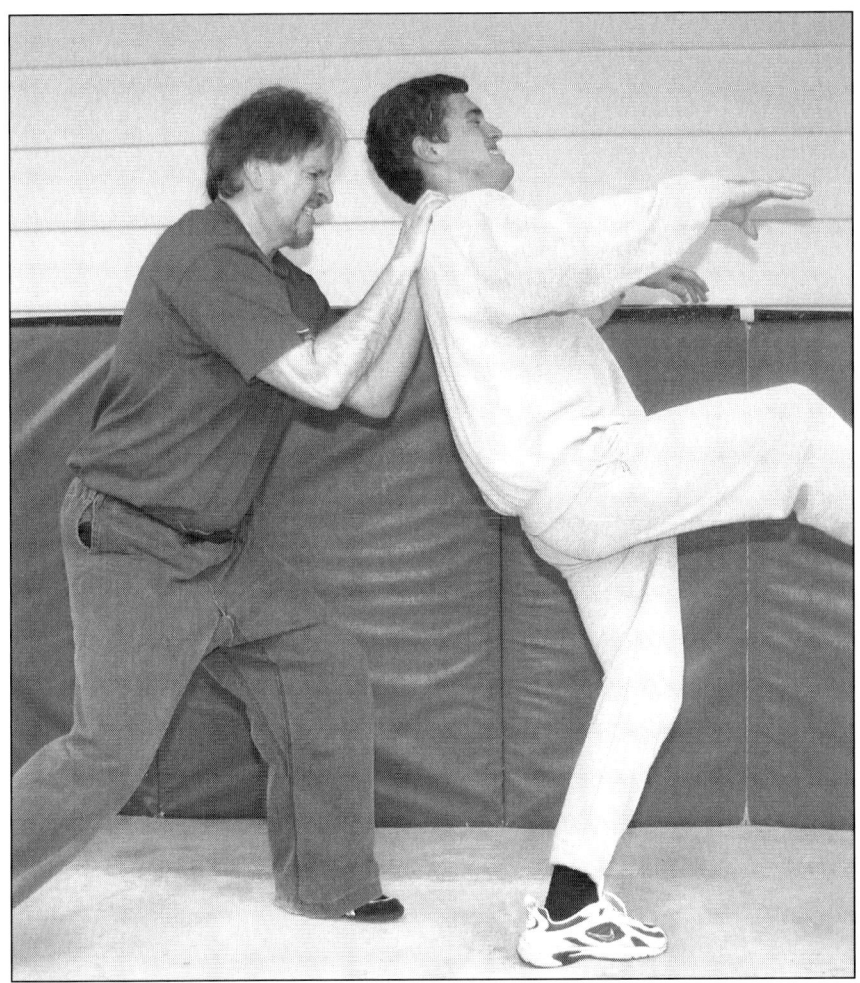

Figure 42

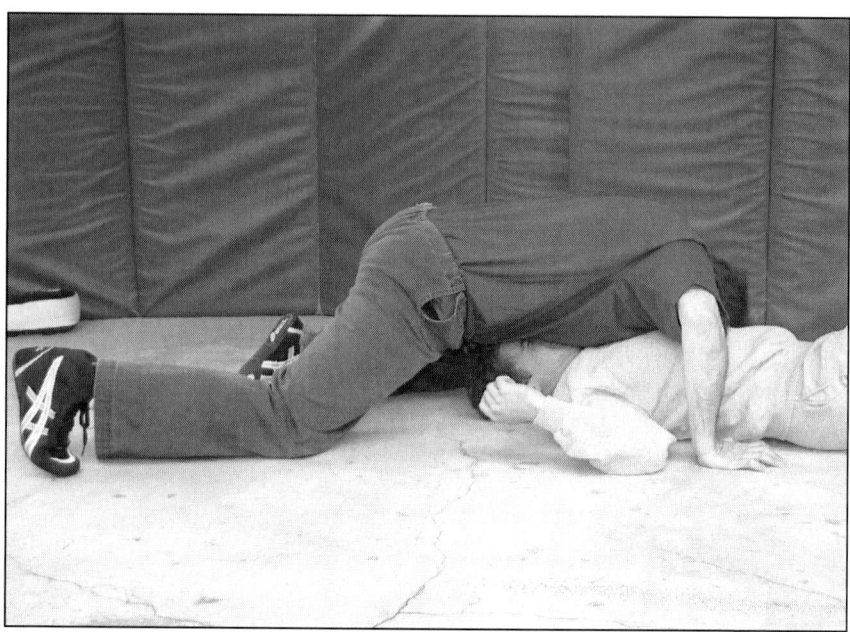

Figure 43

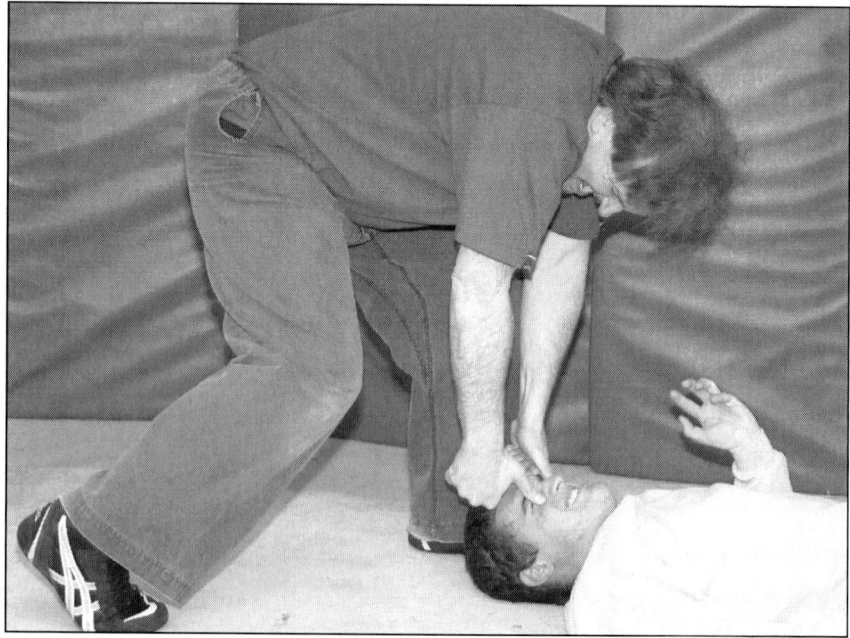

Figure 44

Long Press Takedown

The attacker attempts to grab your neck with one hand.

- Swat his arm aside. (Fig. 45)

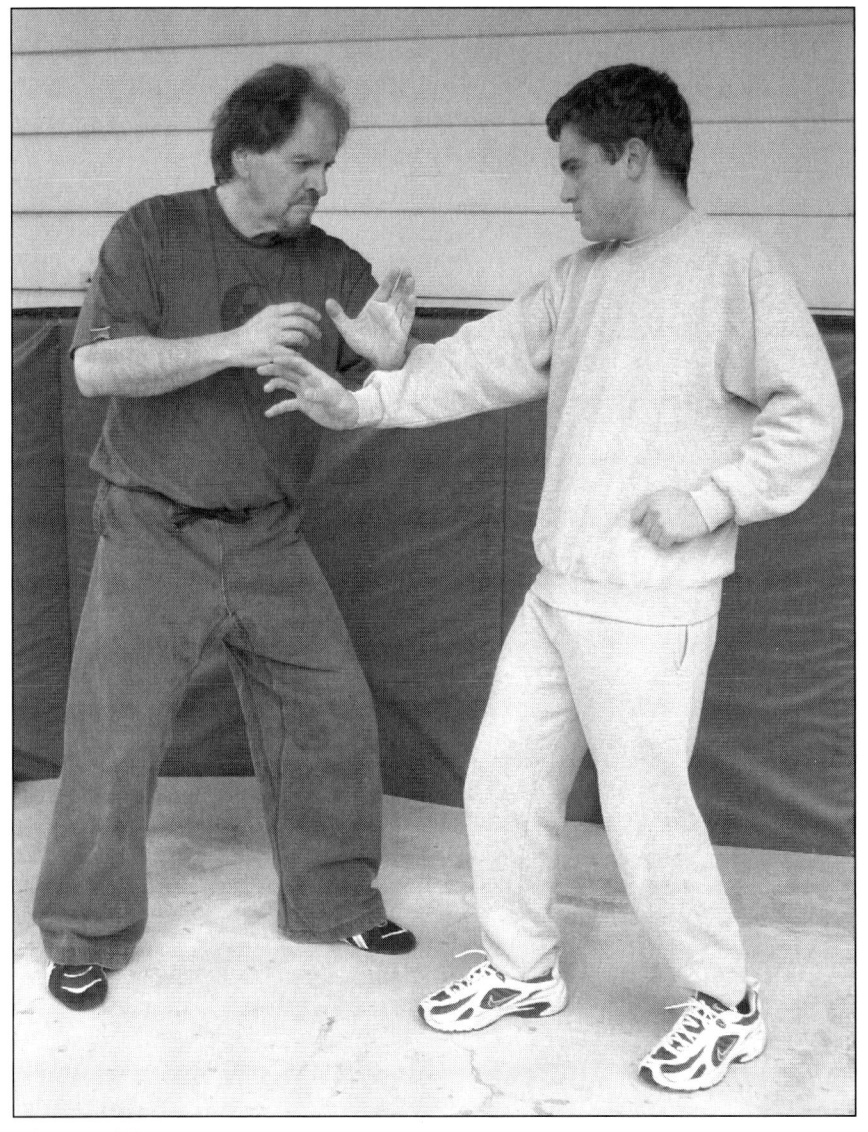

Figure 45

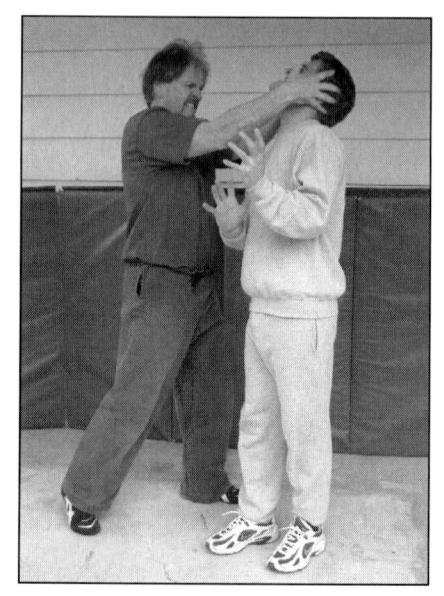

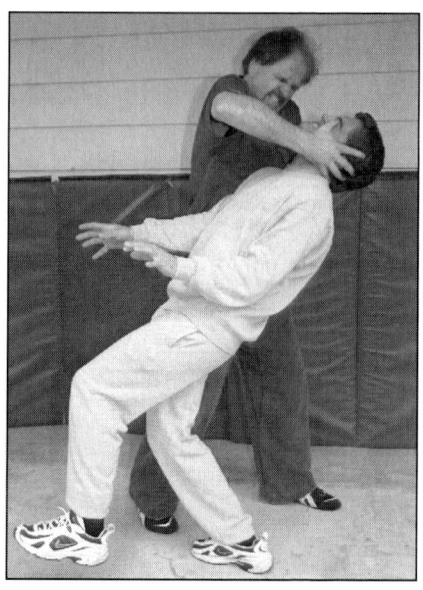

30 *The Brutal Art of Ripping, Poking, and Pressing Vital Targets*

Figure 46

Figure 47

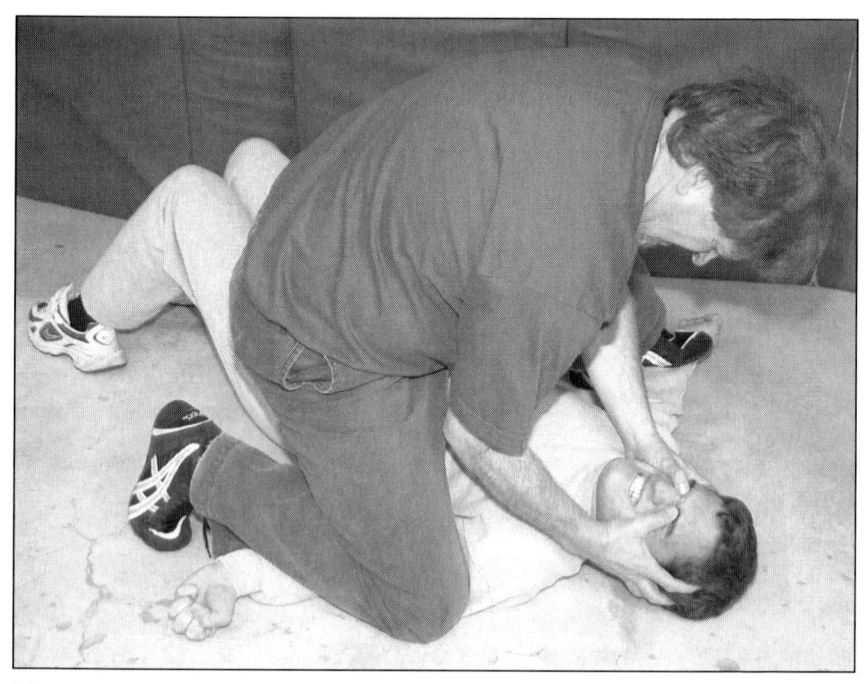

Figure 48

Head

- Ram your thumbs into his eyes and drive him back. The average person will jerk his head upward, which is a good thing because it makes it easier to take him down. Continue to press as you step off to his right or left side. This prevents you from tripping over him and falling down, too. (Figs. 46, 47)
- Once he lands, you can straddle his upper torso, pinning his arms under your legs, and continue to press into his eyes. (Fig. 48)

Variation:

- The instant he lands on his back, quickly move around behind him (you have to release his eyes momentarily). Then press his eyes again with your thumbs. He can still reach you, but it's harder, especially when his overwhelming concern is the agony in his eyes. (Fig. 49)

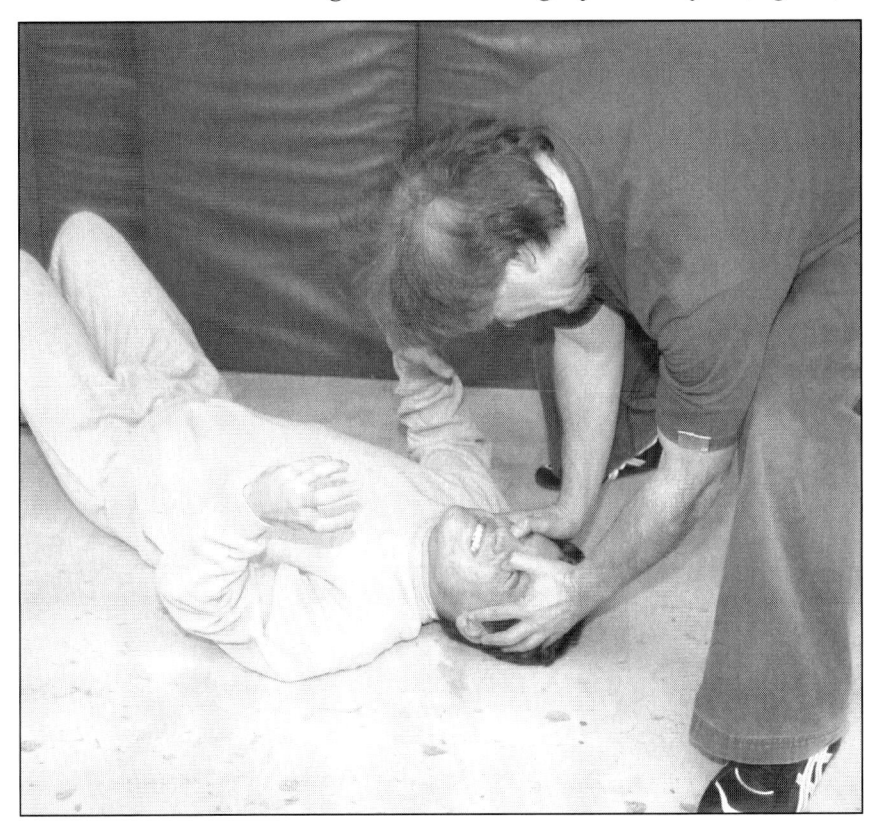

Figure 49

You Got Him Down, Now What?

Many of the techniques illustrated in this book conclude with the attacker on the floor. Sometimes follow-up techniques are suggested, sometimes not.

You have three options after you've taken someone down:

- Run away.
- Follow up with a restraint technique.
- Follow up with kicks and punches.

The first option is the best one in the eyes of the legal system. If there is no avenue of escape for you, a restraint hold is the second best option. If that is impossible, hitting him with your fists or feet is the last choice, but only do so enough to allow an opportunity for you to escape or apply a hold.

Practice all three options when you train.

Long Press Defense Against a Top Mount

Practice this one on a live person or a mannequin-style bag.

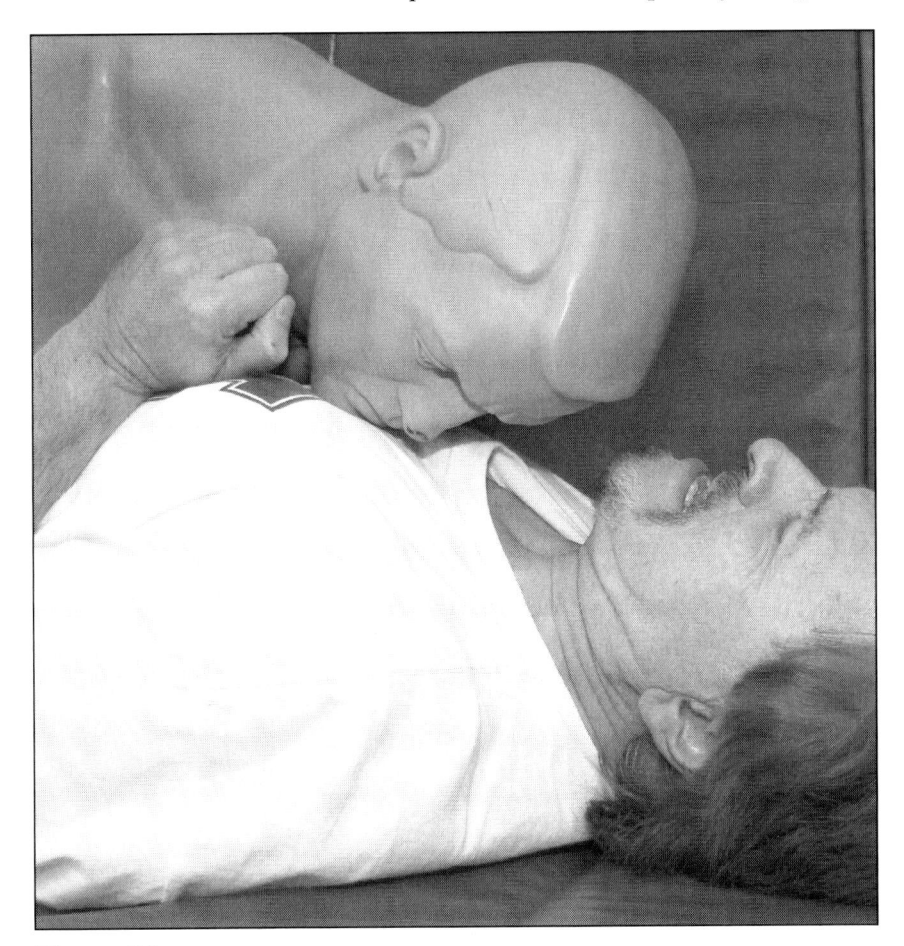

Figure 50

- The attacker is on top of you. (Fig. 50)
- Grab his head or hair at the back. Press your fingers into his eye sockets and pull his head into your one-hand eye press. (Fig. 51)
- Pull his head to one side a little and buck him off in the same direction. (Fig. 52)

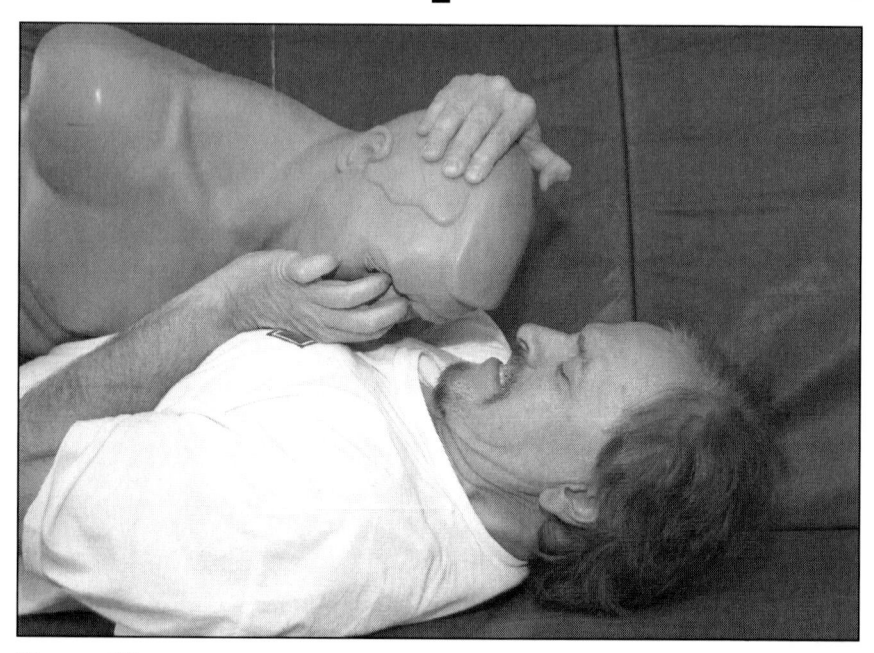

Figure 51

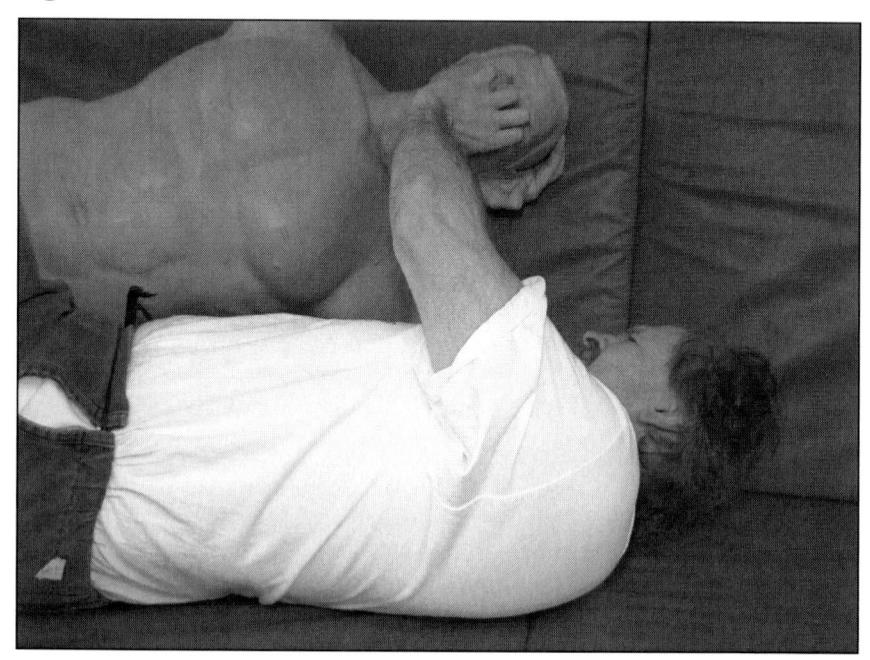

Figure 52

Long or Short Press

The fight has gone to the ground and you have your attacker in a headlock.

- You have one of his arms trapped but he's starting to wiggle it free. His other arm is grabbing at you, too. (Fig. 53)

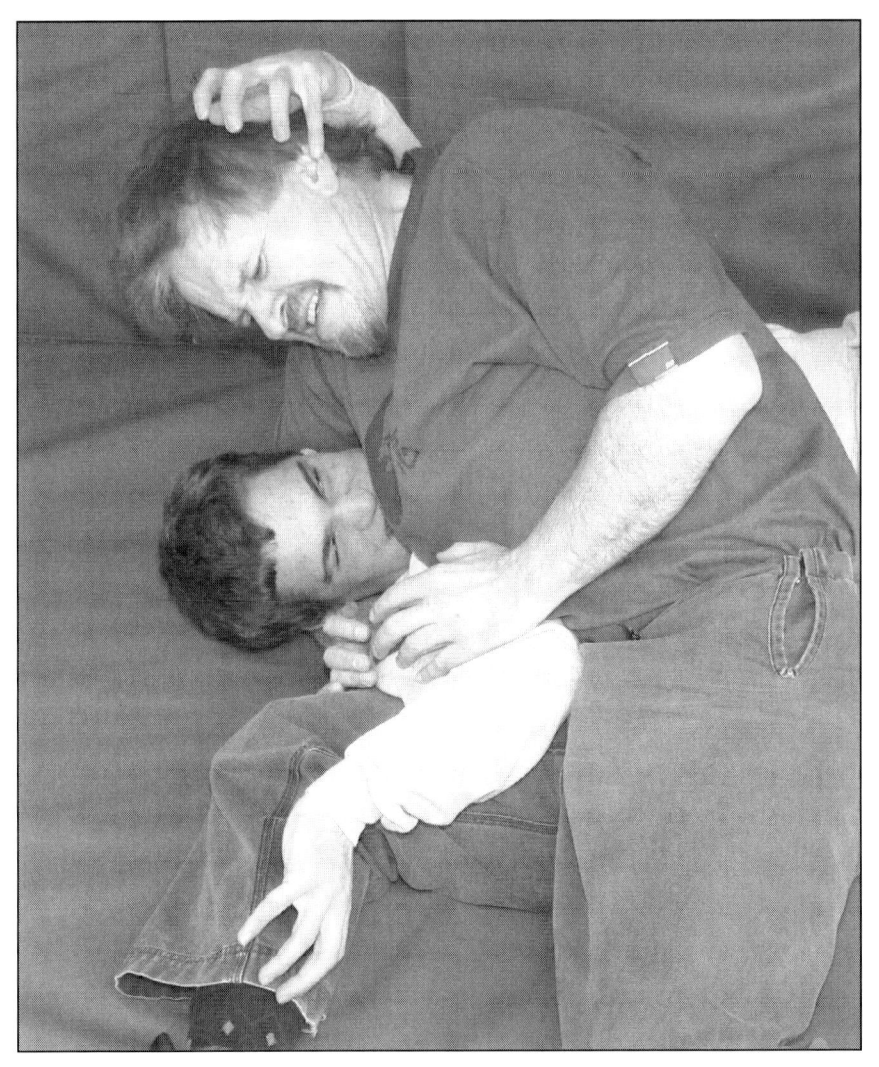

Figure 53

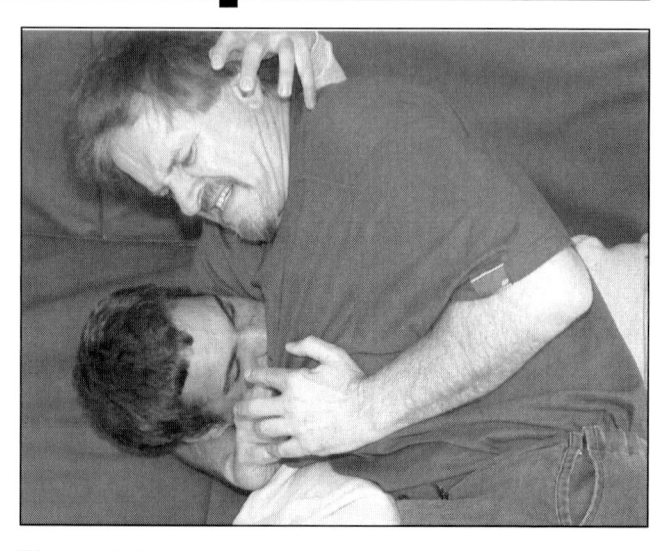

Figure 54

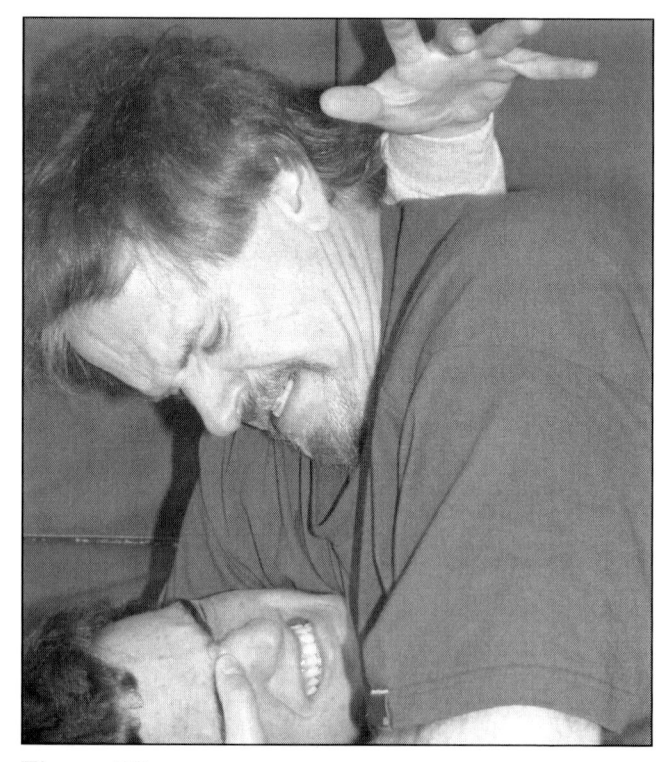

Figure 55

Head

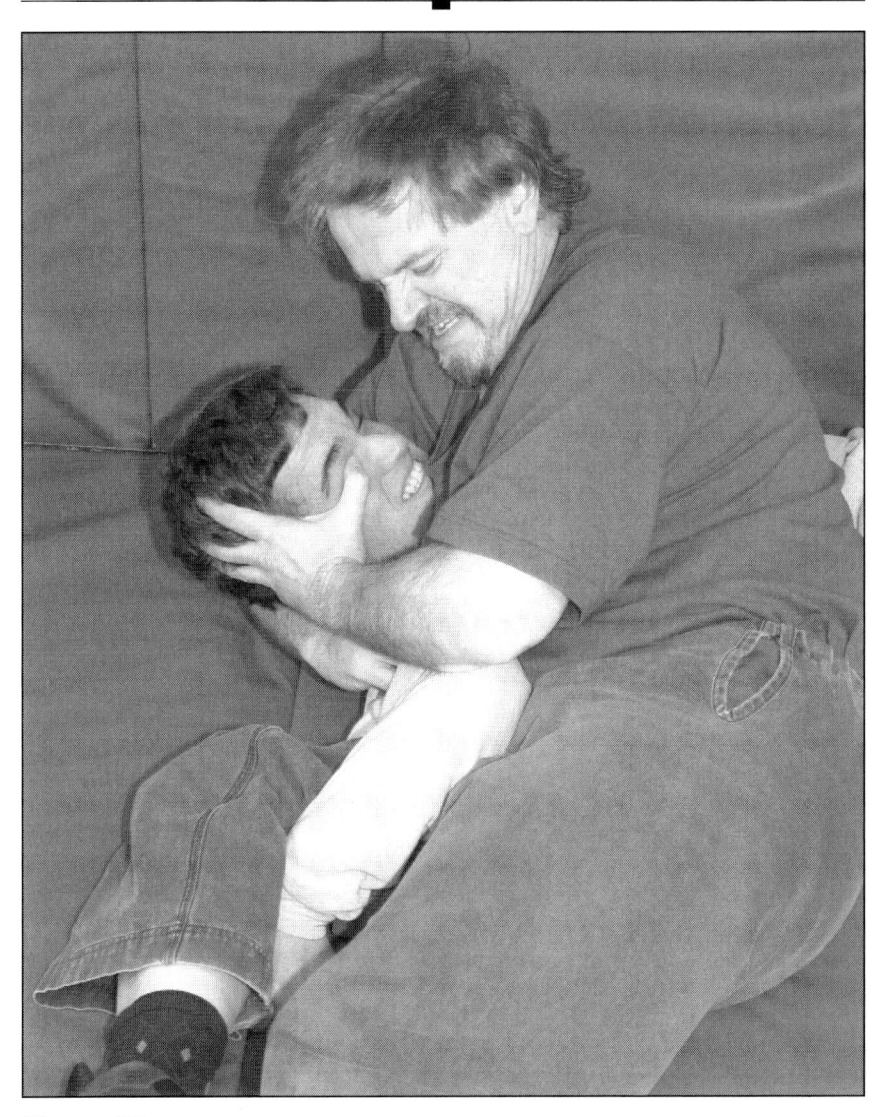

Figure 56

- Secure the neck hold by grabbing your clothing. (Fig. 54)
- Press your thumb into an eye and secure it by gripping his head with your other four fingers. (Fig. 55)
- Pull his head forward to painfully stretch his neck, and continue to press your thumb into his eye. Press for however long it takes to get what you want out of the hold. (Fig. 56)

Long or Short Press with Elbow

You're lying perpendicular on top of your attacker.

- Apply a figure-four lock on his arm. (Fig. 57)
- Scoot your knee in close to prevent your attacker from turning his head away. (Fig. 58)
- Place your elbow into his eye socket and crank his shoulder by lifting your arm. (Fig. 59)

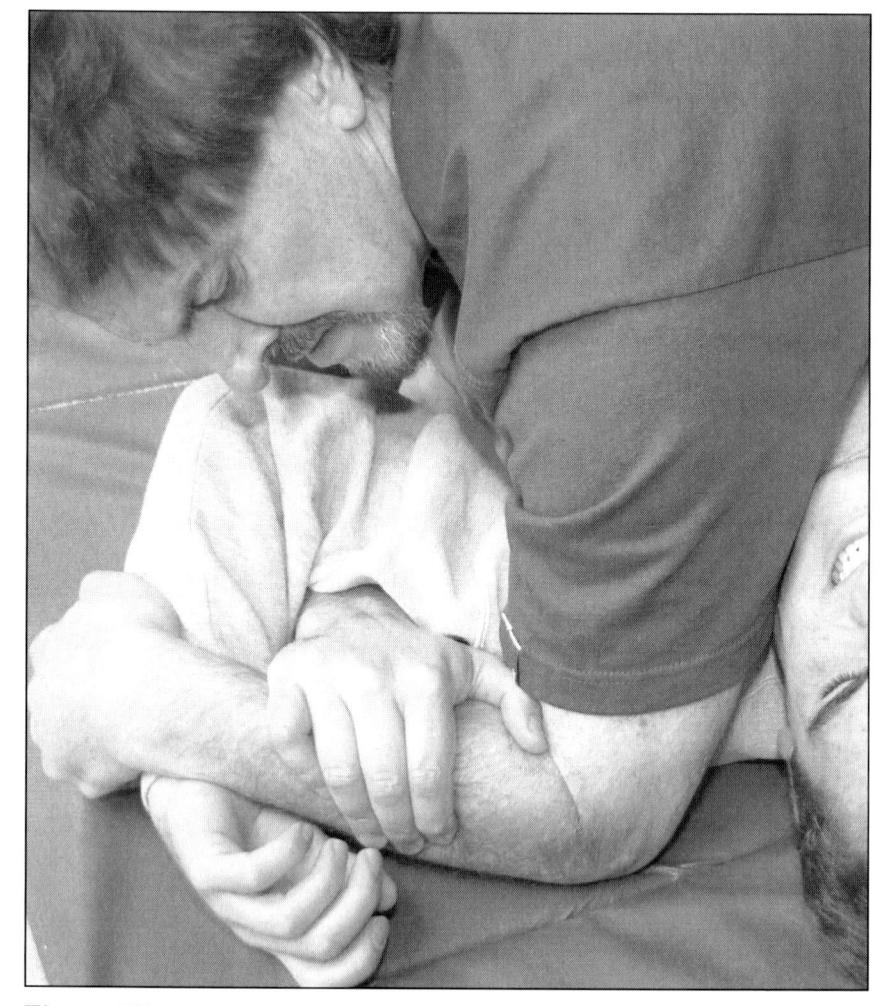

Figure 57

Head 39

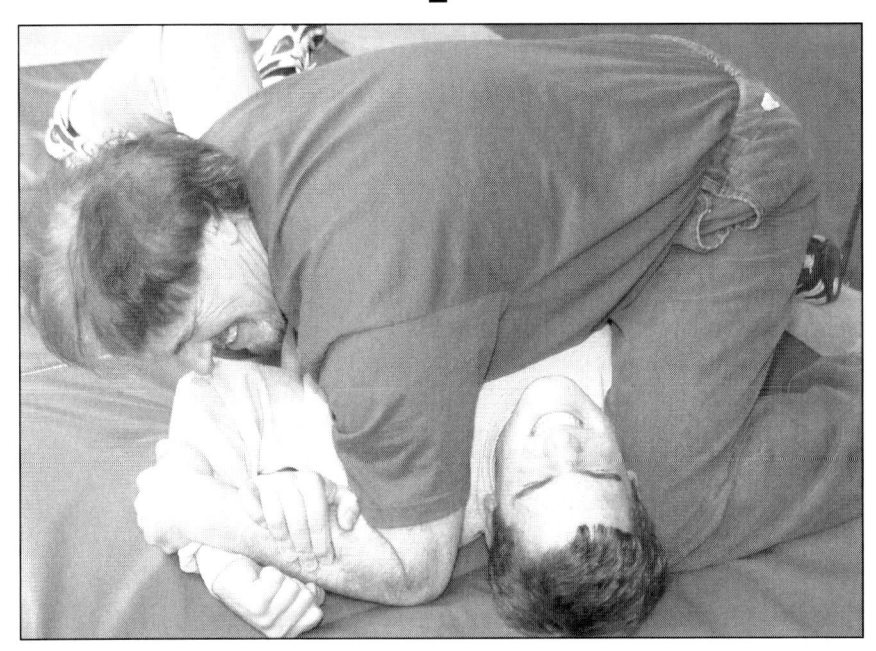

Figure 58

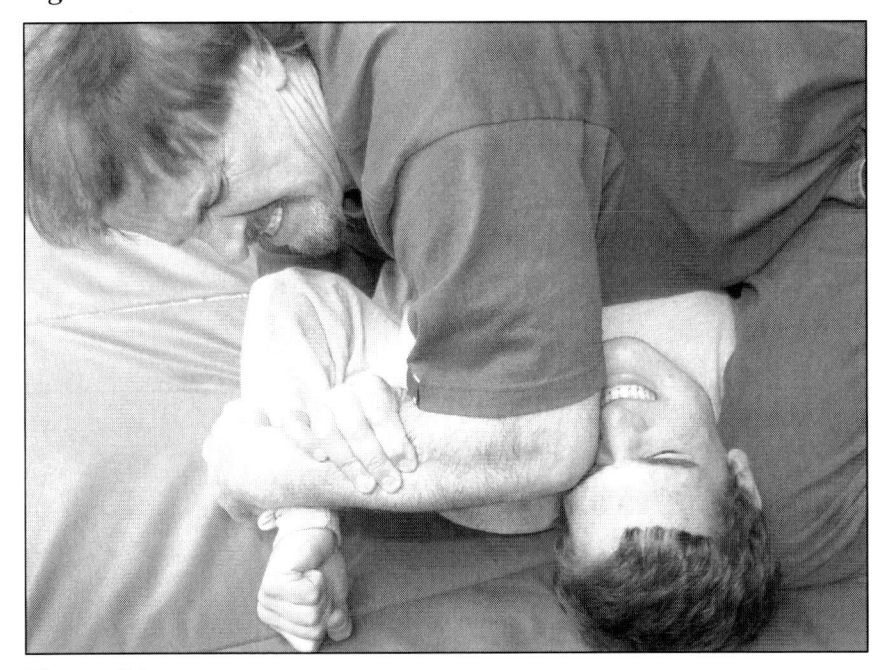

Figure 59

Long or Short Press with Wrist Bone

You're both on the ground and you've gotten behind your attacker. Practice on a real person or a mannequin-style bag.

- Slip your right arm around his head and place the thumb side of your wrist into his right eye socket at the outside corner. Brace the back of his head against your upper chest or shoulder. (Fig. 60)
- Join hands. Pull with your left hand so the pressure from your wrist goes inward, upward, and slightly across his eye toward the left. (Fig. 61)

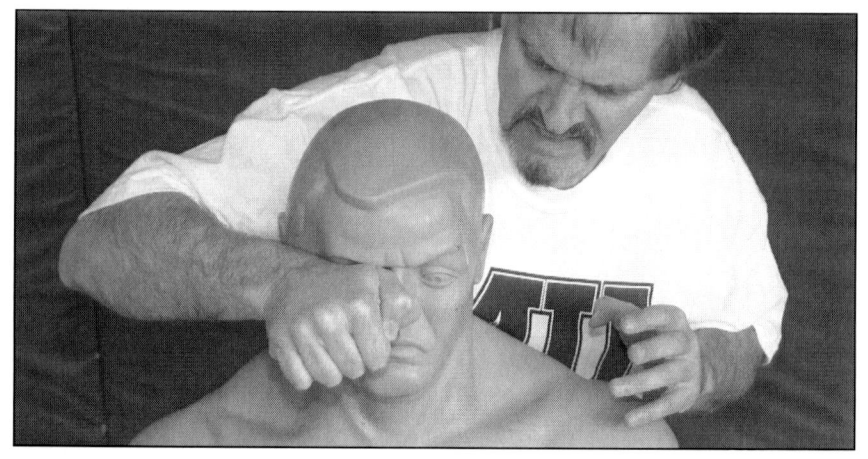

Figure 60

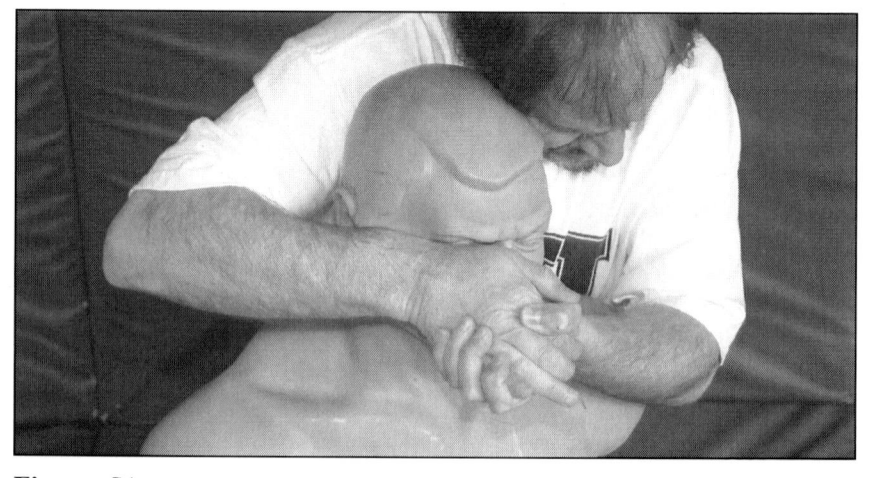

Figure 61

RIPPING

Ripping might not actually rip anything, though in most cases your attacker will think it did. There is great potential for injury with this, so it's important that you're justified to use this level of force.

Rip as You Fall

In the course of the fight, you step back and trip over something.

- The attacker immediately lunges toward you. (Fig. 62)

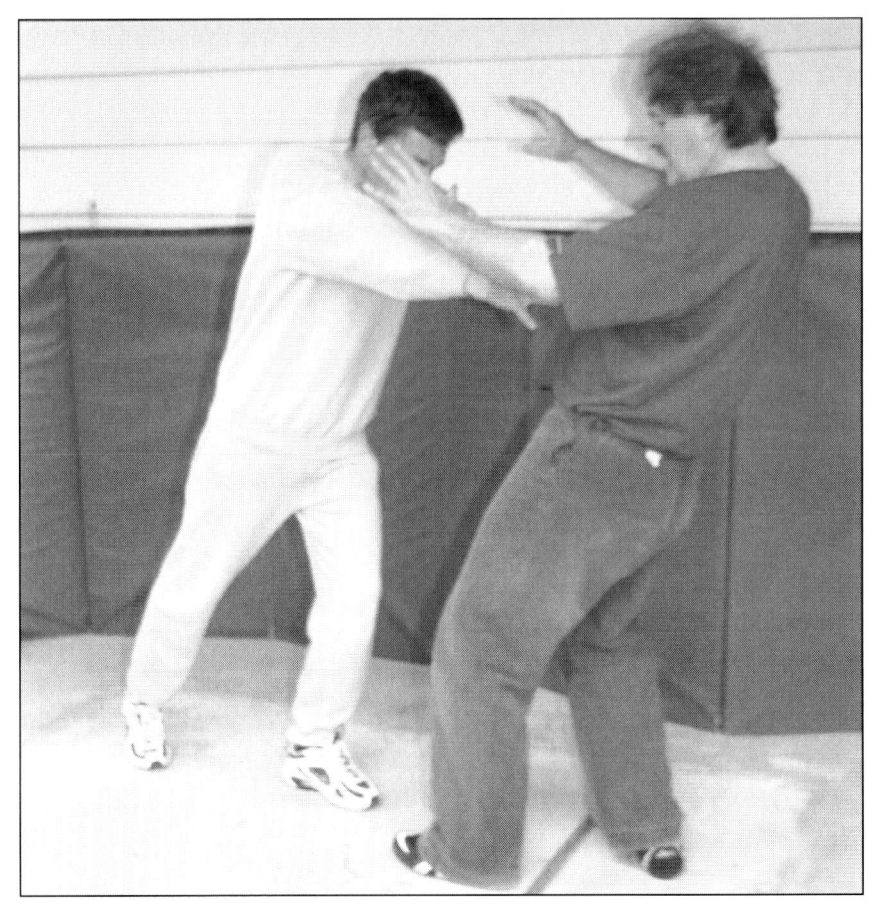

Figure 62

Figure 64

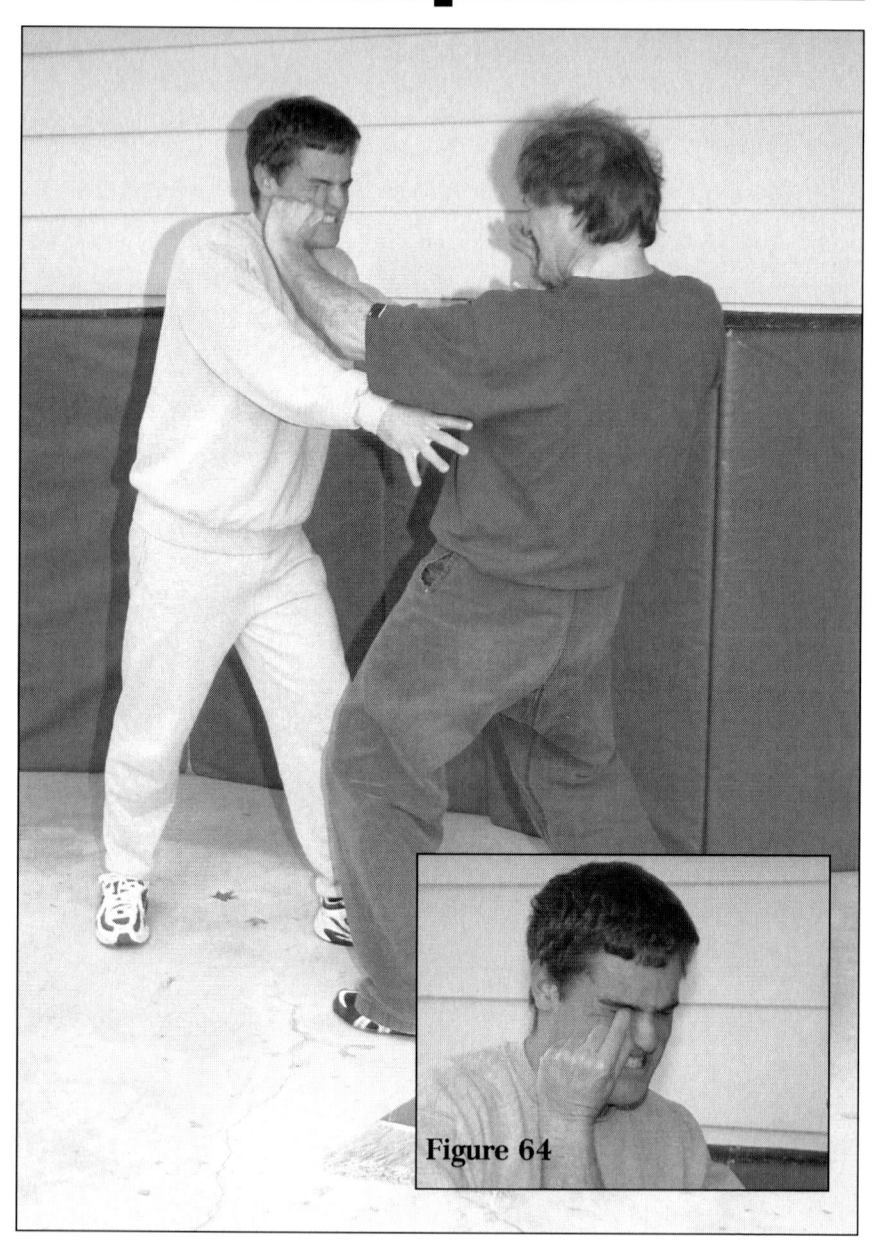

Figure 63

- As you fall, hook his eye with your mantis finger. (Figs. 63, 64)

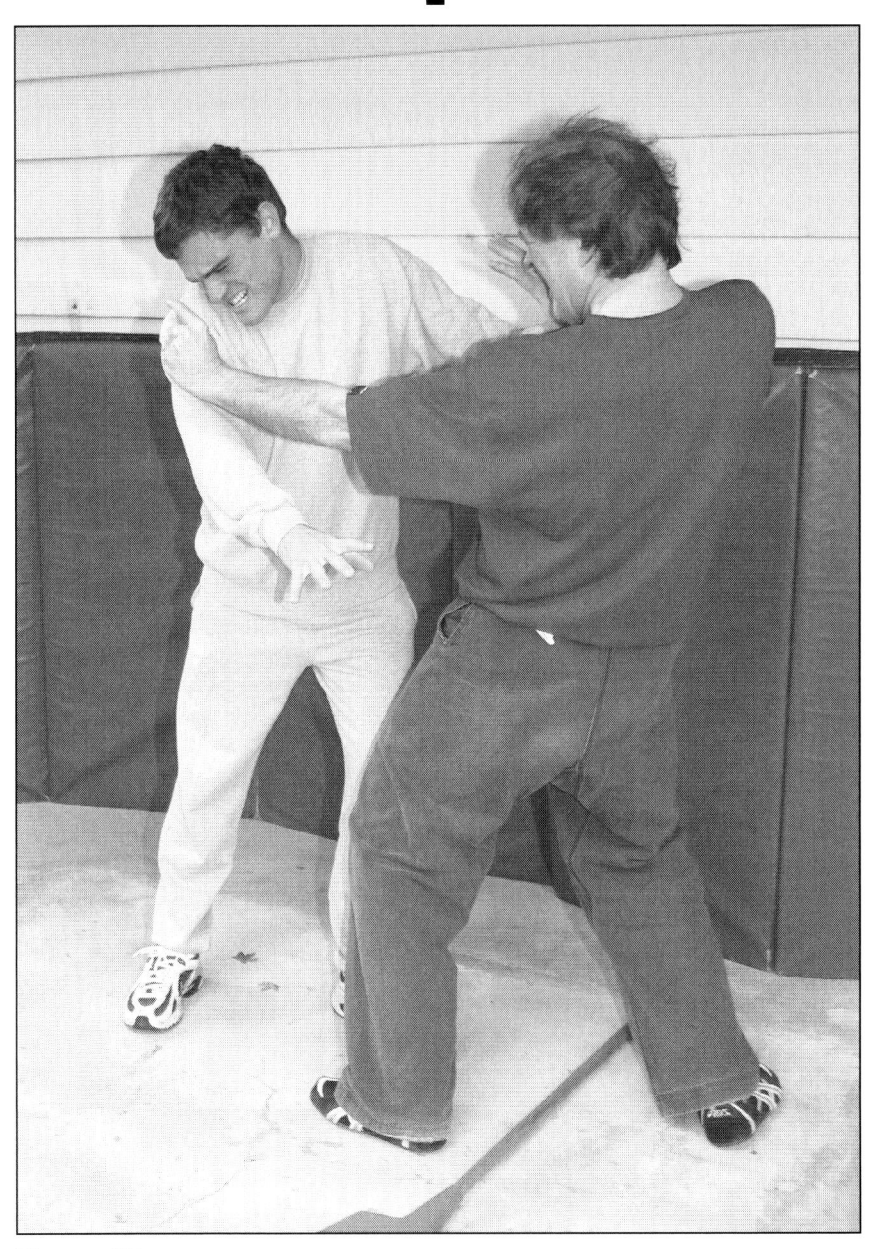

Figure 65

- Rip it to the side. (Fig. 65)

Block and Rip

An assailant jabs at you.

- Sweep his punch with your closest forearm. This isn't a power smash but a mere glancing motion made so that your arm sort of kisses his just enough to force it off course. (Fig. 66)
- Without hesitation and in one fluid motion, press your thumb into his eye. (Fig. 67)
- Snap your hand to the side in a quick, ripping motion. (Fig. 68)

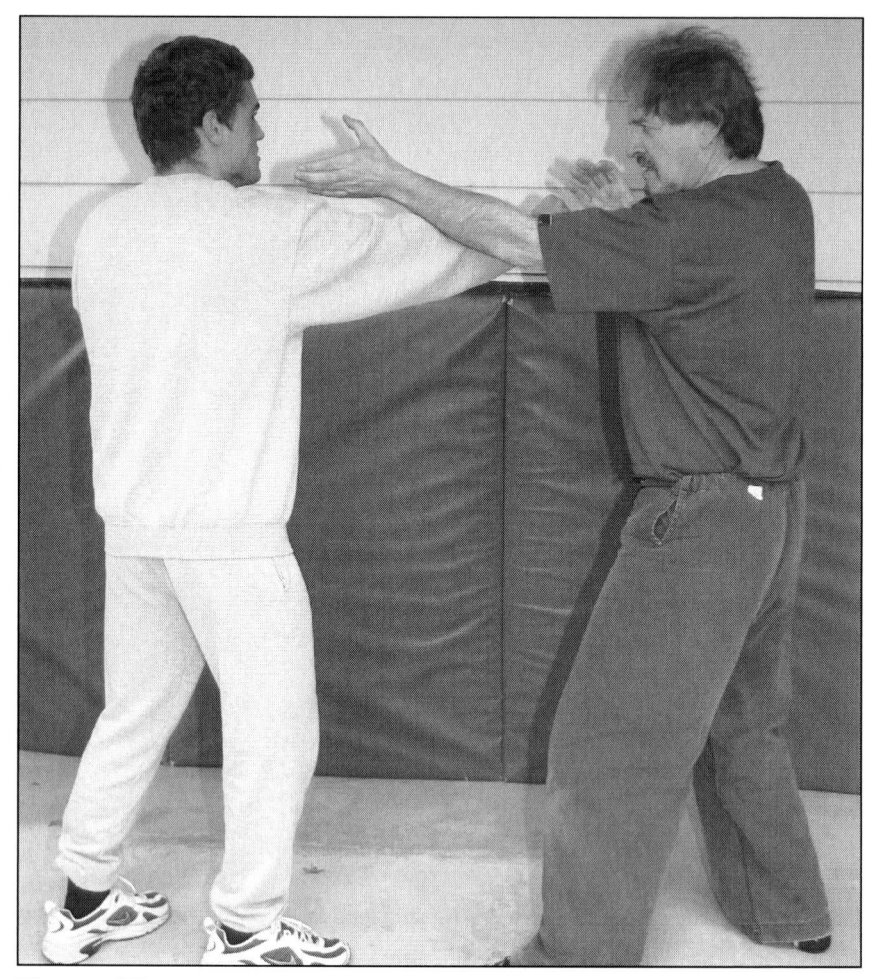

Figure 66

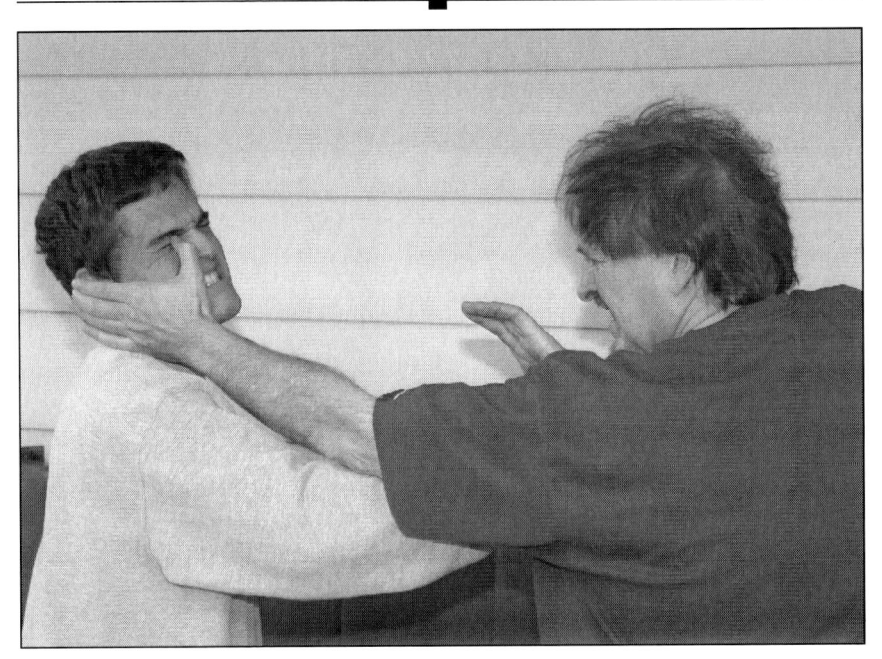

Figure 67

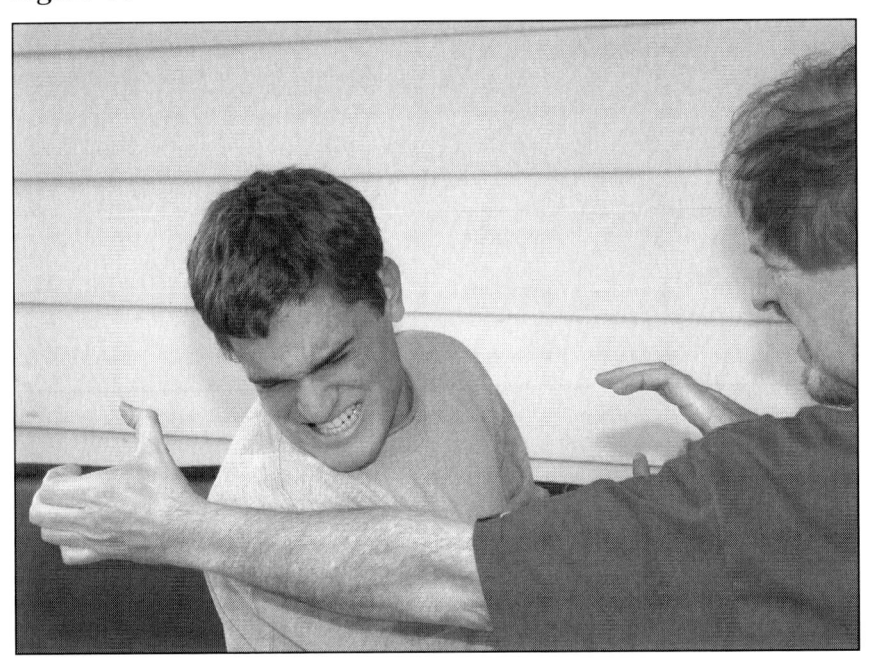

Figure 68

Hook and Rip

An attacker thrusts a 2 x 4 board at you.

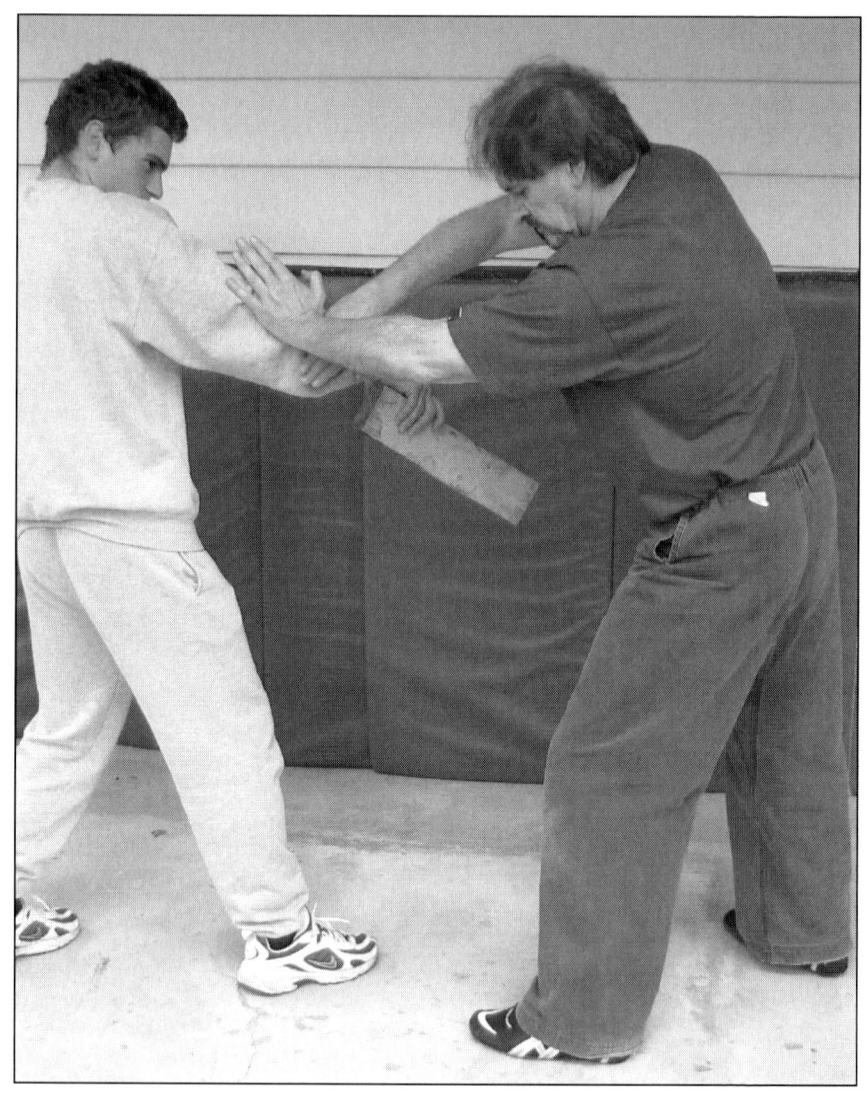

Figure 69

- Swat the board to his inside so that he turns part way around. Step a little to the outside in the event he doesn't turn far enough. (Fig. 69)

Head

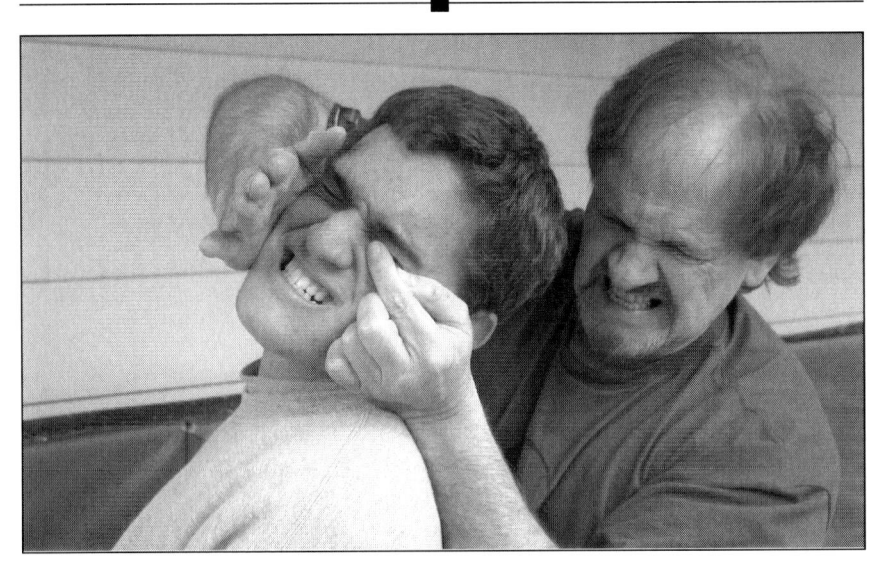

Figure 70

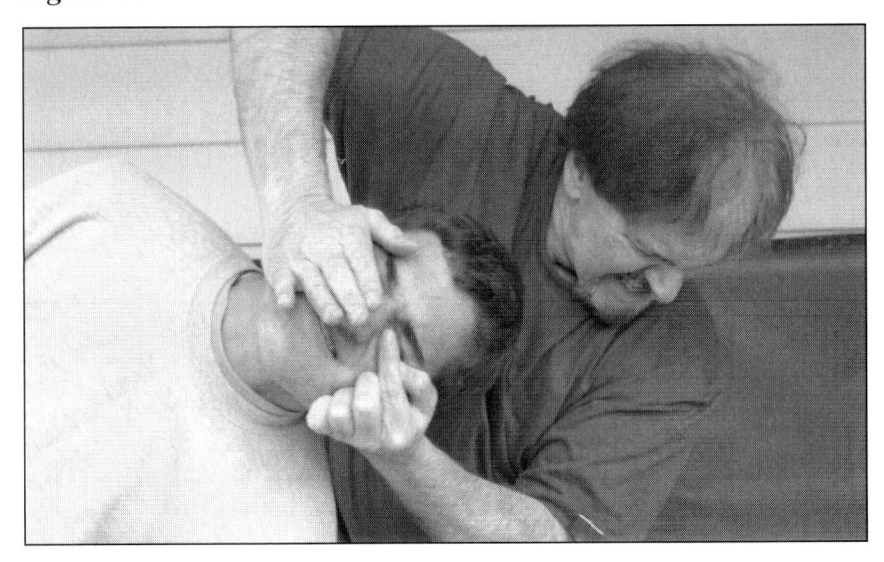

Figure 71

- Reach around the side and back of his head to his face and hook your mantis finger into his eye. Slap your other hand against the other side of his face. (Fig. 70)
- To spin him around, push with your open hand as you pull his eye socket with your finger. (Fig. 71)

Figure 72

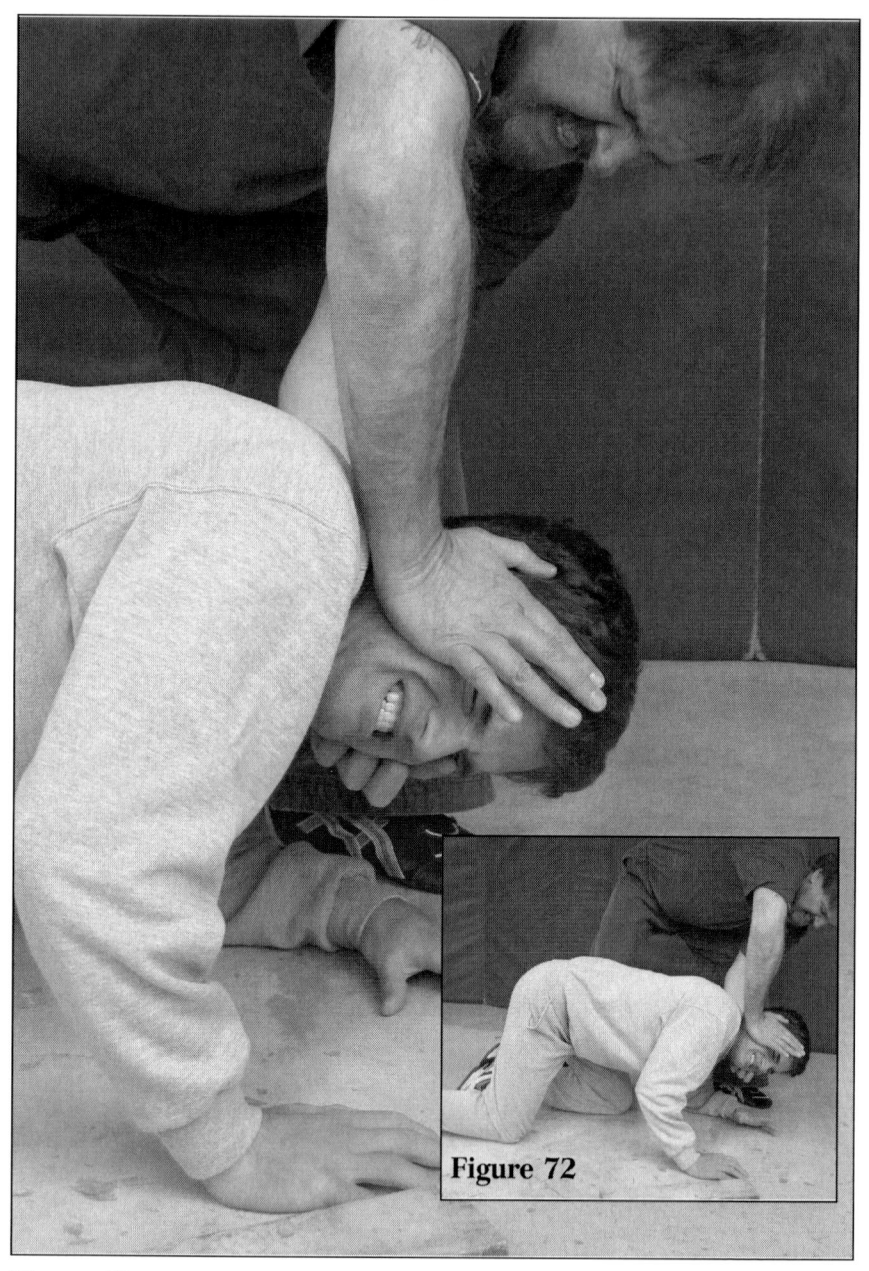

Figure 73

- Take him down. (Figs. 72, 73)

FLICKING

Flicking might not seem like much, and it isn't when you do it against an attacker's shoulder or leg. But when it's delivered to the eye, it's intensely painful and potentially injurious. As always, be legally justified.

When Restrained on the Ground

You can't move your arms to punch or grab, but at least one of your fingers is a couple of inches away from your attacker's eyeballs.

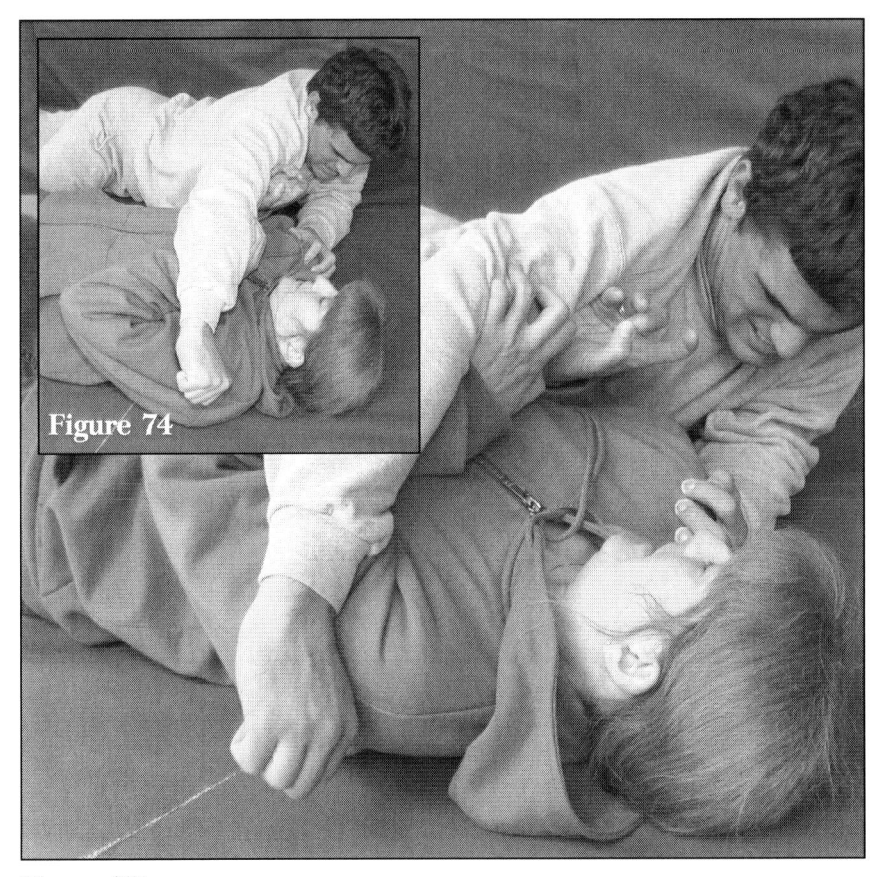

Figure 74

Figure 75

- Chamber your finger. (Figs. 74, 75)

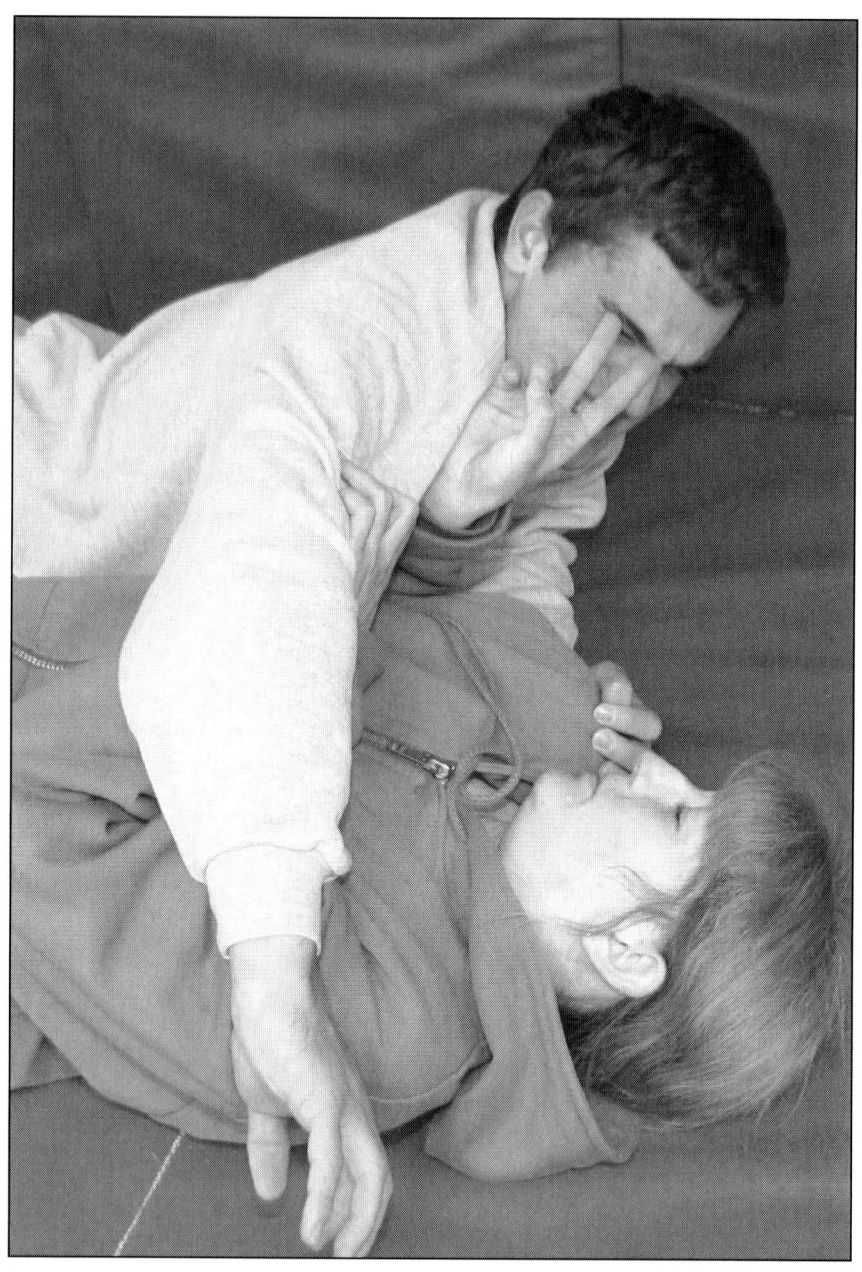

Figure 76

- Flick it into his eye. (Fig. 76)

When Restrained While Standing

Your attacker grabs you so that your arms are restrained against your chest.

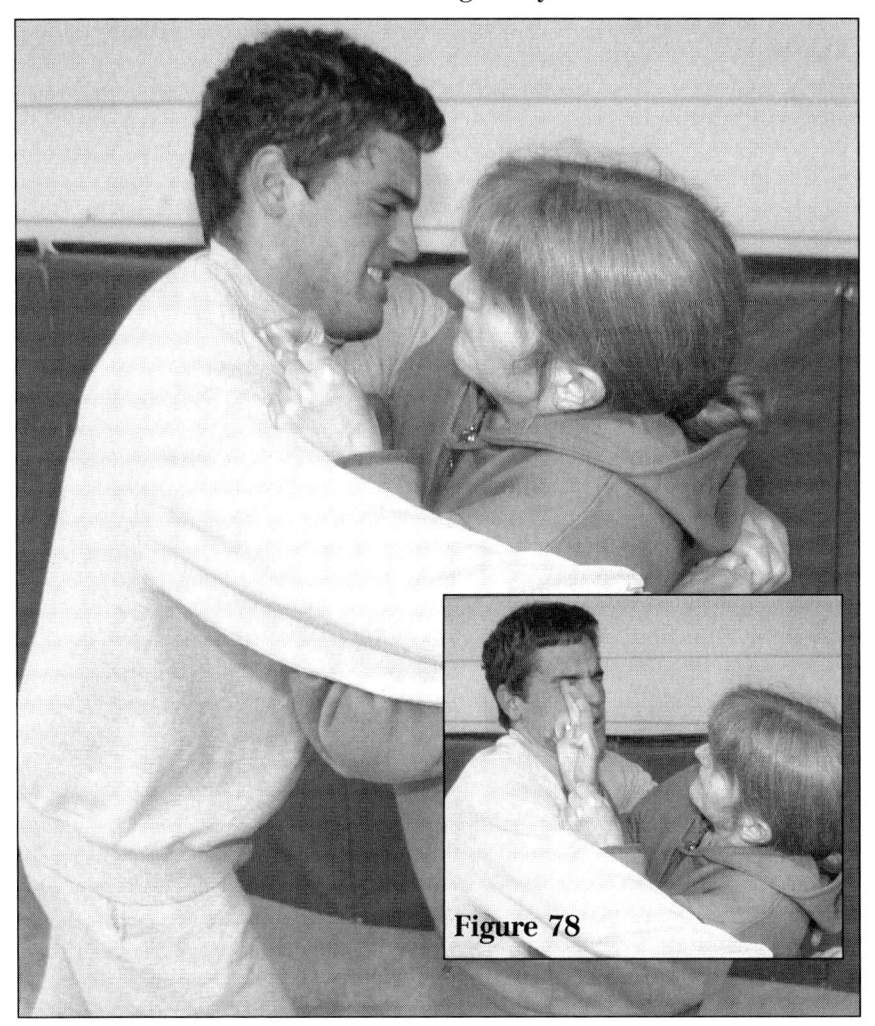

Figure 77

Figure 78

- You can barely move your arms but at least one of your attacker's eyes is within reach of your flick. (Fig. 77)
- Flick his eye and then make your escape when he releases his hold. (Fig. 78)

Eyelid Pinching

This shocks and frightens its recipients. It hurts, too, but the shock and fear factors just might be more intense.

When you reach for someone's eye, he will likely close it and jerk his head away. This is good, because by dropping his lid, he sort of "hands" you the target.

Pinch his eyelid between your thumb and pointy finger. Experiment to see which of the following grips you like best.

- Pinch with the pads of both the thumb and index finger.
- Pinch with the pad of the thumb pressed against the middle section of the index finger.

A pinch can be done several ways:

- Pinch and squeeze.
- Pinch and pull.
- Pinch and rip.
- Pinch and shake (like a dog with a rabbit).
- Pinch and twist (like turning a key in a door).

In most situations, you can use any one of these methods, or you can combine them for added effectiveness. Let's look at a simple attack, the jab, and see how you can apply each method as a counter.

THE ATTACKER JABS
Pinch and Squeeze

- Deflect his jab with the back of your hand. (Fig. 79)
- Shoot your hand toward his closest eye. Secure a nice pinch and squeeze. (Fig. 80)
- As his hands jerk toward his face, drive your palm into his ear or cheek while maintaining the pinch. (Fig. 81)

Head

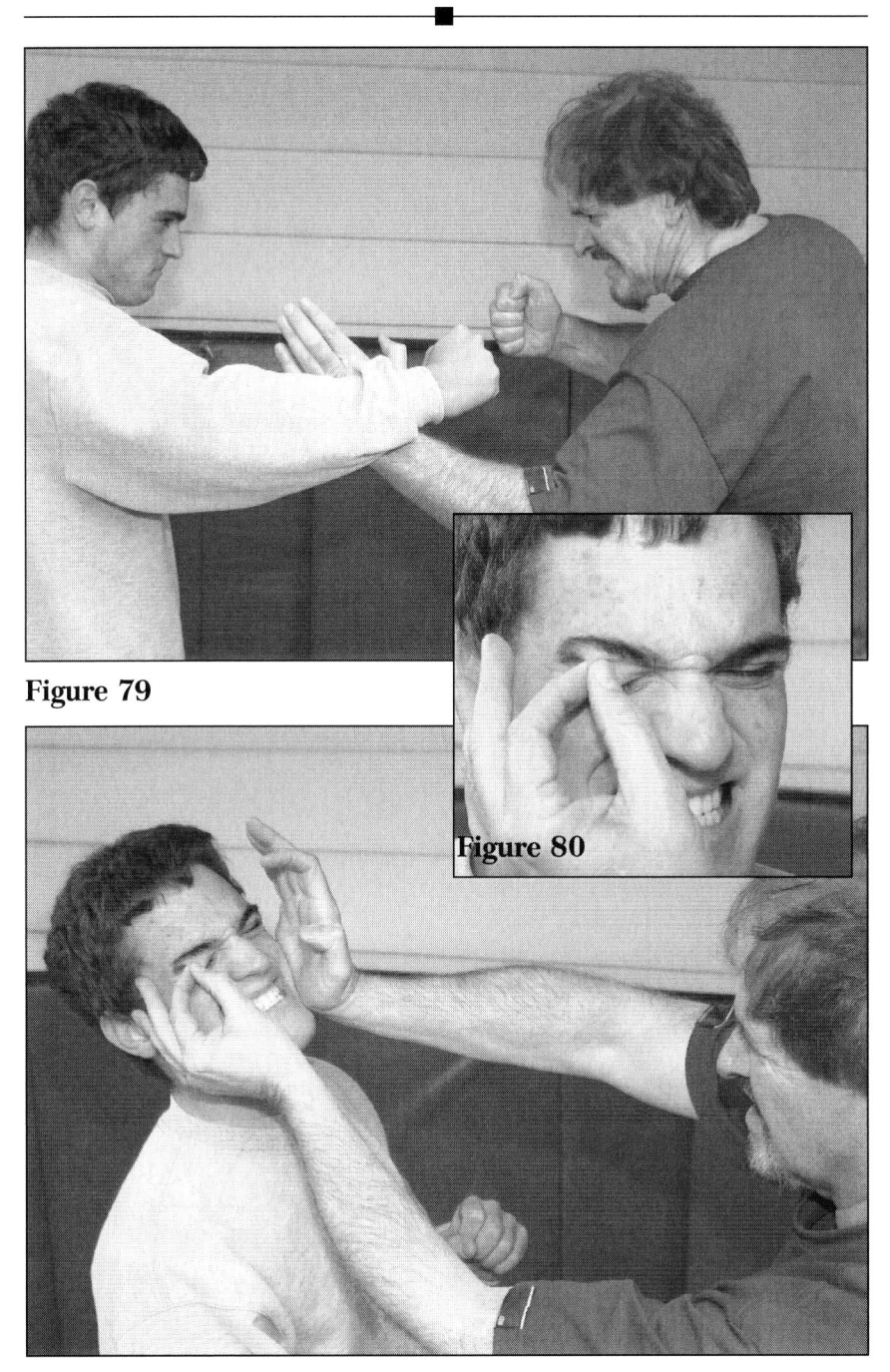

Figure 79

Figure 80

Figure 81

Pinch and Pull

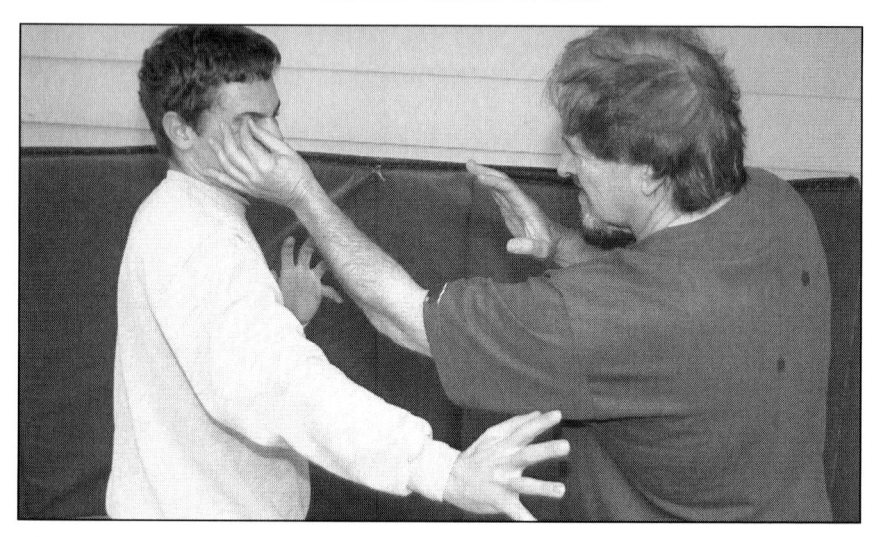

Figure 82

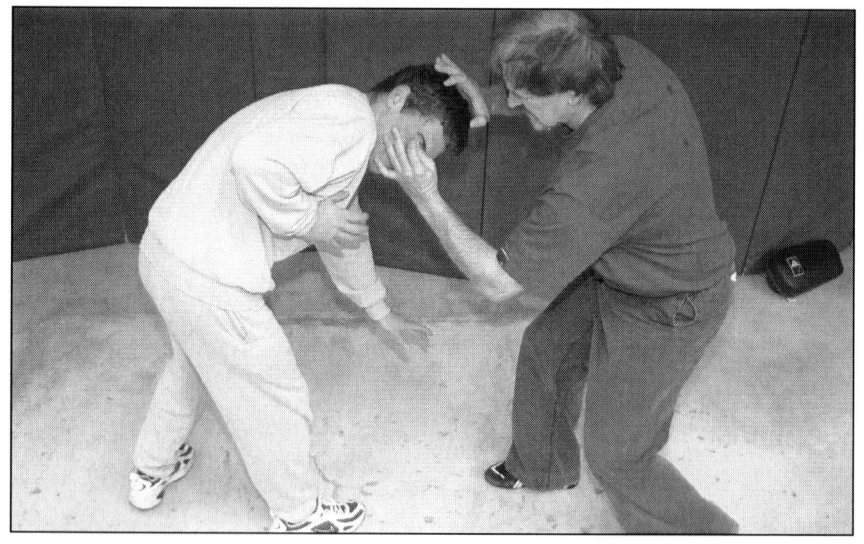

Figure 83

- After you block, shoot your hand toward his closest eye and pinch the eyelid. (Fig. 82)
- Jerk your elbow straight down as you step back to give him space to fall. (Fig. 83)

Pinch and Rip

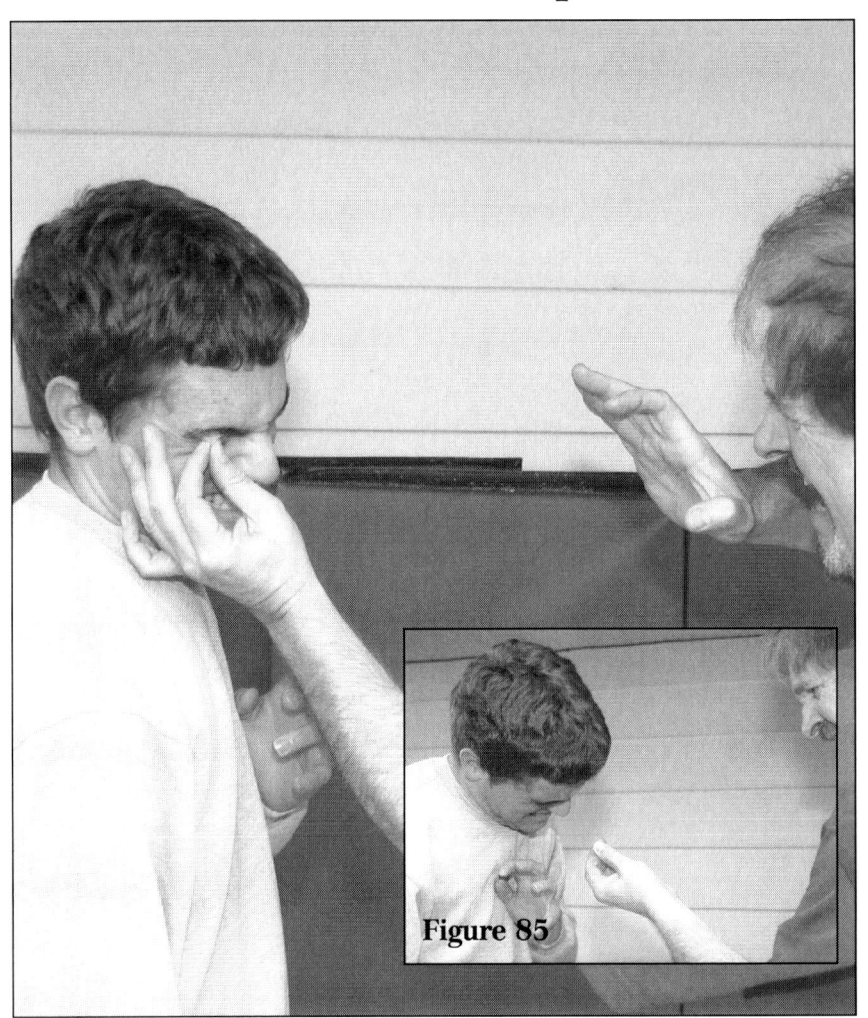

Figure 84

Figure 85

- After you block, shoot your hand toward his closest eye and pinch the eyelid. (Fig. 84)
- As if quickly ripping a bandage off a wound, snap your hand back toward yourself. His eyelid will only stretch a half inch or so, but to him it will feel as if it traveled a foot. You might even rip the flesh. (Fig. 85)

Pinch and Shake

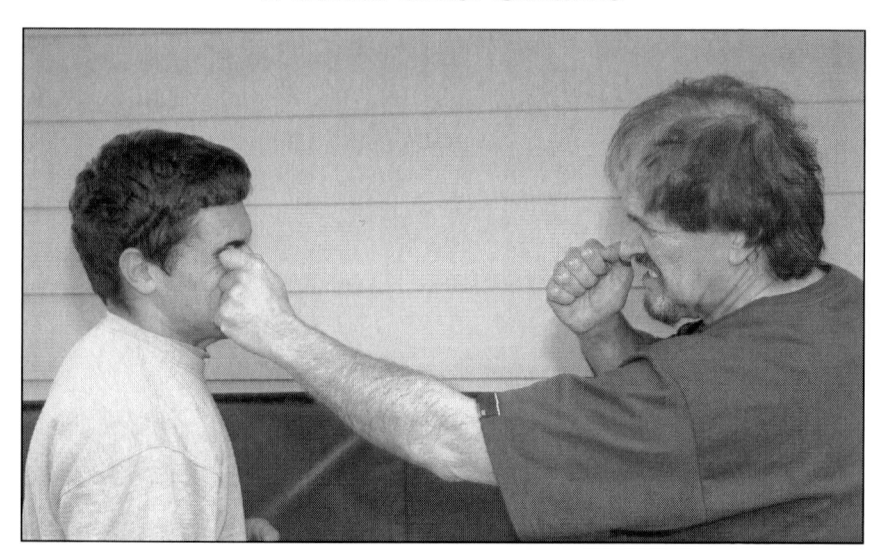

Figure 86

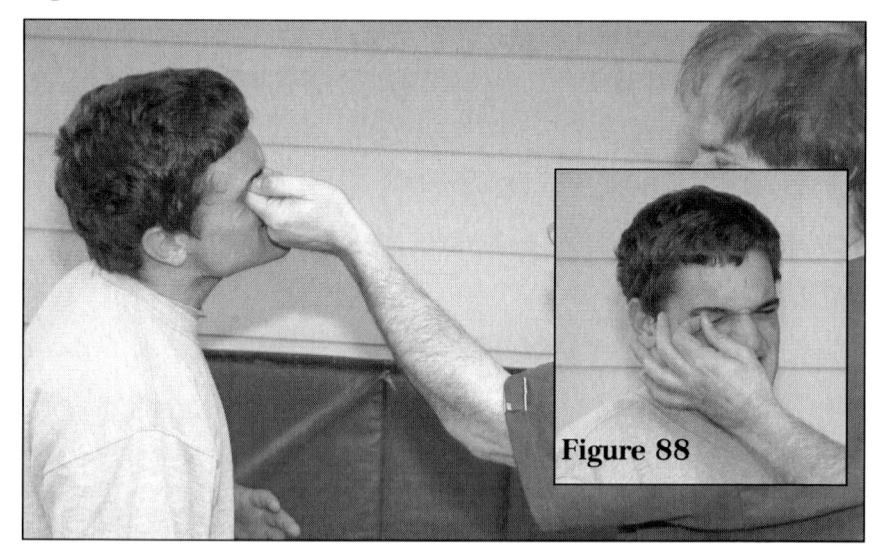

Figure 87

Figure 88

- After you block, shoot your hand toward his closest eye and pinch the eyelid. (Fig. 86)
- Shake it vigorously in little back-and-forth motions. (Figs. 87, 88)

Pinch and Twist

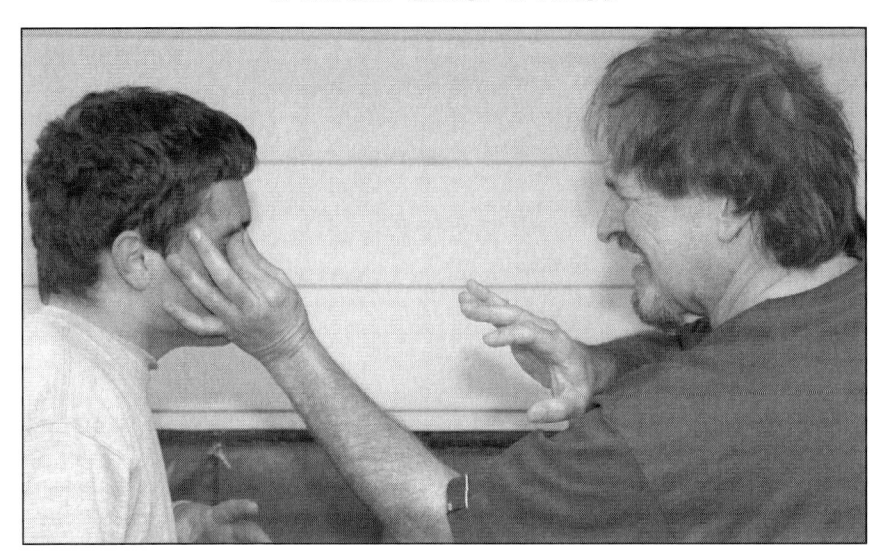

Figure 89

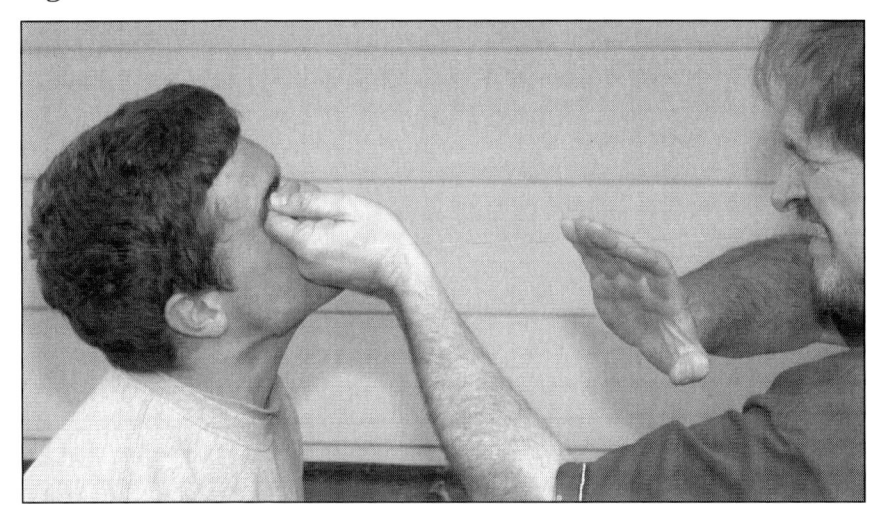

Figure 90

- After you block, shoot your hand toward his closest eye and pinch the eyelid. (Fig. 89)
- Twist the lid with a sharp snap of your wrist, as if quickly turning a key in a door. (Fig. 90)

Here are two examples of how to combine these techniques:

Pinch, Twist, and Pull

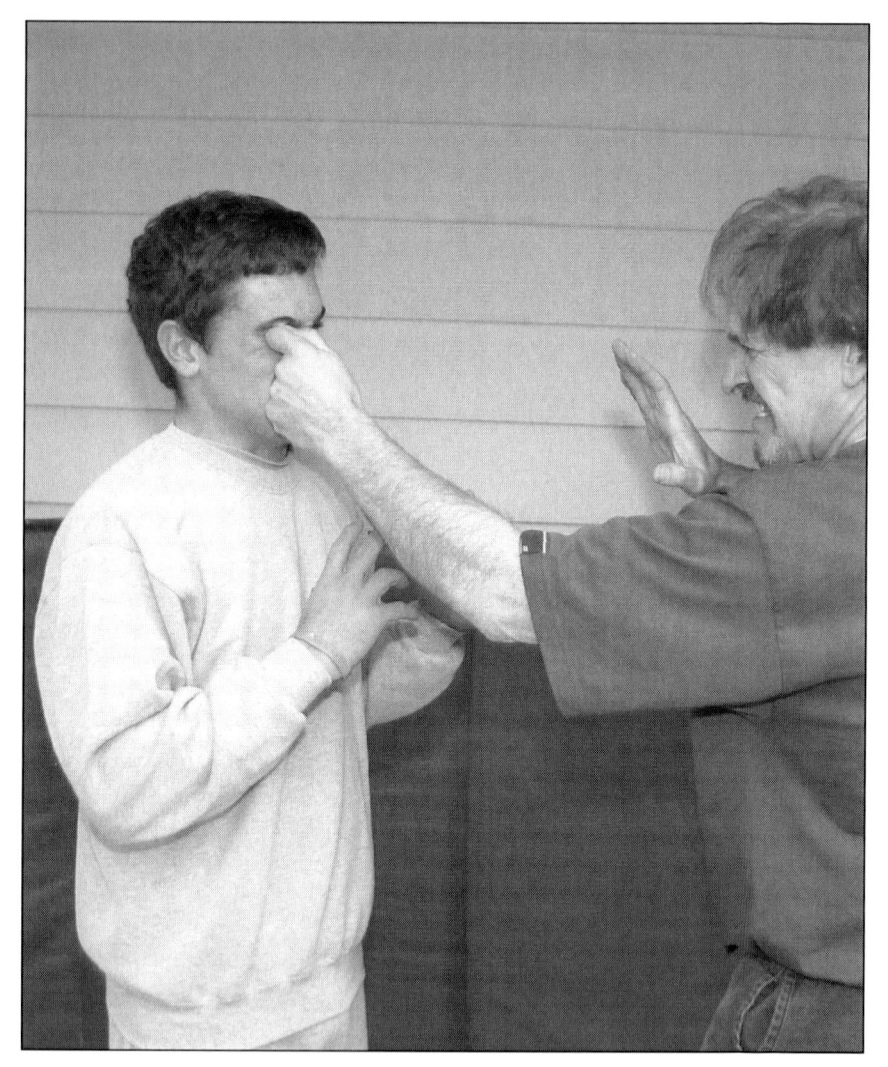

Figure 91

- Pinch the eyelid. (Fig. 91)
- Twist and tuck your elbow. (Fig. 92)
- Pull the lid and the attacker to the floor. (Fig. 93)

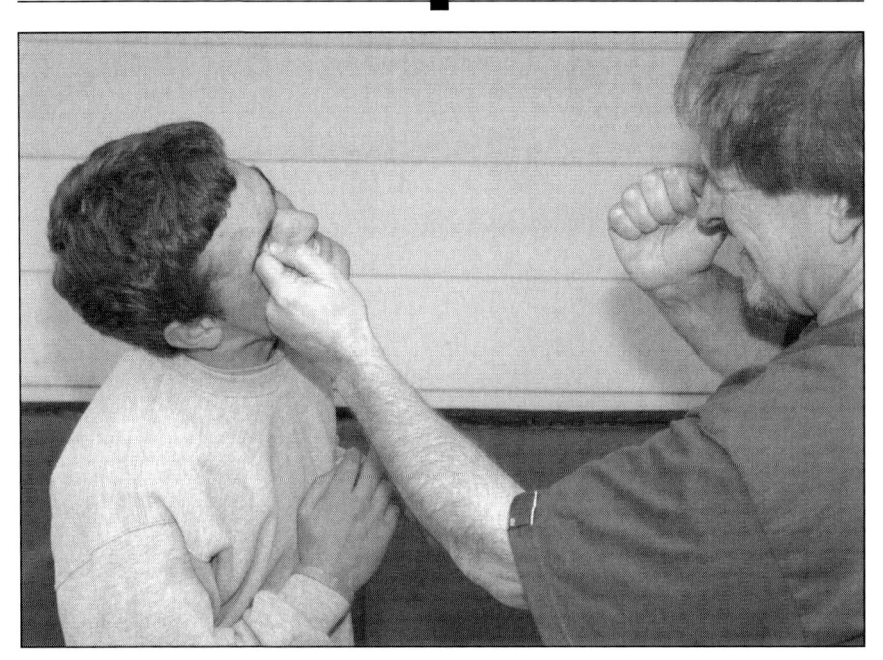

Figure 92

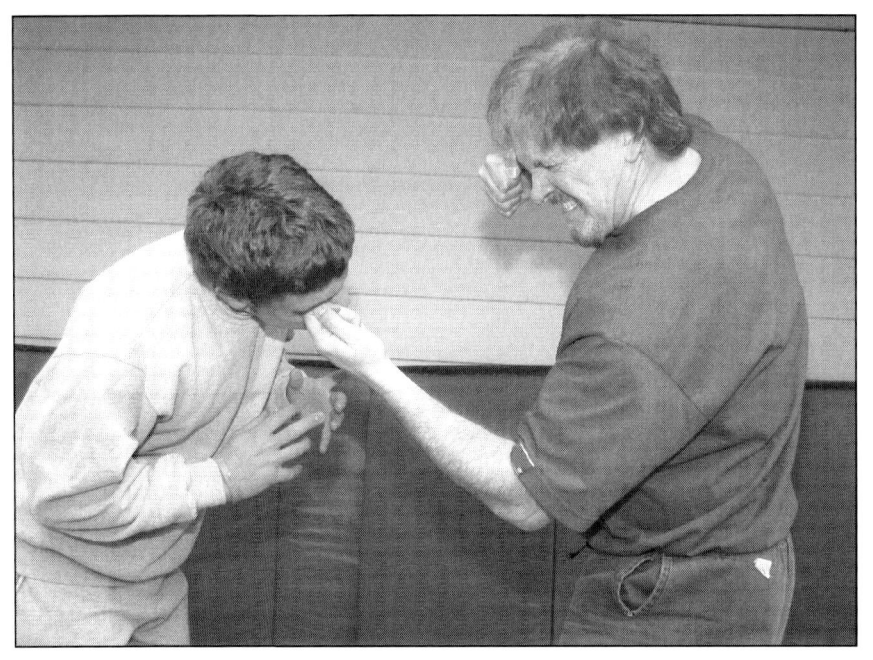

Figure 93

Pinch, Twist and Rip

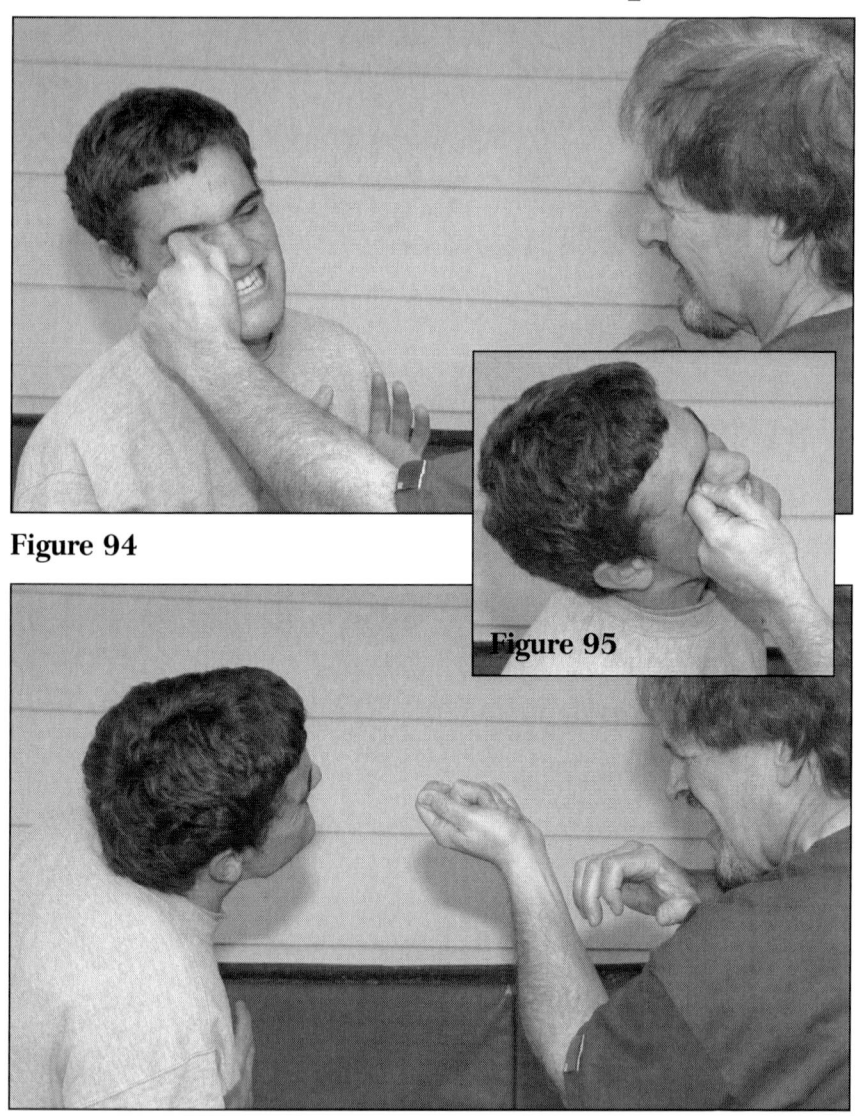

Figure 94

Figure 95

Figure 96

- Pinch the eyelid. (Fig. 94)
- Pinch and twist. (Fig. 95)
- Rip. (Fig. 96)

Here are a few others:

- Pinch, shake, and twist.
- Pinch, pull for the takedown, and rip.
- Shake it three or four times and then rip it to the side.
- Pinch, pull for a takedown, and twist.

We have used defense against a jab as an example, but you can apply the eyelid pinch anytime a window of opportunity allows you access.

Eye Techniques: One Last Warning

Although techniques delivered to the eyes carry less risk than those delivered to an attacker's throat, there is still an inherent danger of causing blindness and even death. These are tragedies that will be carefully examined in court. Many attorneys agree that juries are uncomfortable with eye techniques because, to the squeamish, violence against someone's eyes is abhorrent to imagine.

Expect to be grilled as to why you chose such brutal methods when there are so many other ways you can defend yourself. One day you're forced to fight for your life in the street, and a year later you're being grilled in court as if you were the attacker. Welcome to our legal system.

Choose an attorney who is savvy to all aspects of self-defense, legal-wise and street reality-wise.

FOREHEAD

The forehead isn't as sensitive as other parts of the head, but pressing there with a hard knuckle or elbow might give you the reaction you want from your attacker, such as to:

- Move or turn his head.
- Release his grip on you.
- Allow you to better your grip on a hold.
- Better position you so you can hit him.

As you read this, take the middle knuckle of your index finger and press it into your forehead about an inch above either eye. Press it in hard and, without losing contact, grind it back and forth a little. Imagine what it would feel like to press the point of your elbow into someone's forehead with your body weight behind it. Poke other places on your forehead to see what they feel like.

Elbow Press on the Ground

You've taken the attacker down onto his back.

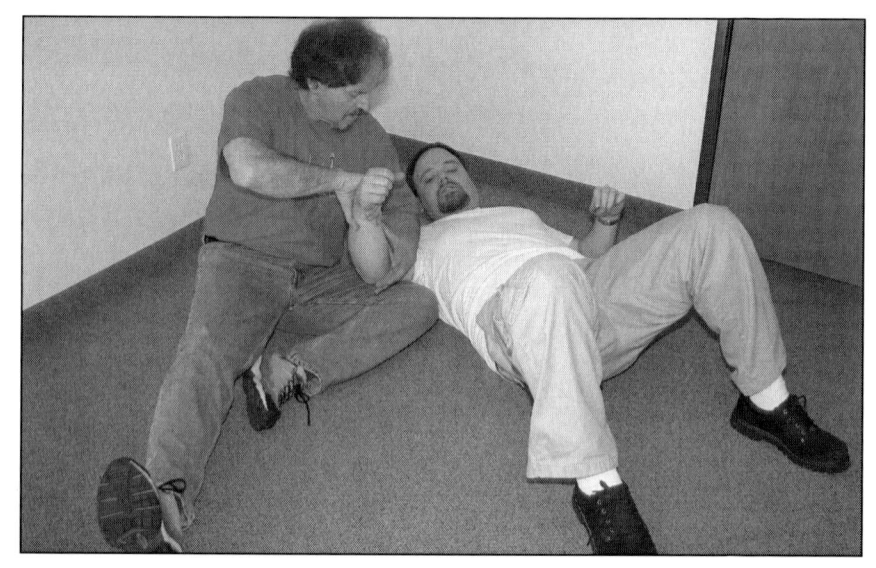

Figure 97

Head

- You're attempting to hyperextend his elbow over your leg but he is lifting his head and trying to defeat your hold. (Fig. 97)
- Press your closest elbow into his forehead and lean into it. (Fig. 98)
- The pain will distract him momentarily and allow you to secure the hold. (Fig. 99)

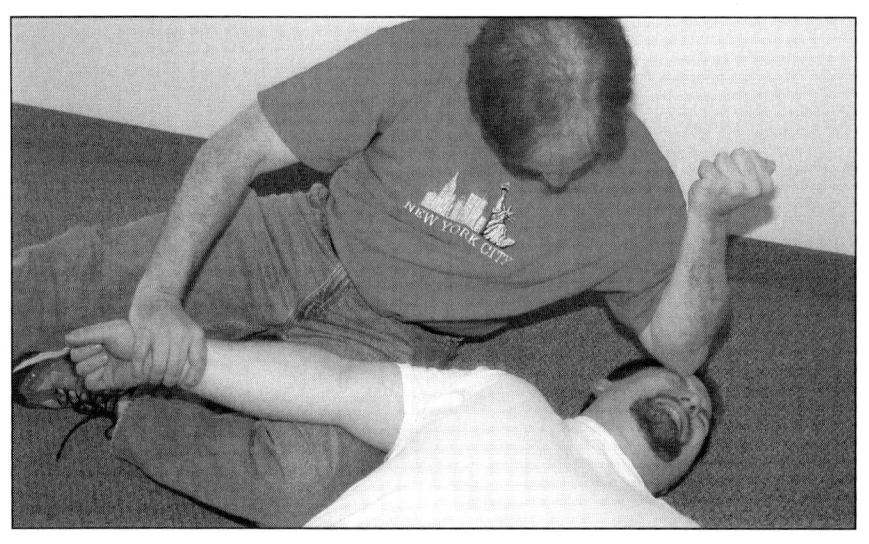

Figure 98

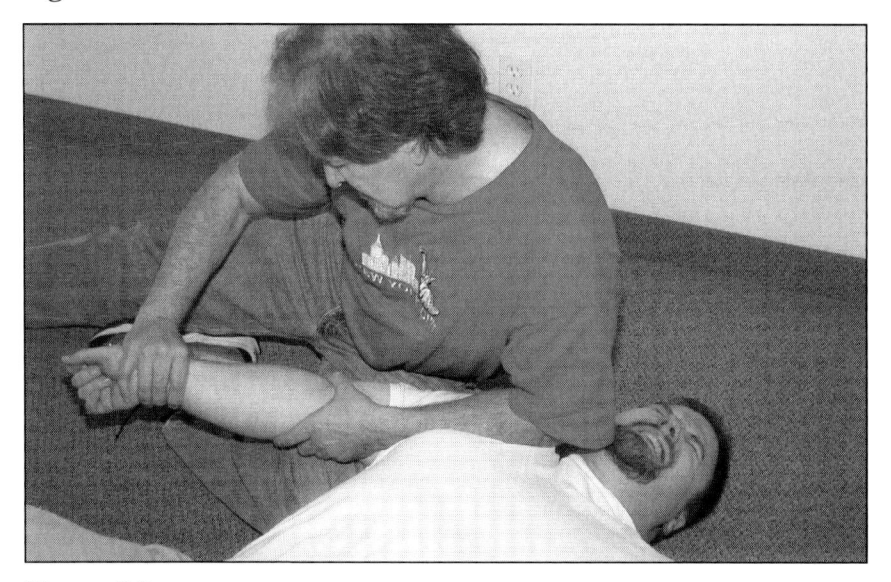

Figure 99

Knee Press on the Ground

You've taken your attacker down onto his belly.

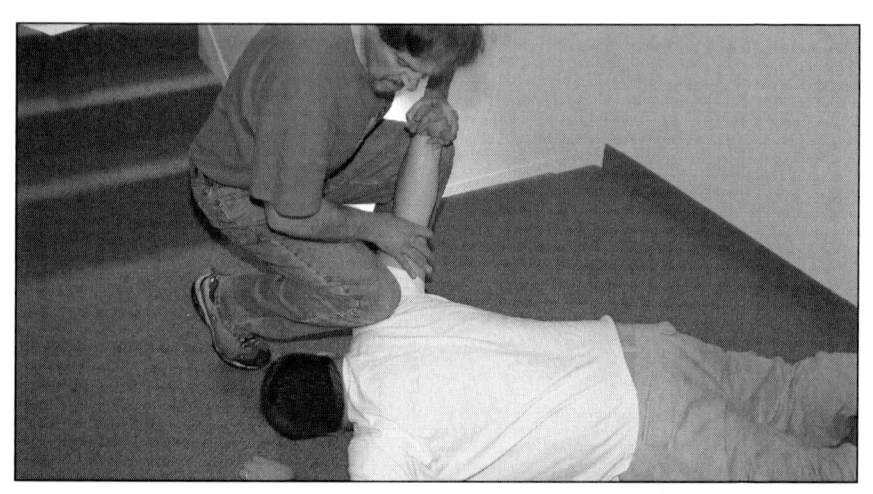

Figure 100

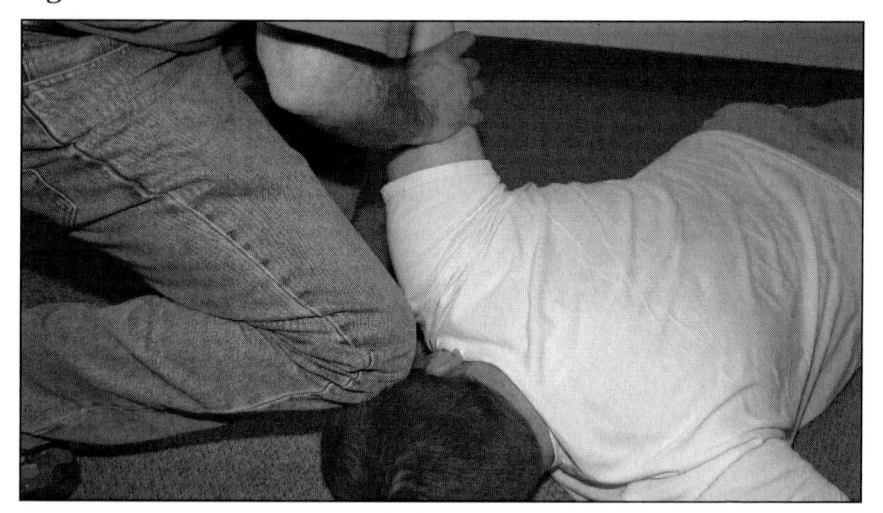

Figure 101

- His face is turned toward you, watching your every move. You order him to turn his head away but he doesn't comply. (Fig. 100)
- Since he might be thinking of a counter, move your knee from his shoulder to the side of his forehead. (Fig. 101)

Head

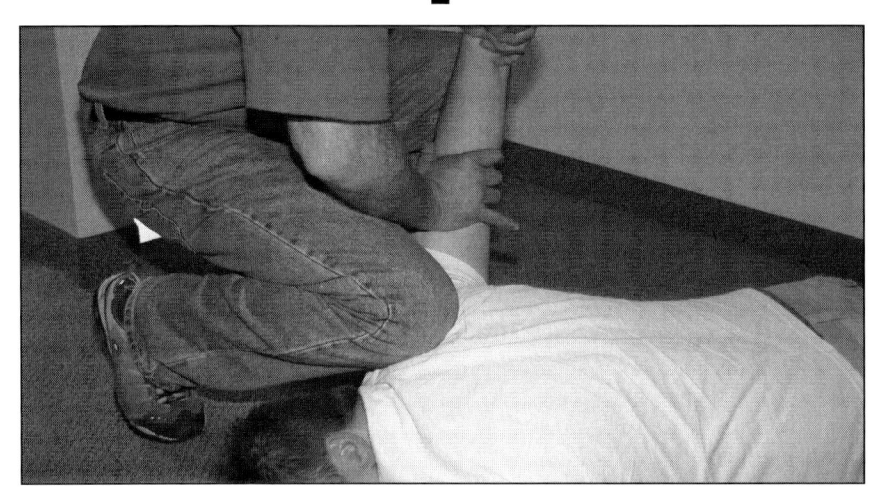

Figure 102

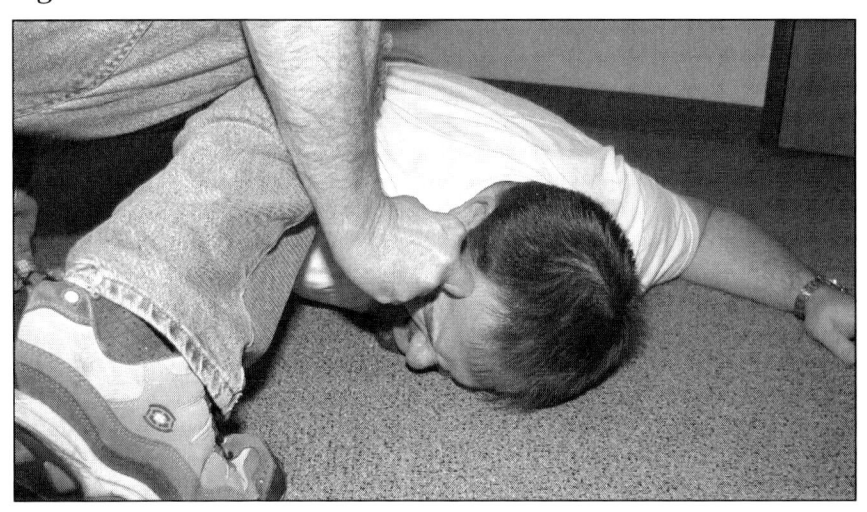

Figure 103

- Press your knee downward with enough force that he turns his head away. (Fig. 102)

    Variation:

- If you can control his arm with one hand, use your middle knuckles to press and rub into the side of his forehead until he turns away. (Fig. 103)

NOSE

While some boxers and other full-contact fighters can take hard hits to the nose and keep fighting, most people can't. They react by jerking their heads, grabbing their faces, and momentarily losing their vision as their eyes flood with tears. Even tough guys who can keep fighting with broken noses will almost always react in some way, at least for a moment. They will snap their heads, blink rapidly, or yelp—wonderful reactions that provide you with the half-second opening you need to execute a follow up.

The following crushing techniques aren't intended to break the nose, though they might. So what do you do if you hear that sickening breaking sound? You keep crushing to take advantage of your attacker's new sensitivity.

Nose Crush from Behind

I used this technique several times when I was a cop. It can be applied in a standing position or on the ground. Practice it on a live partner or a mannequin-style bag.

Your attacker pushes with both hands.

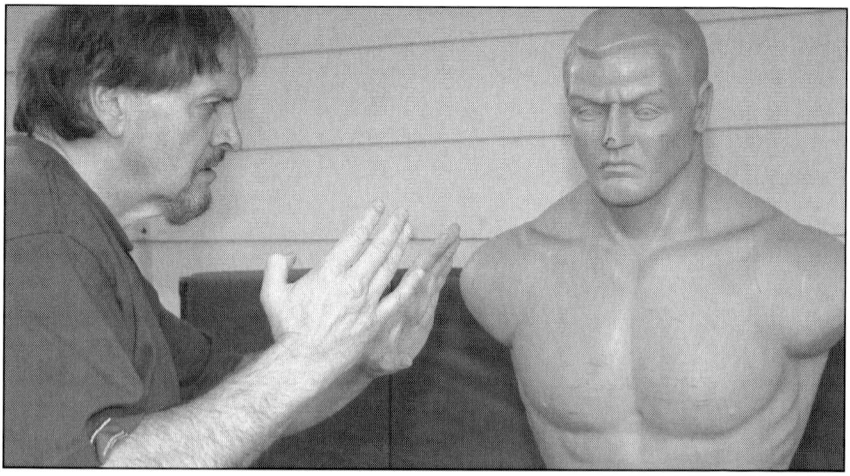

Figure 104

- Swat his arms aside. (Fig. 104)

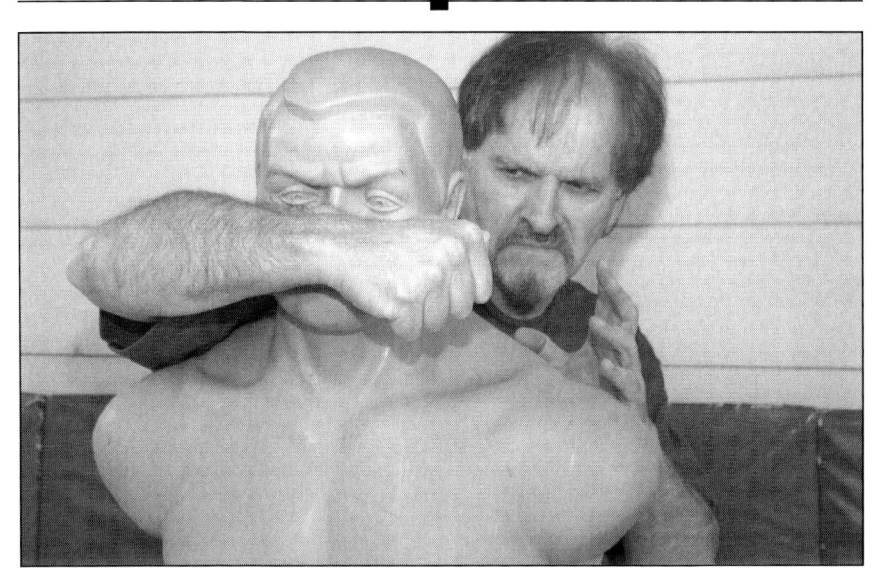

Figure 105

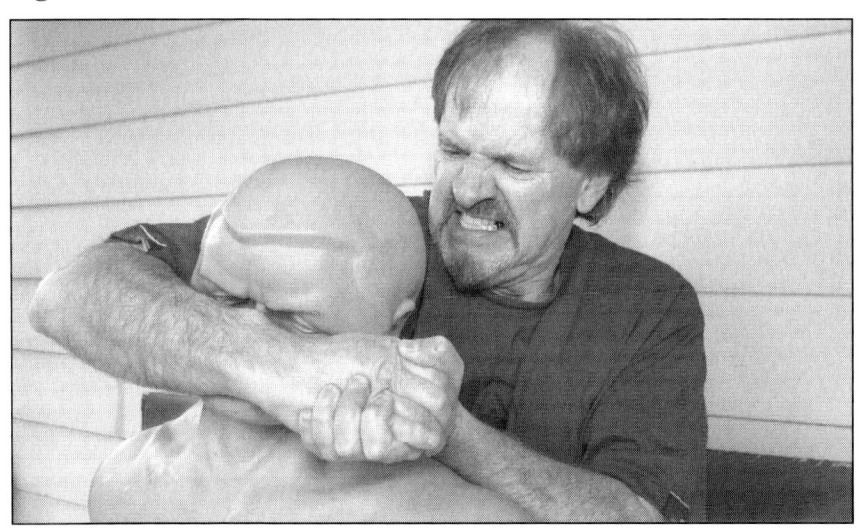

Figure 106

- Move behind him and whip your right forearm across his nose. (Fig. 105)
- Clasp your hands and pull your right thumb-side wrist into his nose. Use your chest or shoulder to brace the back of his head and squeeze your arms toward your chest for added power. (Fig. 106)

Nose Crush When He's on Top of You

You're on your back and your attacker is on top of you, face up. Practice on a live partner or a mannequin-style bag.

- Apply the nose crush as you did in the standing variation. (Fig. 107)

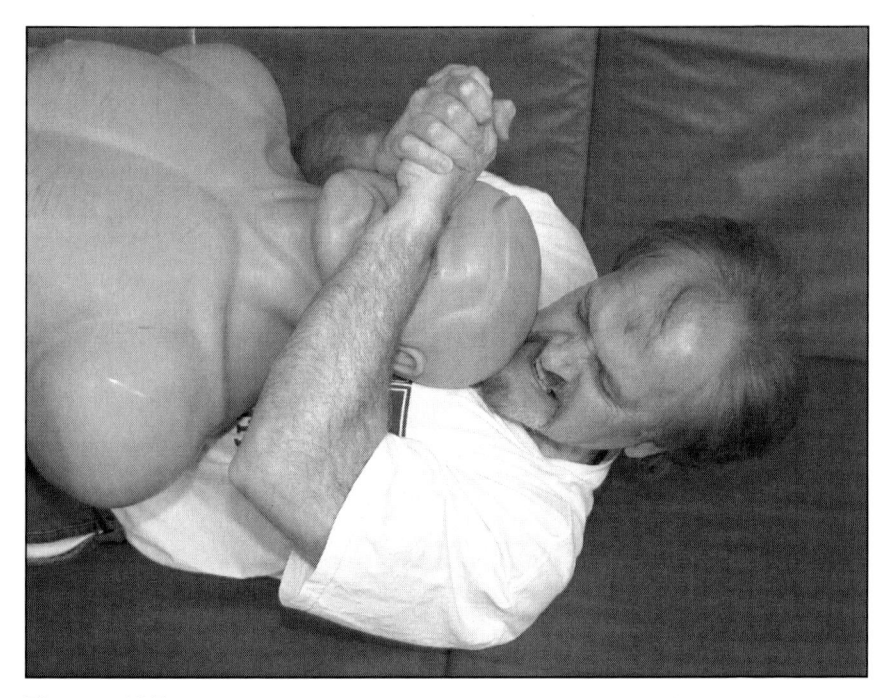

Figure 107

Nose Crush When He's in the Mount

This is an easy hold for your attacker to get out of since you can only sustain it for a second or two. Think of it as a transition move and be ready with a good follow-up.

- Your attacker is crawling up between your legs, intending to punch or choke you. (Fig. 108)
- Draw up your knee so that it's in front of his face and reach for the back of his head with one or both hands. (Fig. 109)

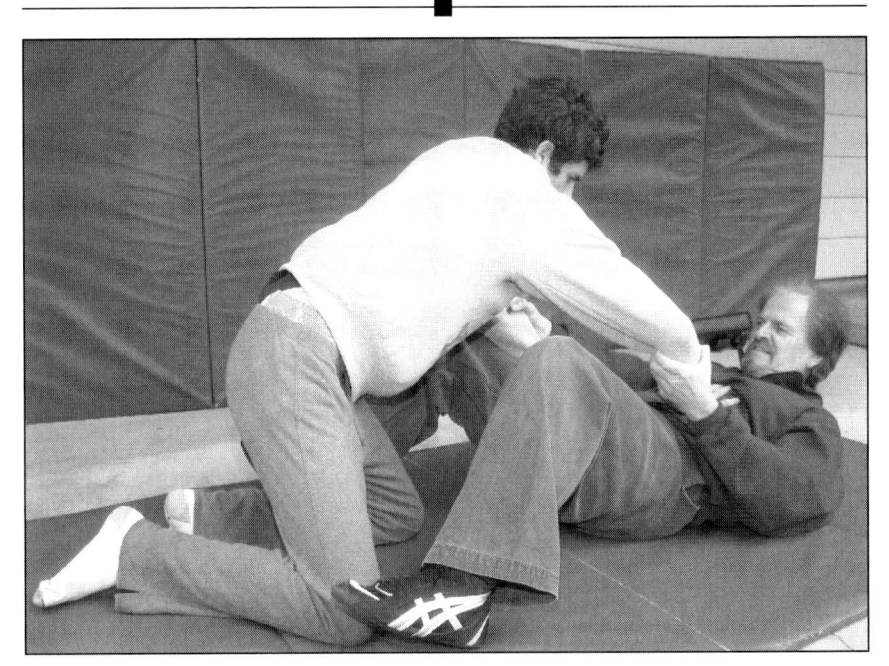

Figure 108

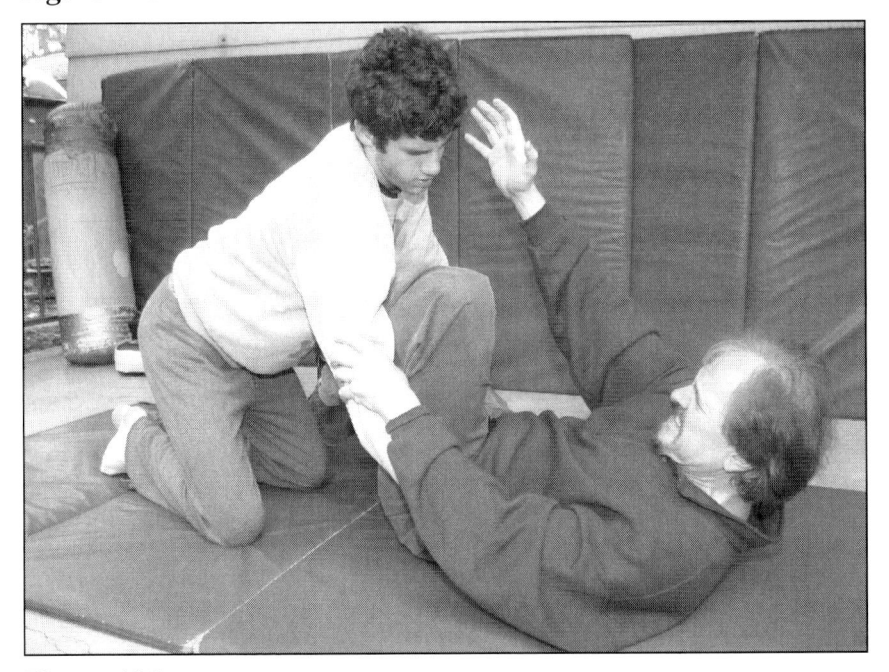

Figure 109

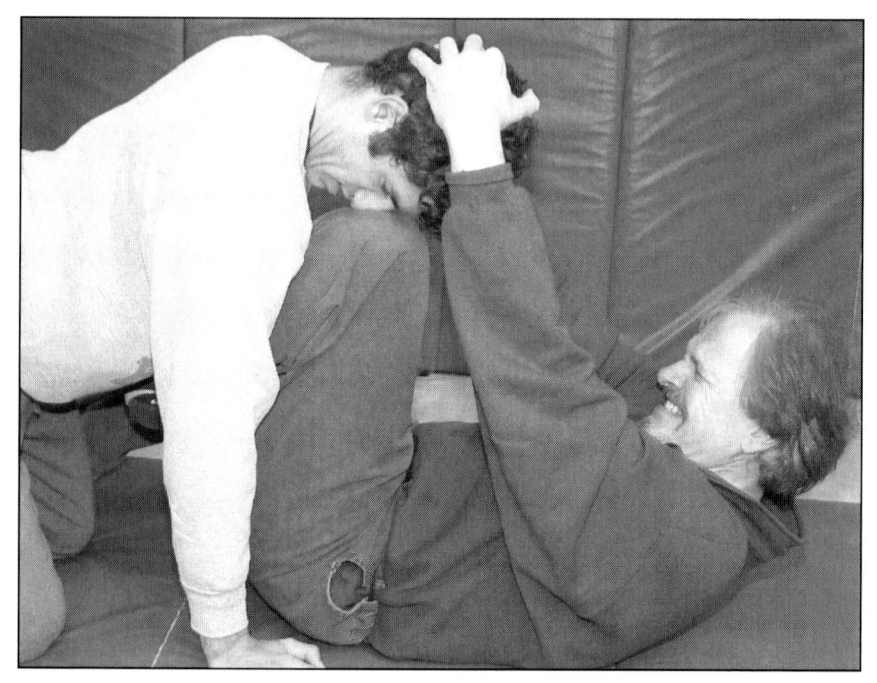

Figure 110

- Pull his head and nose into your knee cap or shin. If possible, jerk his head forcefully so that his nose slams into your leg. Then, as he grunts or screams in pain, rub your leg into his injured nose. (Fig. 110)

Nose Crush When You're on Top of Him

Practice with a live opponent or on a mannequin-style bag.

- You've maneuvered your attacker around until he is face down and you're on his back. Use your arms to pin his head, with your left wrist directly under his nose. (Fig. 111)
- Press your chest and body weight onto the back of his head, squishing his nose into your arm. Move your chest back and forth a little to rub in the pain. (Fig. 112)

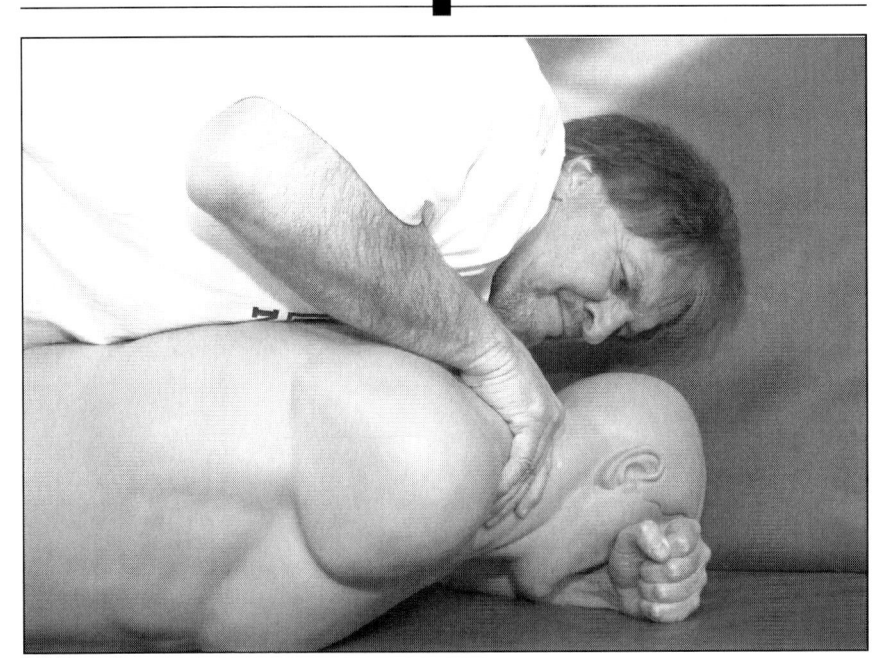

Figure 111

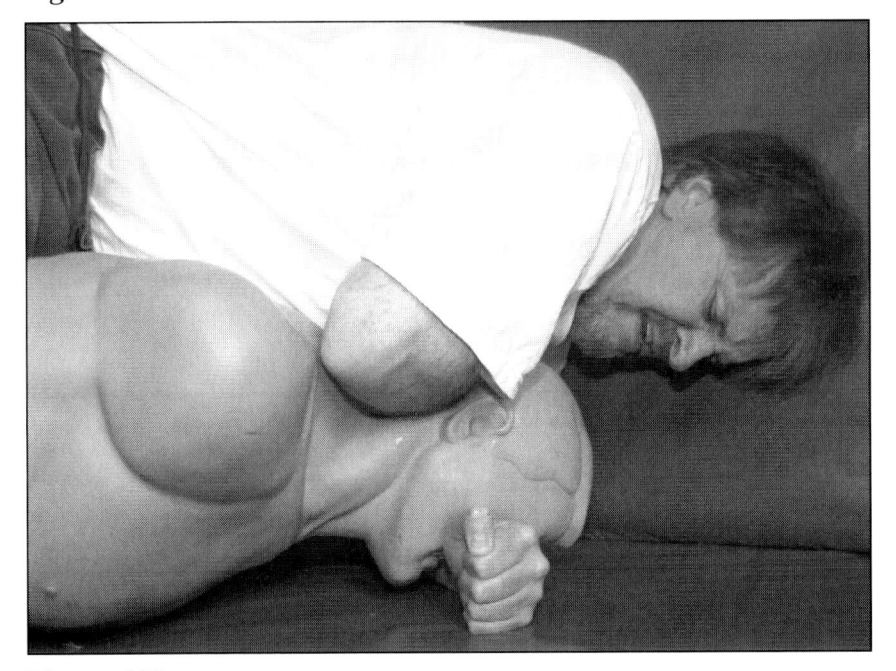

Figure 112

Nose-Rip Counter

This is quick, simple, effective, and disgusting. Practice on a mannequin-style bag when your partner has a cold.

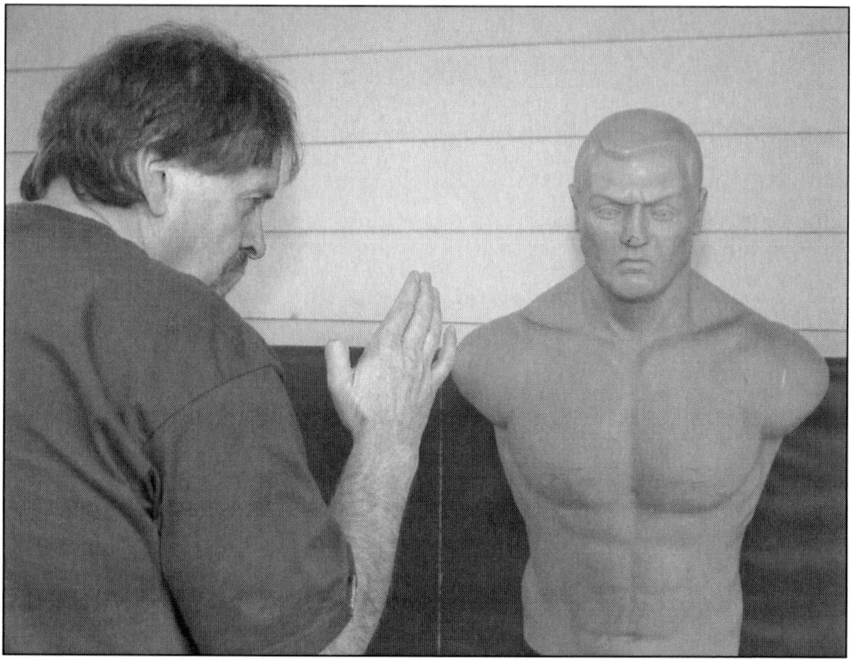

Figure 113

- Your attacker thrusts his fingers toward your eyes, which you block with a backhand block (though any block will work with this counter). (Fig. 113)
- Jab your mantis finger up his nostril. (Fig. 114)
- Jerk your hand to the side. (Fig. 115)

Variation:

- Insert your index and middle fingers into both his nostrils. (Fig. 116)
- Rip upward or to the side. (Fig. 117)

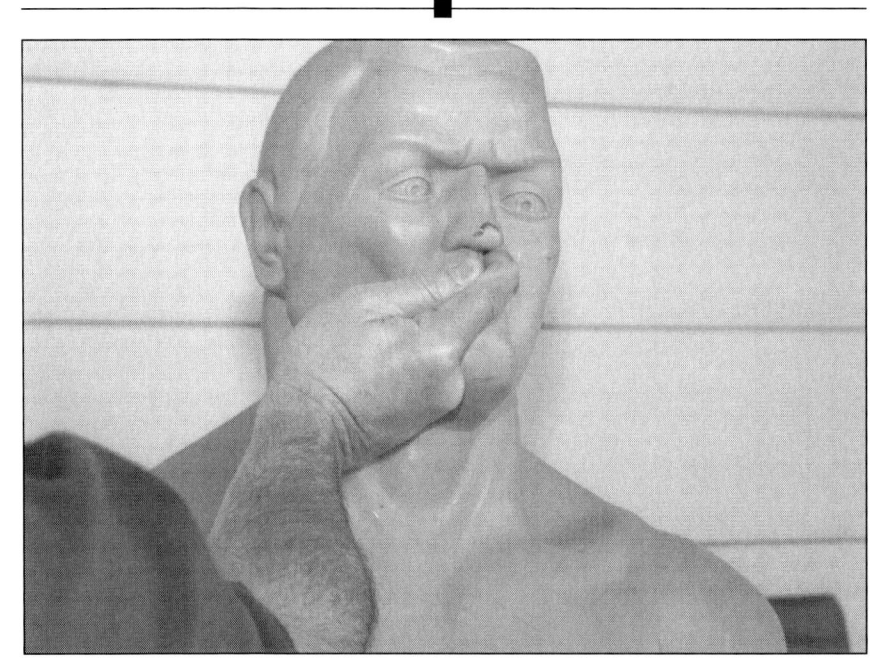

Figure 114

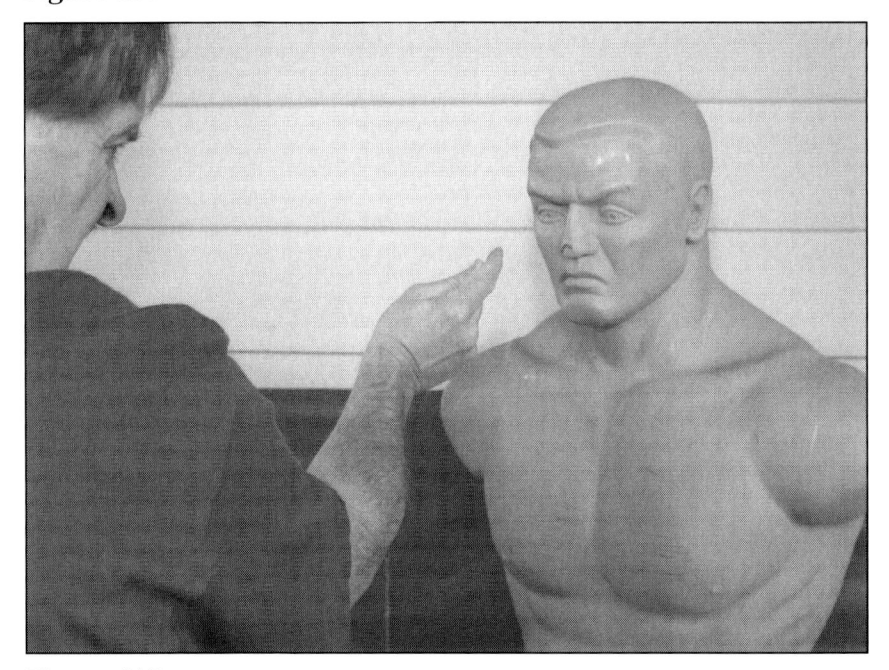

Figure 115

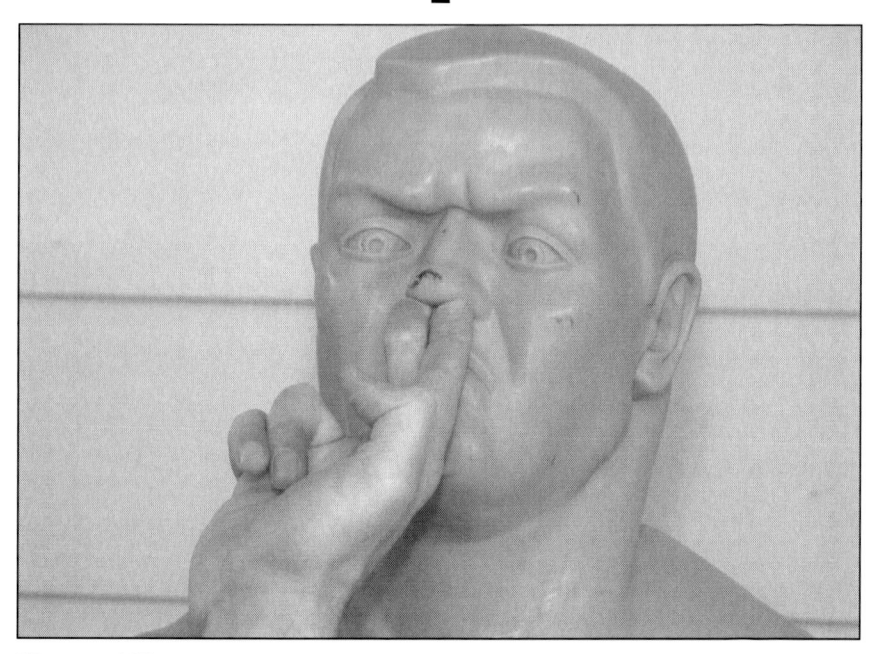

Figure 116

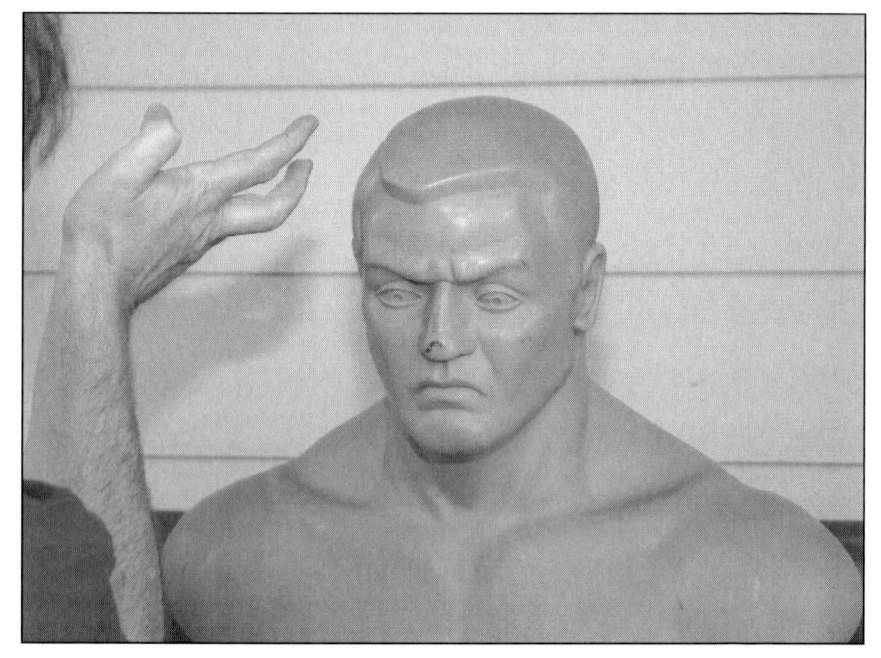

Figure 117

Nose Rip to Reestablish a Hold

You're controlling your attacker on the floor with a wrist flex.

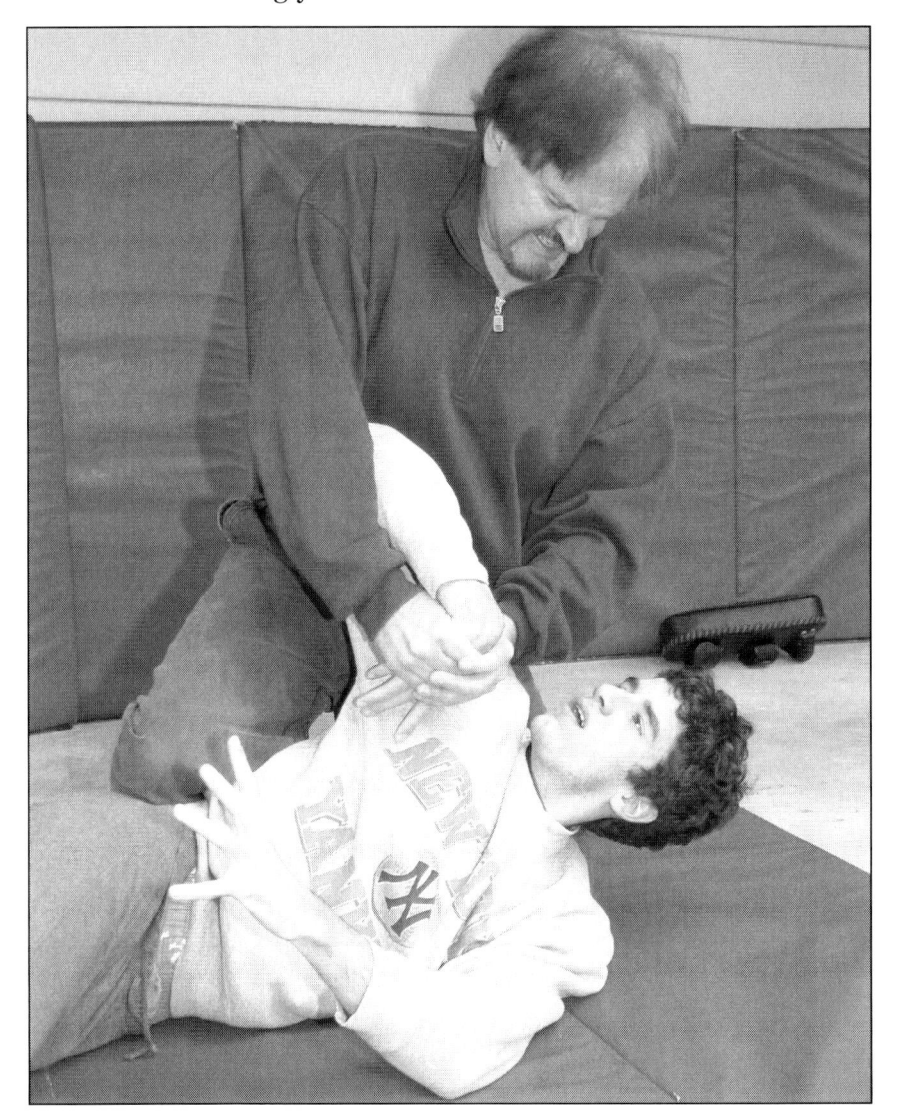

Figure 118

- Your knee has inadvertently slipped off his head and he is starting to sit up. (Fig. 118)

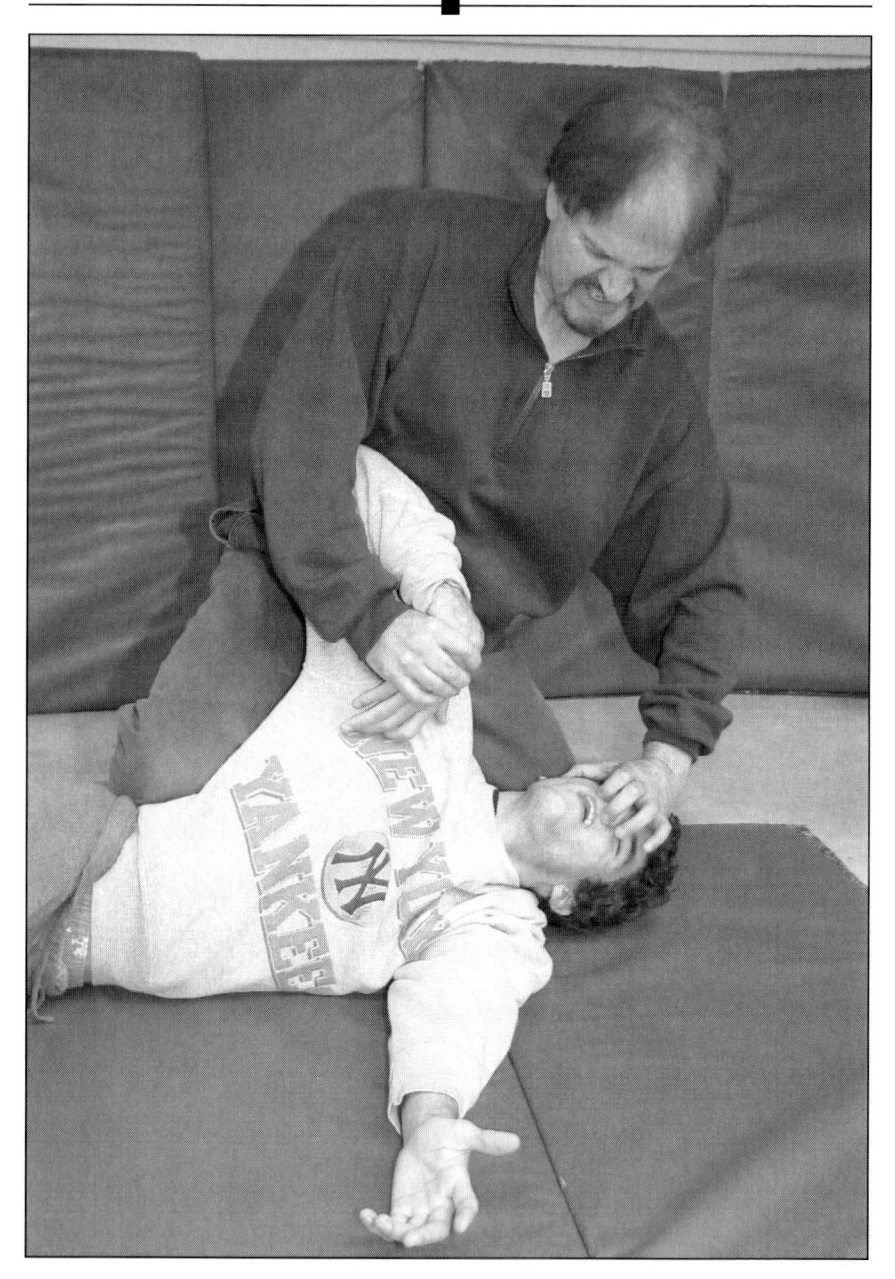

Figure 119

- Quickly jab one or two fingers into his nostrils. (Fig. 119)

Head

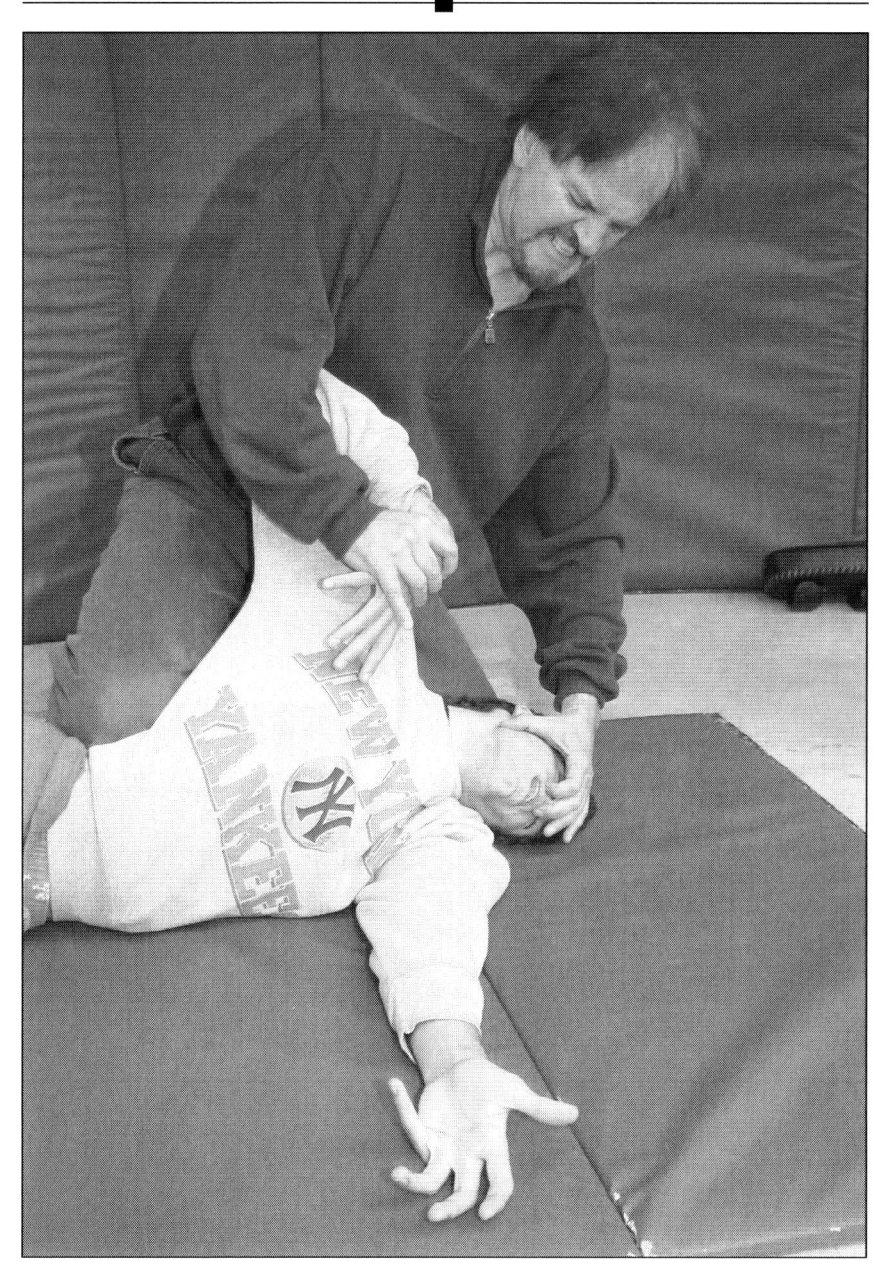

Figure 120

- Rip back to force his head to the floor. (Fig. 120)

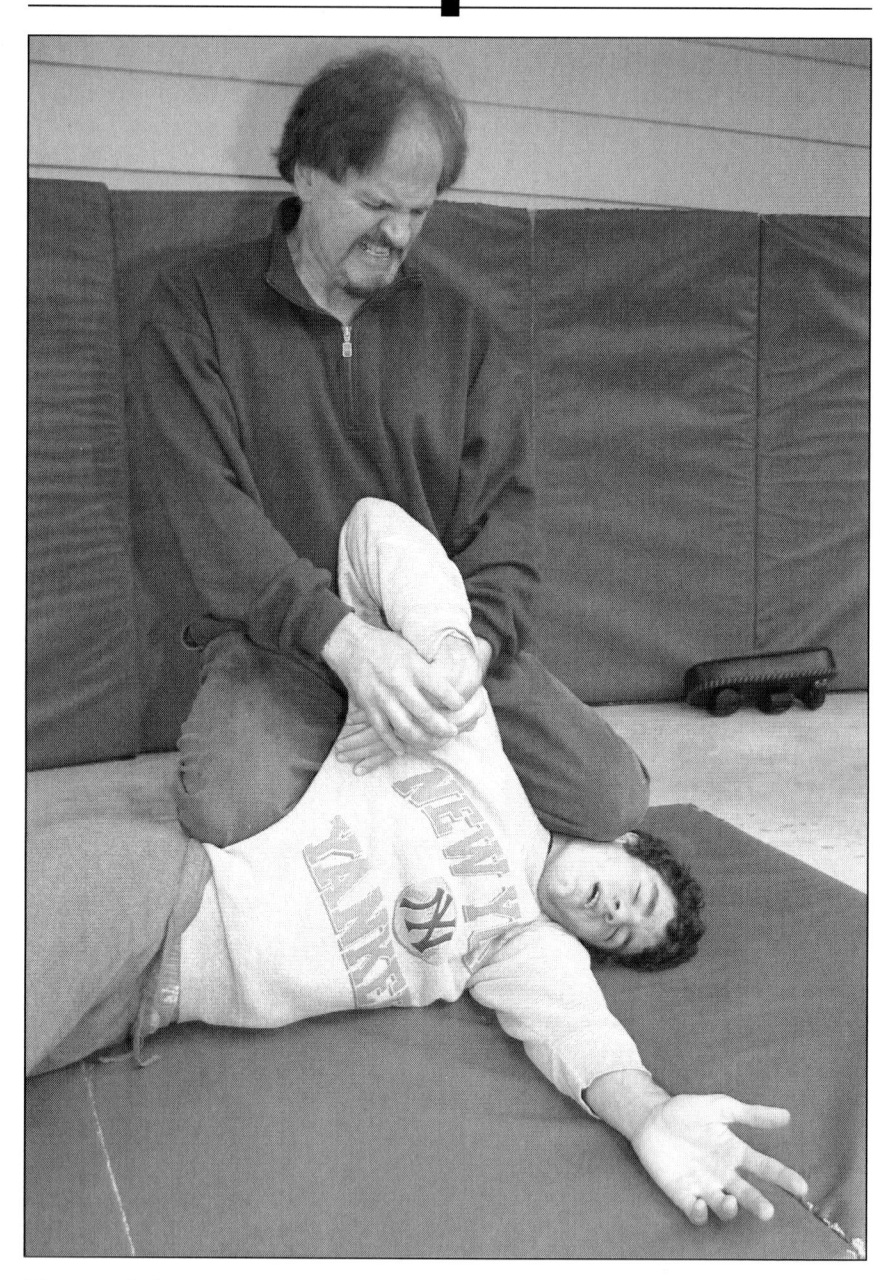

Figure 121

- Once his head is down, replace your knee more securely. (Fig. 121)

Nose Rip to Help with a Choke Hold

You have taken your attacker to the floor from behind.

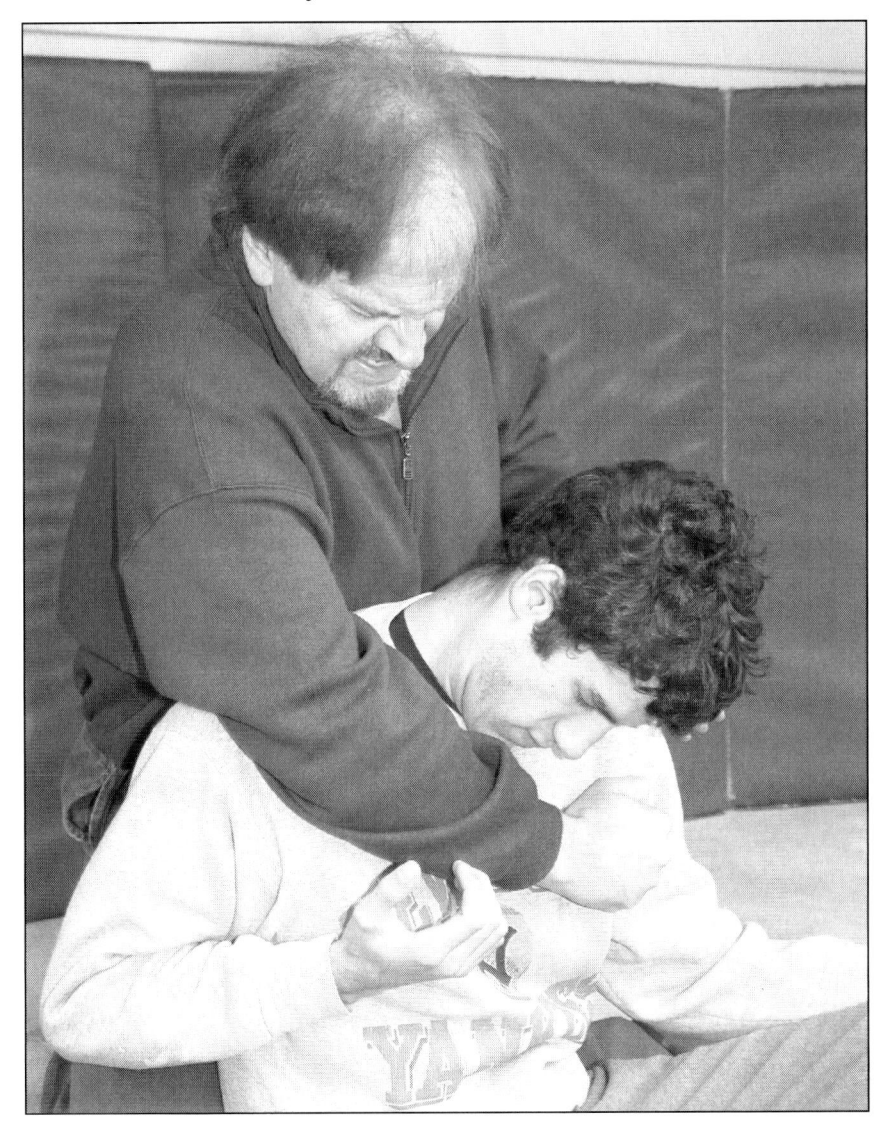

Figure 122

- When you move in for a choke, he tucks his chin. (Fig. 122)

Figure 123

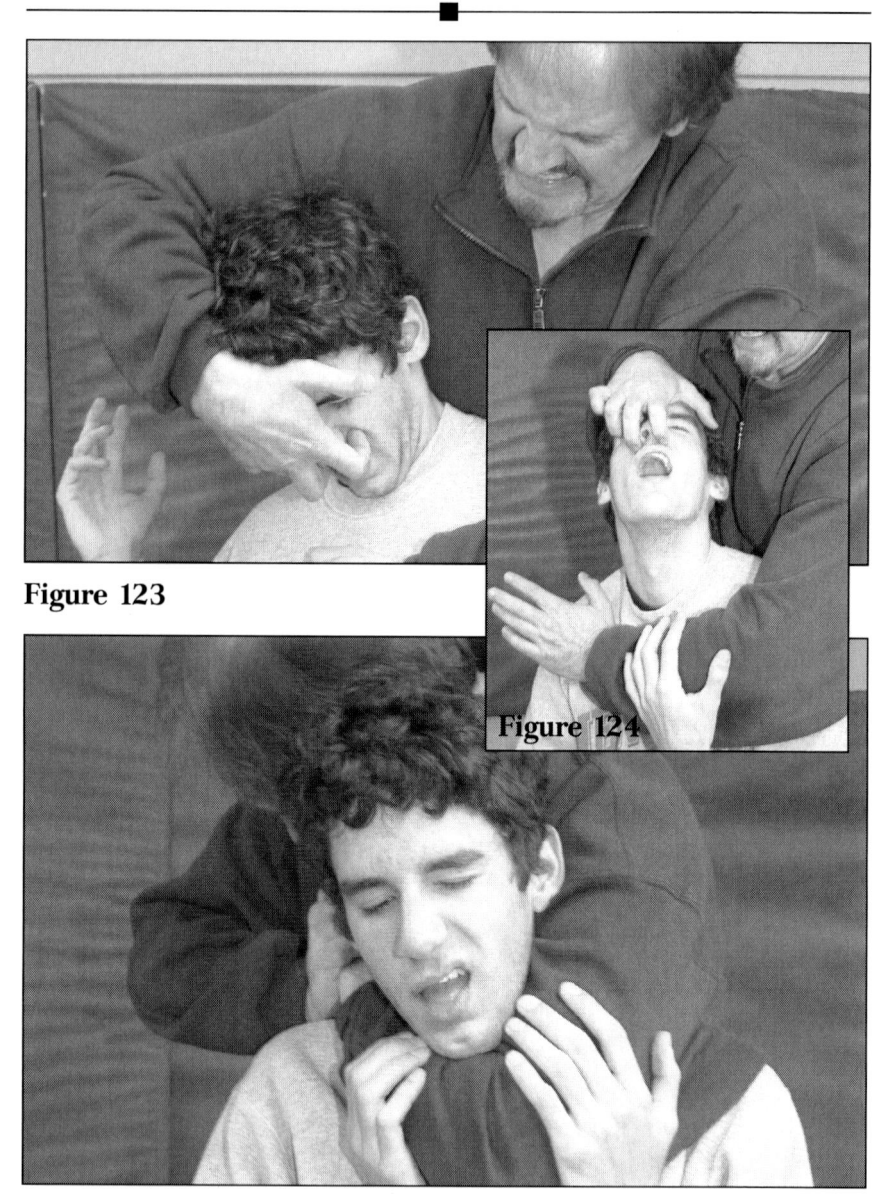

Figure 124

Figure 125

- Snag his nostrils with one or two fingers of the same hand. (Fig. 123)
- Yank his head back. (Fig. 124)
- Slip your other arm around his neck and apply a carotid constriction hold or a windpipe choke. (Fig. 125)

MOUTH

In these days of AIDs, hepatitis, and other highly transmittable diseases, targeting an attacker's mouth is a risk. But when it's the only window of opportunity you have, here are a few techniques.

Mantis Finger Hook

The attacker is in a fit as he dances about in front of you, waving his arms and making verbal threats. Practice on a live partner or a mannequin-style bag.

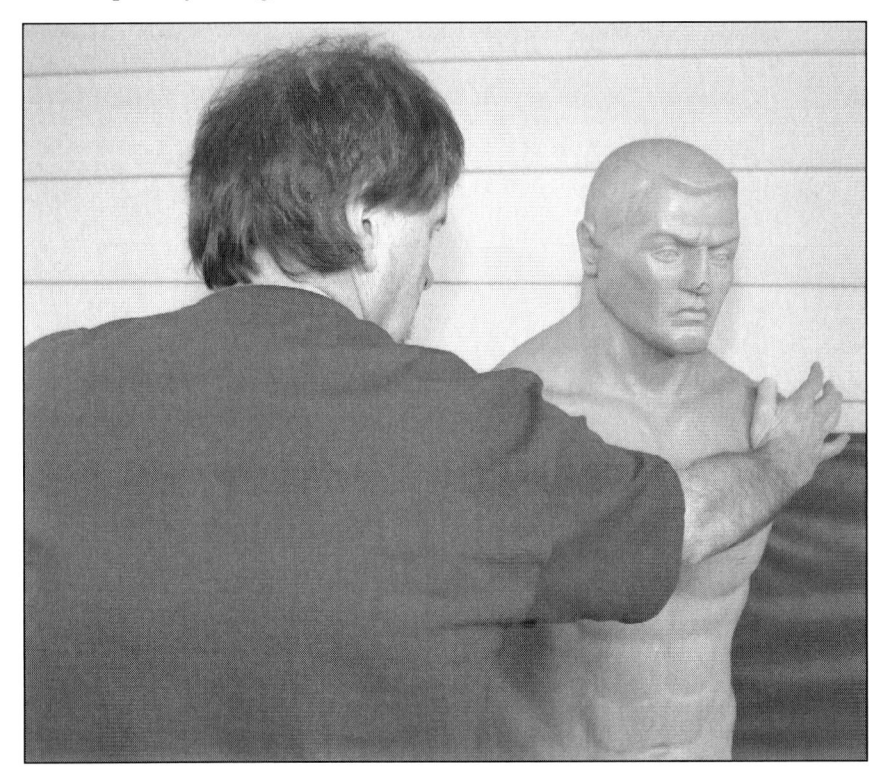

Figure 126

- The instant his flapping arms drop to his side, twist him around by pushing on his left shoulder and pulling on his right. (Fig. 126)

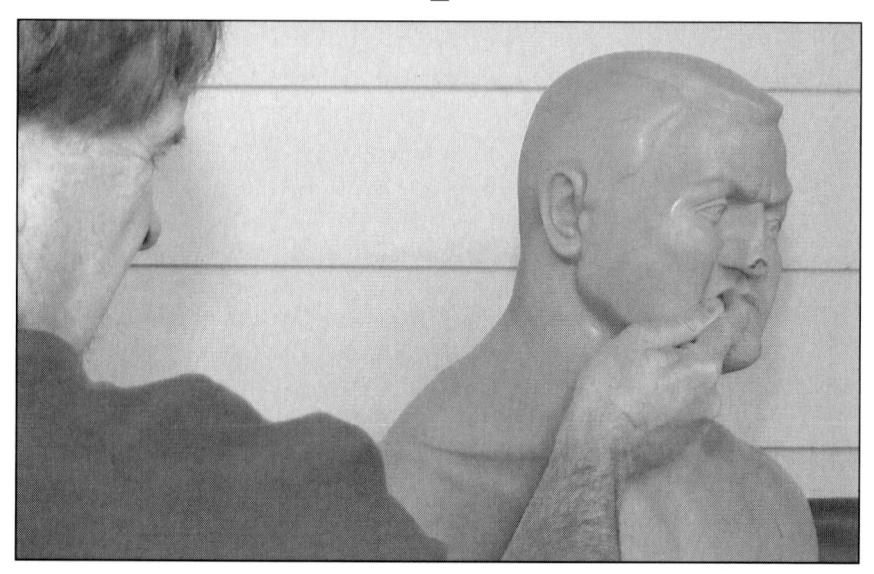

Figure 127

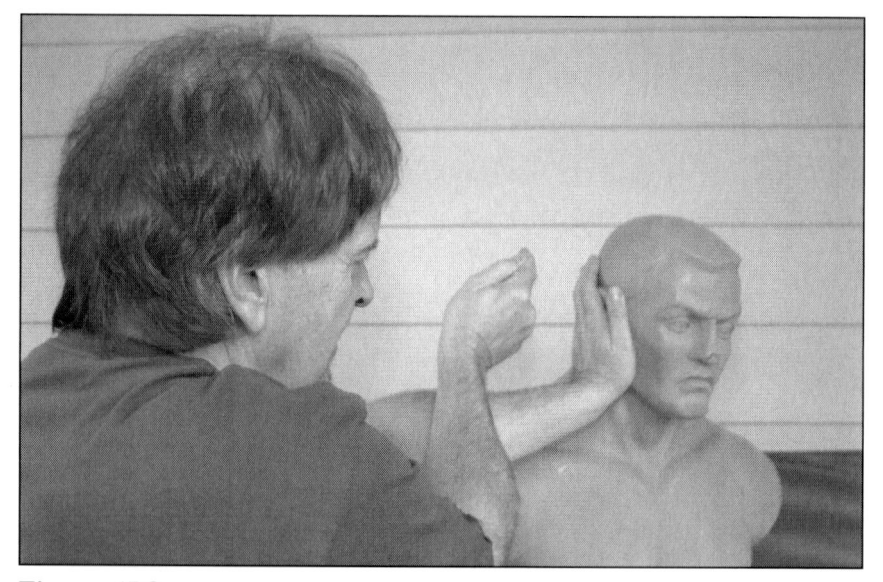

Figure 128

- Hook your mantis finger into the corner of his mouth. (Fig. 127)
- Rip it toward you as you simultaneously push his head with your other palm. (Fig. 128)

Armlock and Mantis Finger Mouth Hook

You have taken the attacker down onto his stomach and into a hammerlock.

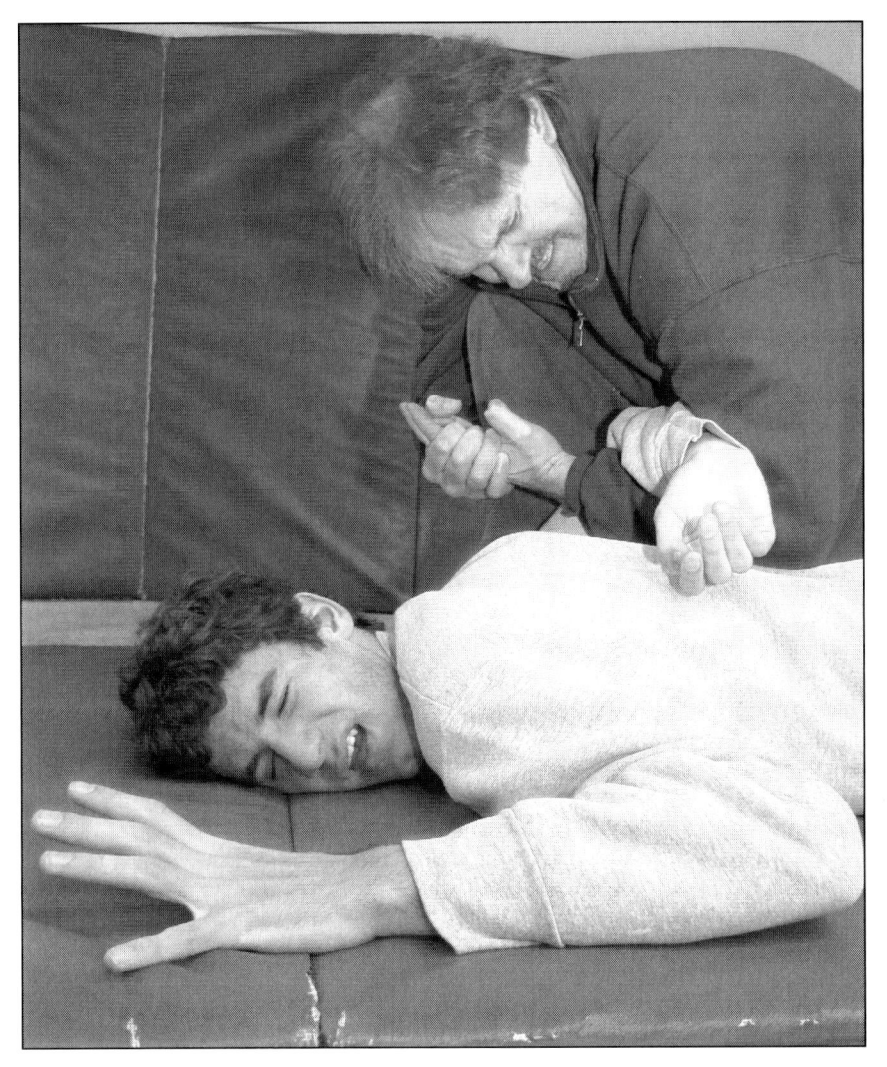

Figure 129

- Pry upward to apply pain to his shoulder. (Fig. 129)

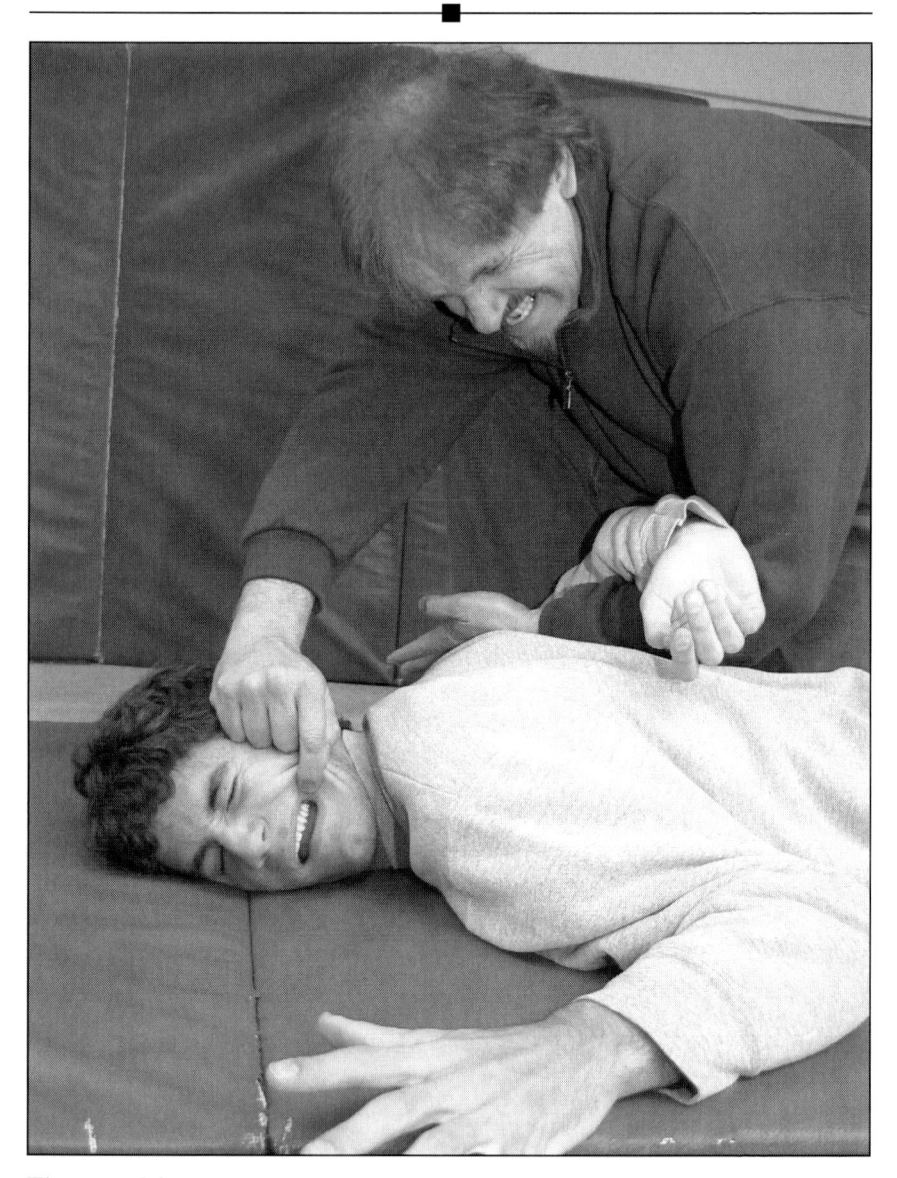

Figure 130

- When he starts wiggling about too much, hook your mantis finger into the corner of his mouth as you simultaneously lift his arm. Tell him to stop resisting. Maintain both holds until he cooperates or until you get help. If he does cooperate, release the mouth pull but continue to apply the shoulder lock. (Fig. 130)

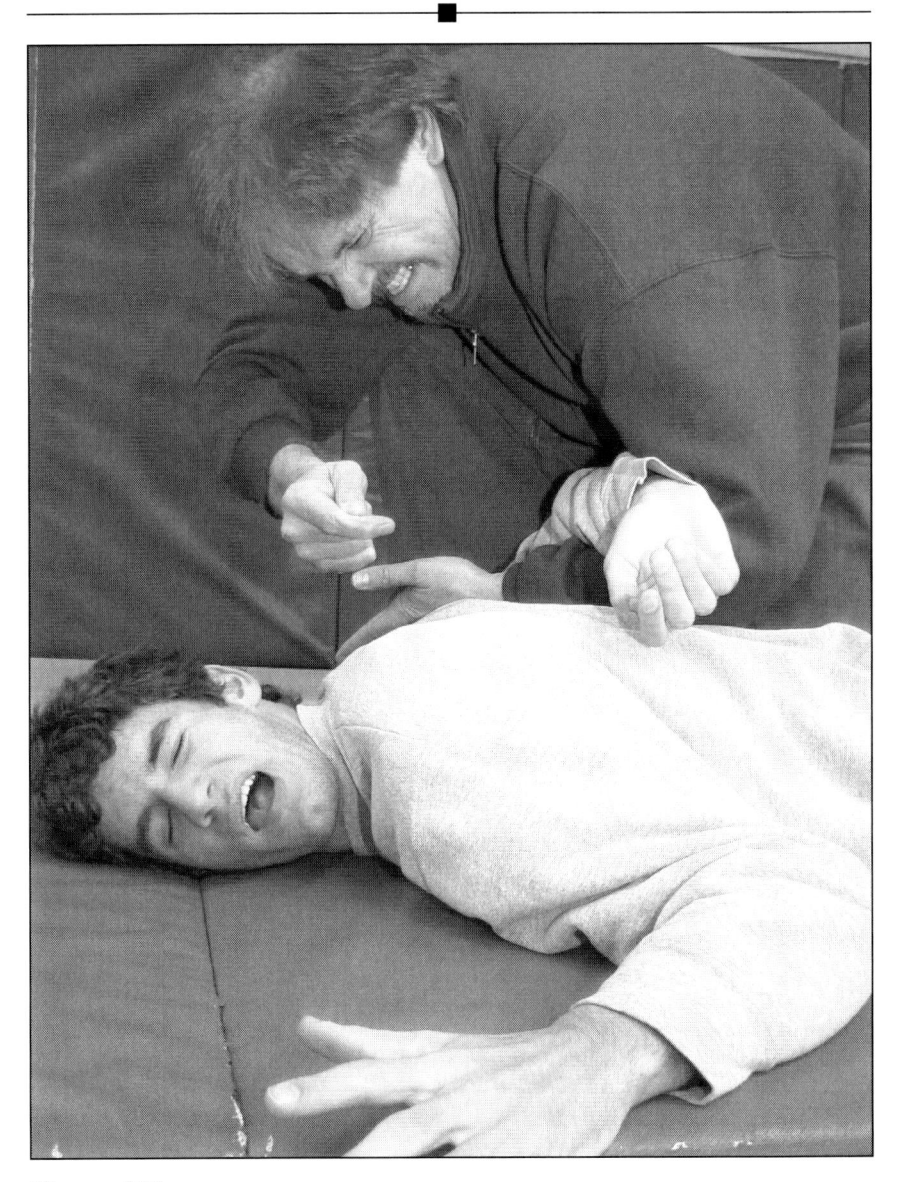

Figure 131

- Should he reach for a weapon on his person or in some way begin to defeat your hold, rip your finger toward you in one swift, excruciatingly painful move. (Fig. 131)

Thumbs Rip

The attacker grabs you in a bear hug with your arms pinned against your chest.

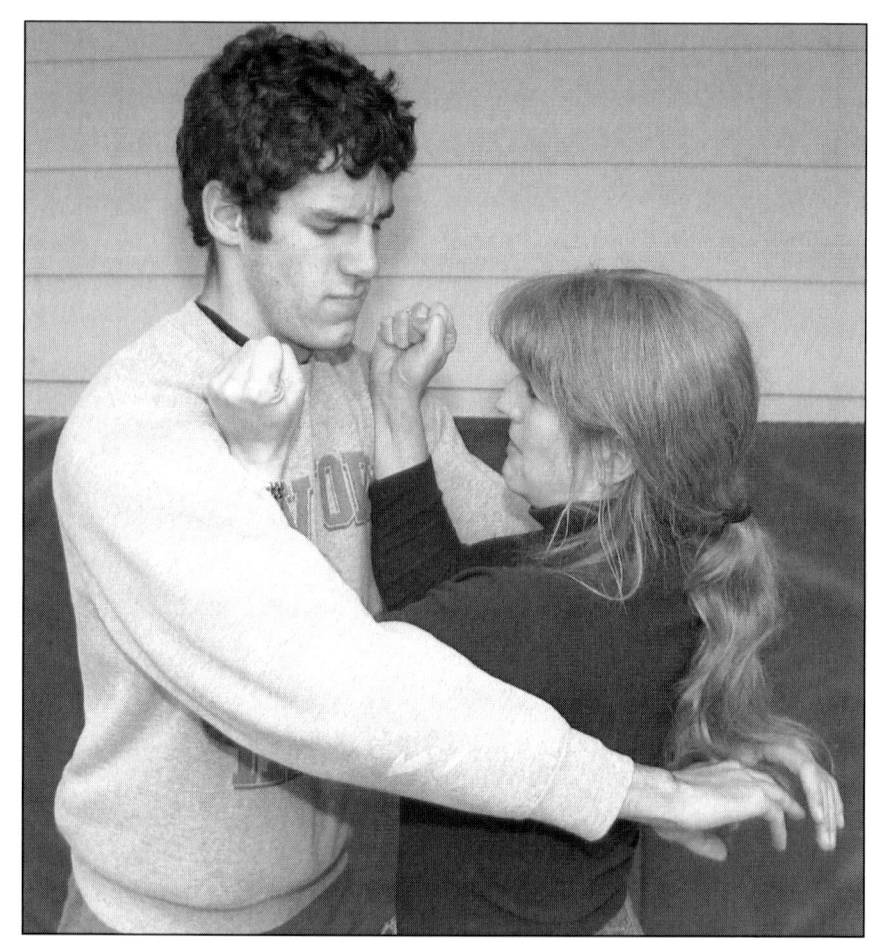

Figure 132

- When his arms relax a little, take advantage of the brief moment to slide your hands up higher. (Fig. 132)
- Before his hug prevents you from moving, ram your thumbs into the corners of his mouth. (Fig. 133)
- Rip outward. (Fig. 134)

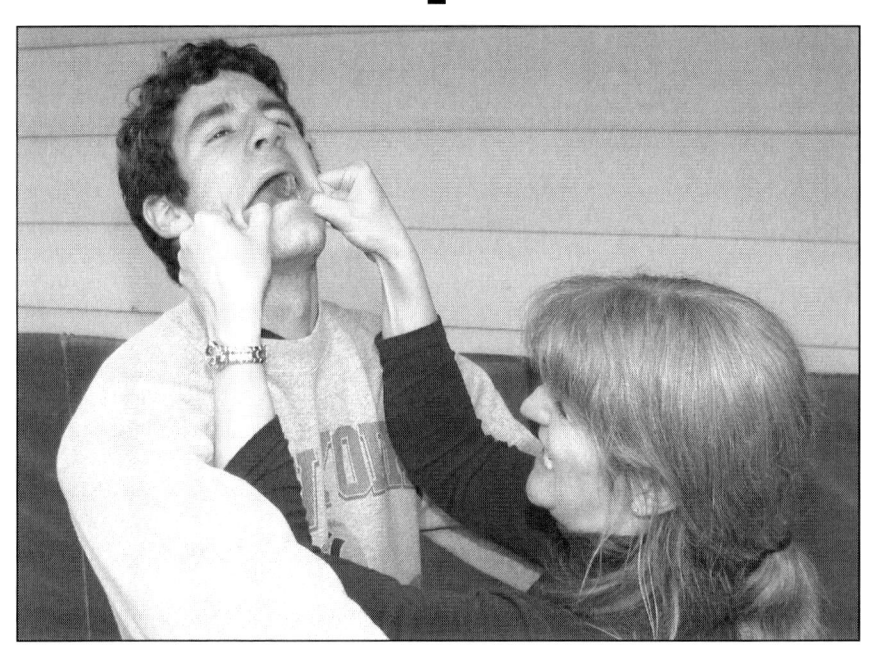

Figure 133

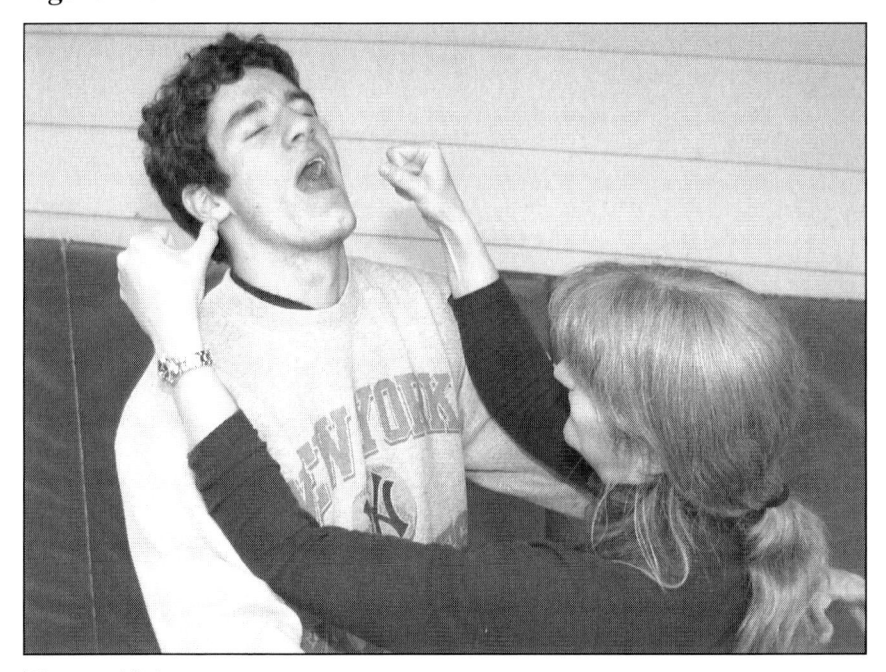

Figure 134

Lip and Mouth Rip with Foot

You have taken your attacker down onto his back.

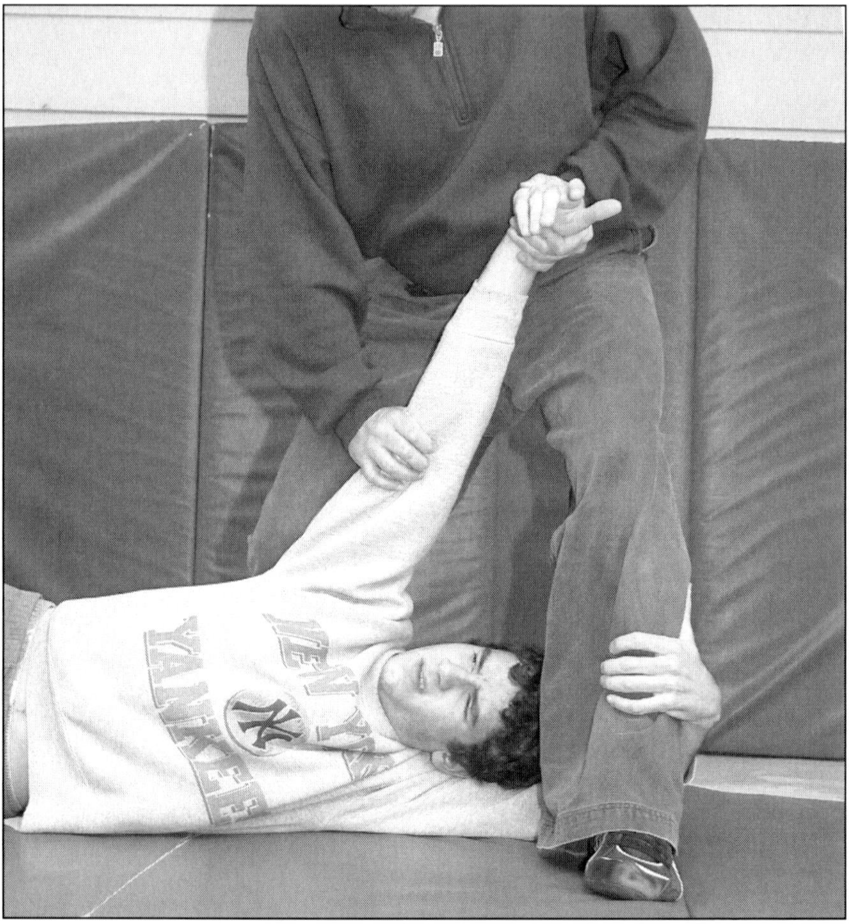

Figure 135

- As you begin an arm drag to turn him over, you accidentally step too close and he grabs your ankle. (Fig. 135)
- Using the edge of the heel of your other foot, step down onto his mouth and then drop your heel forcefully to the floor to rip his lips and gums. This will weaken his grip on your ankle and allow you to continue with your move. (Fig. 136)

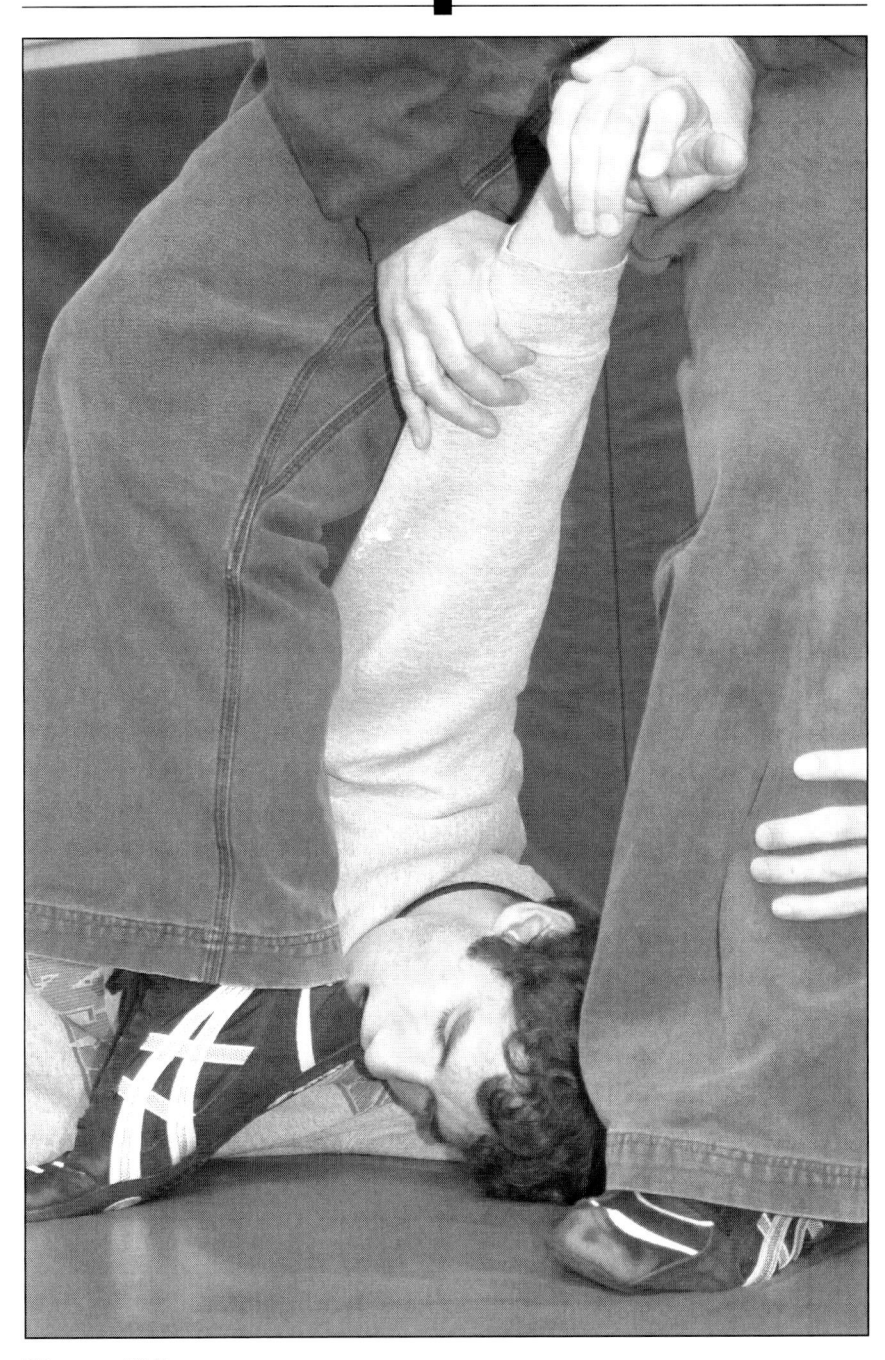

Figure 136

CHIN AND JAW

Not only do these techniques hurt, but they may dislocate the attacker's jaw and even break it.

Chin Press

This technique can be done on an attacker who is standing, sitting, or on the ground. Let's do it on a seated person who is refusing to leave the premises.

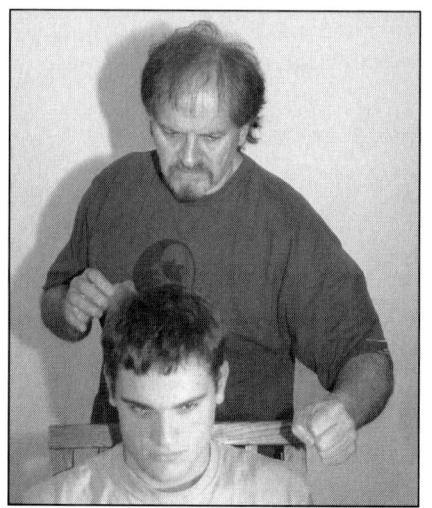

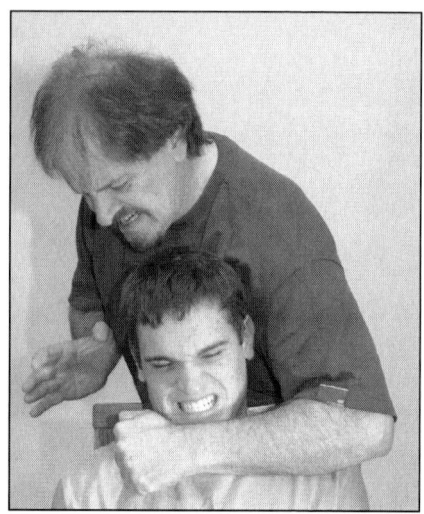

Figure 137

Figure 138

- Approach from behind. (Fig. 137)
- You can either slip your left forearm across his chin or slam your forearm against it. Position your arm just below his lower teeth at the gum line. (Fig. 138)
- Place your upper chest against the back of his head to provide a base to allow the full energy of your technique to go into the target. Clasp hands and pull your left arm so the thumb side of your wrist crushes into his gum, lower teeth, and chin. Inflate your chest to increase the pressure and saw your arm back and forth an inch or two in both directions for added pain. (Fig. 139)

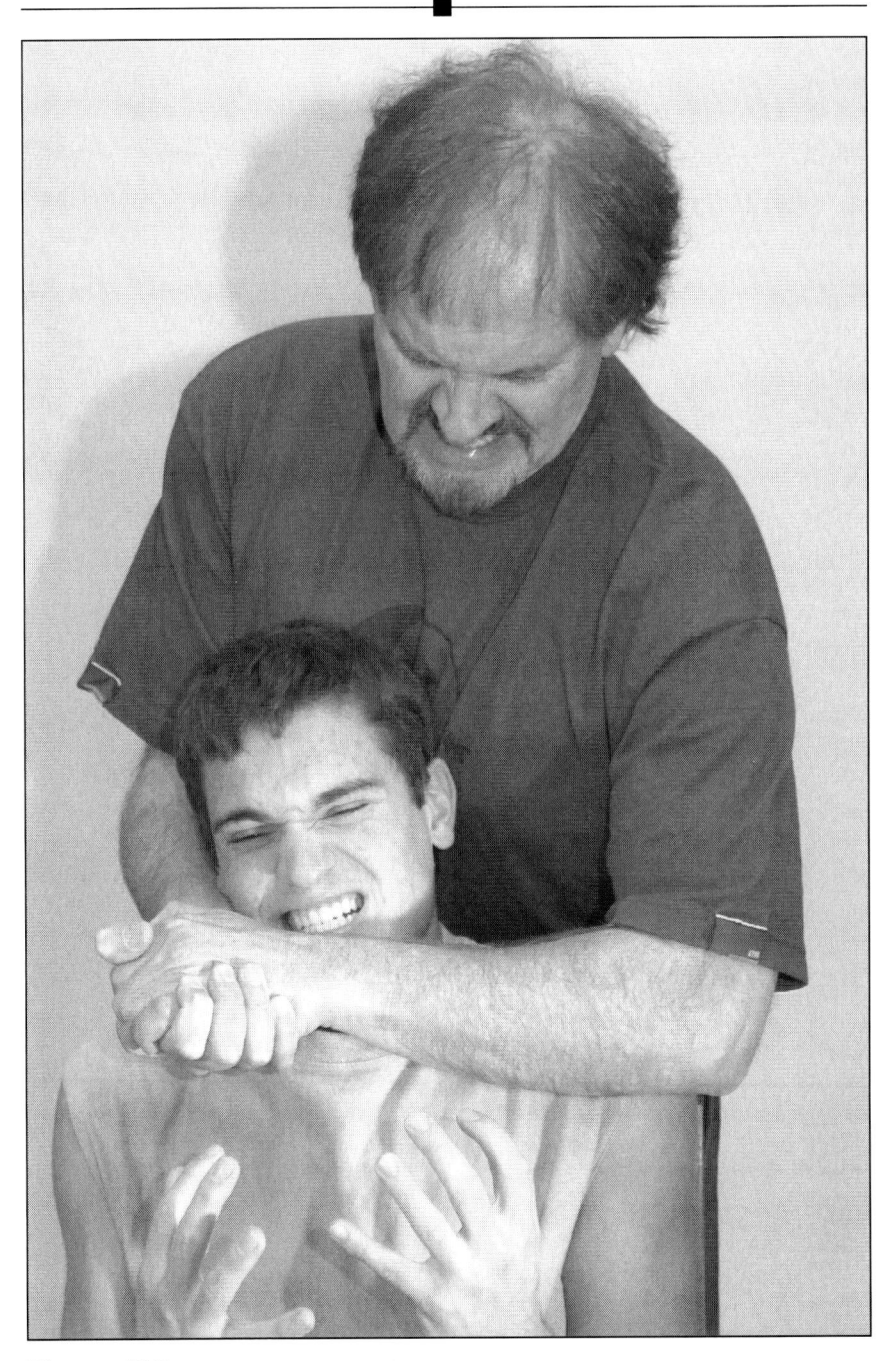

Figure 139

Jaw Press

This technique is done on the floor, which provides a solid base for added pressure. It's a painful move that can break his jaw. Be justified. You have taken your attacker to the floor onto his stomach.

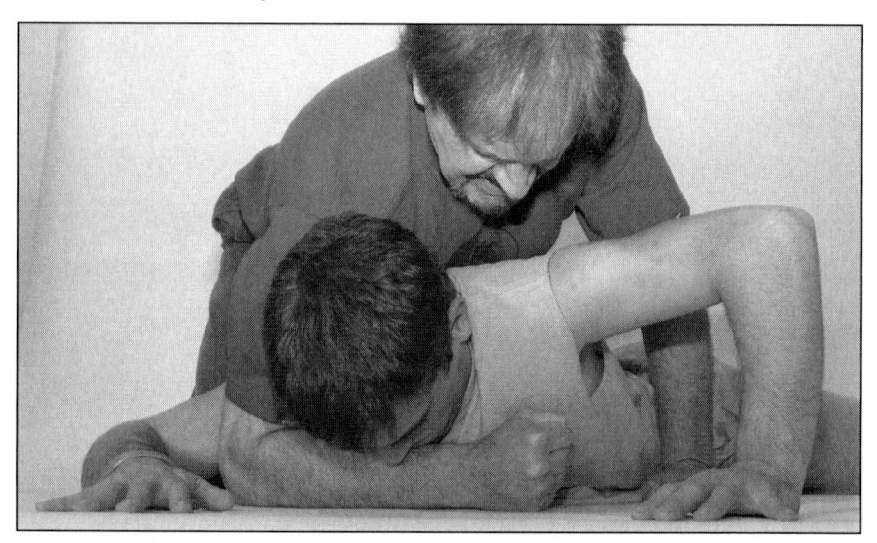

Figure 140

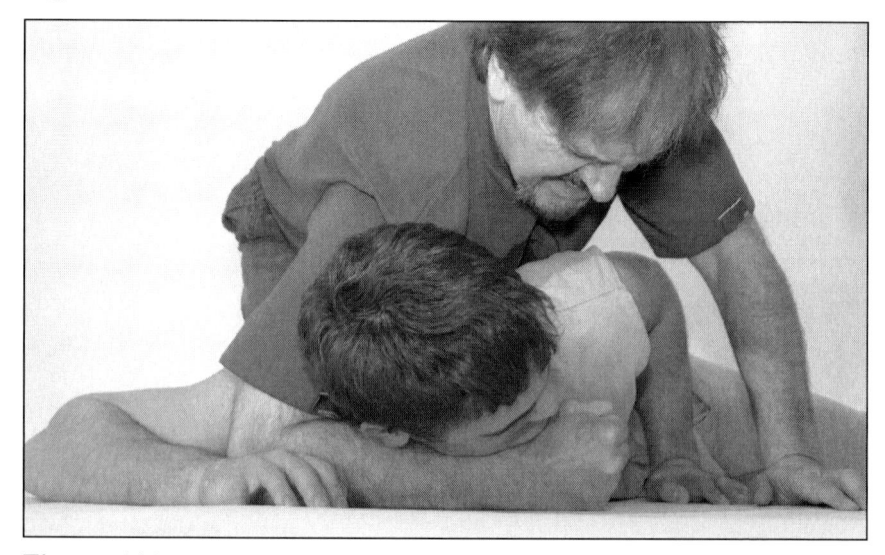

Figure 141

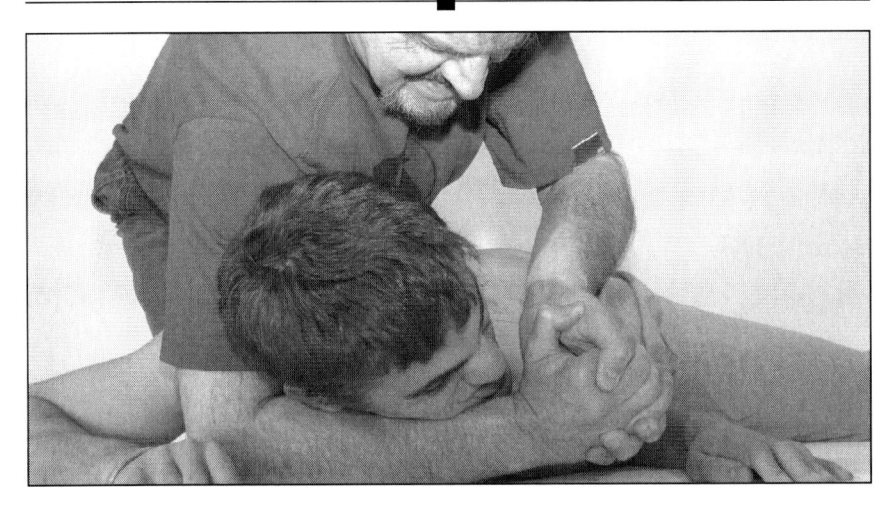

Figure 142

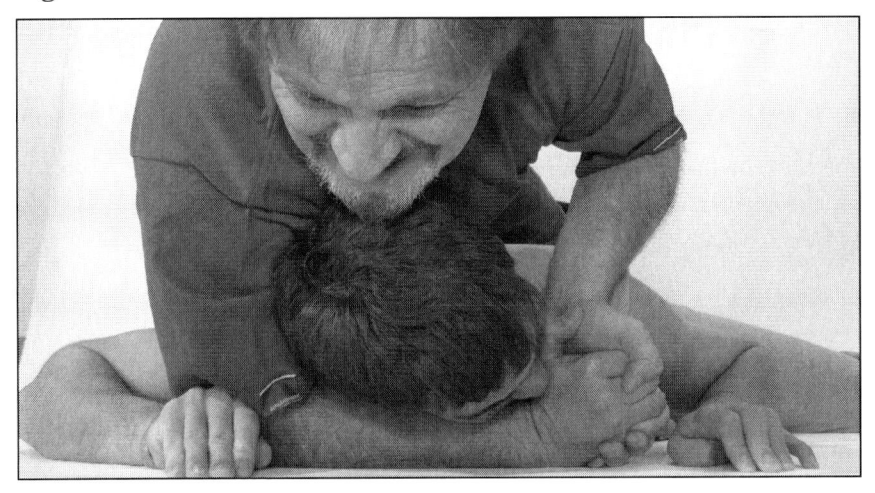

Figure 143

- When you slip your arm around his neck for a choke, he quickly tucks his chin. (Fig. 140)
- Forcefully push the side of his jaw with your wrist so that his head turns to the side. (Fig. 141)
- Place your other wrist on his other shoulder, clasp your hands firmly, and begin to pull your forearm against his jaw. (Fig. 142)
- To create a base, squirm forward until your upper chest is on the back of his head and then squeeze your arms inward as you continue to pull against his jawbone. (Fig. 143)

Jaw Hinge

Slide your fingers from the front of your jaw to just in front of your ear where you feel a rounded section of bone that curves upward. That is your jaw hinge. Now dig under it and then press upward. Feel that strange and unpleasant sensation in your throat? Push harder and the pain escalates.

When you push this vulnerable spot on an attacker, he usually moves in the same direction to escape the pain. Keep in mind that intoxicated people might not react at all.

Lifting people by their jaw hinge was a favorite technique of mine to move seated protestors, people refusing to get out of chairs, and handcuffed people refusing to get out of my police car. It's true. Some of the same people officers have to fight to get into their backseat they must fight again to get out. Pressing the jaw hinge works great.

Press to Encourage the Attacker to Come with You

You want your attacker out the door but he is lying down, refusing to move.

- Squat down behind his head and dig your four fingertips into and under the jaw hinge. (Fig. 144)
- Press and pull so that he scoots himself toward you in an attempt to escape the pain. Scoot backwards until he is out the door. (Fig. 145)

Head 95

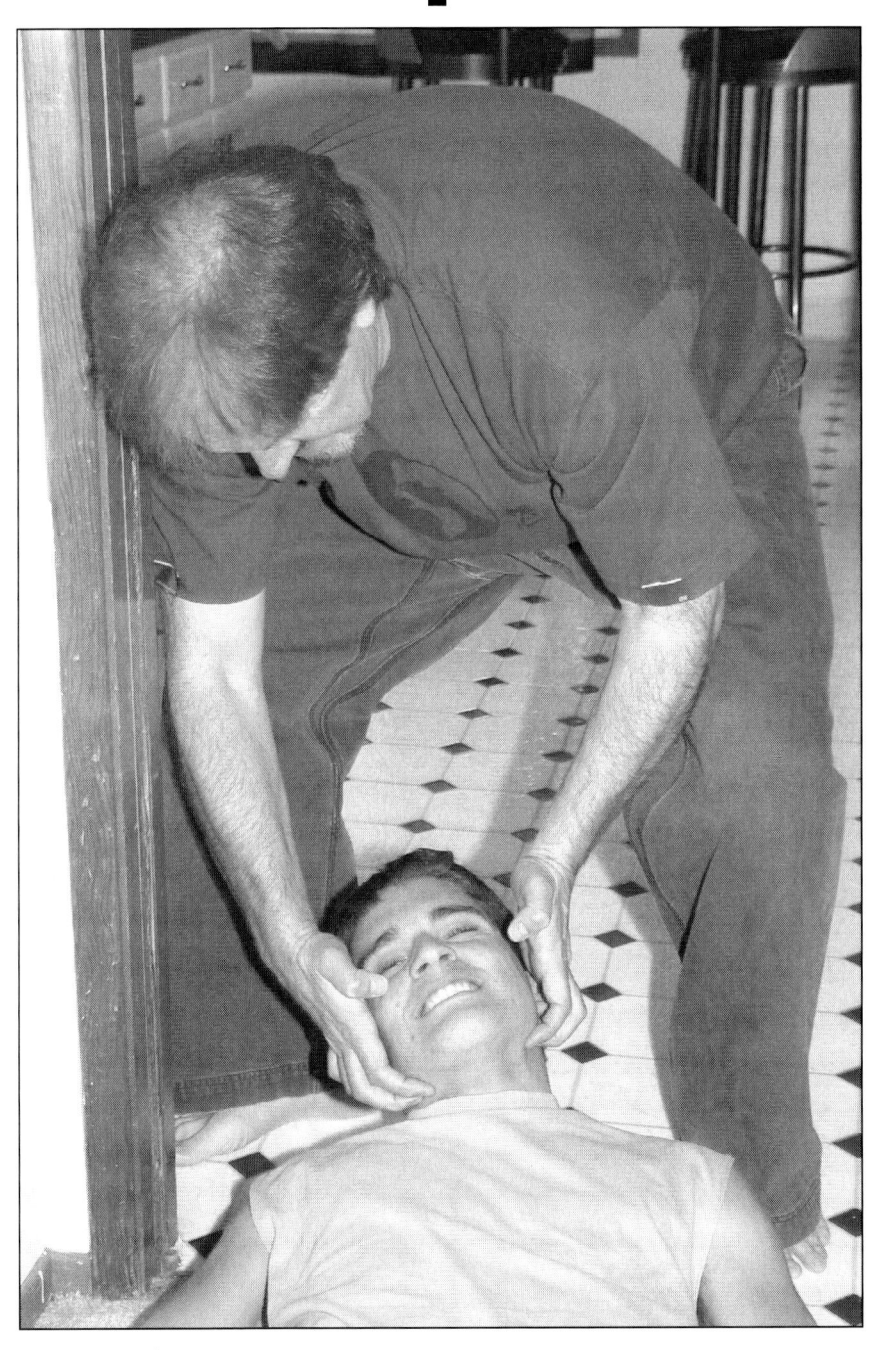

Figure 144

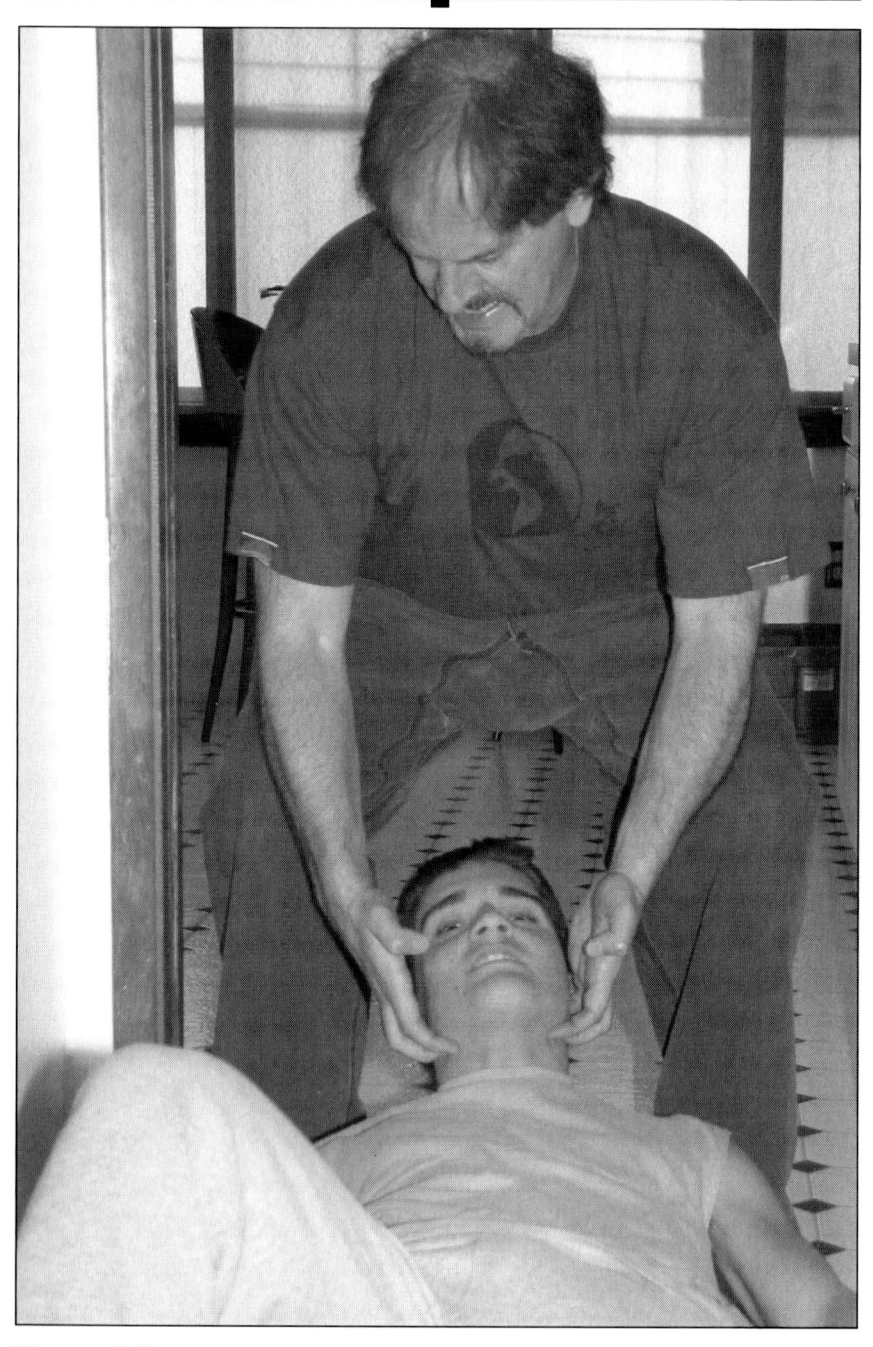

Figure 145

Press to Release from a Headlock

The attacker is lying on your chest trying to apply a headlock.

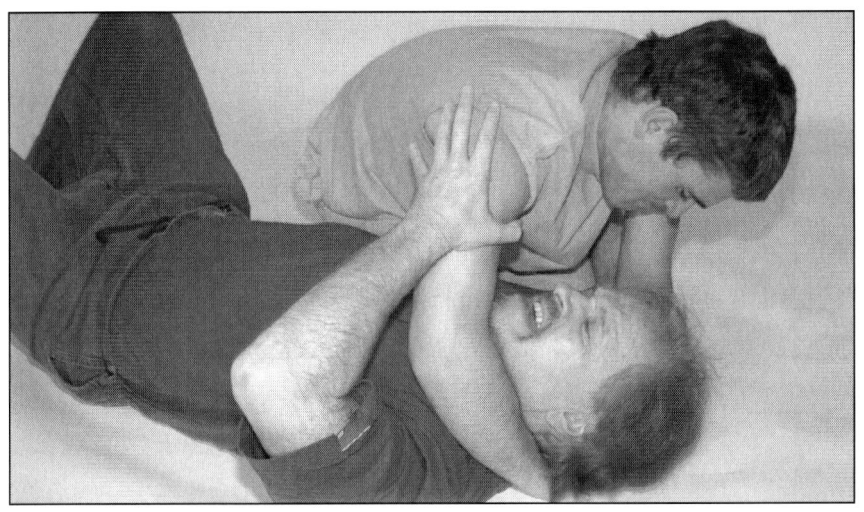

Figure 146

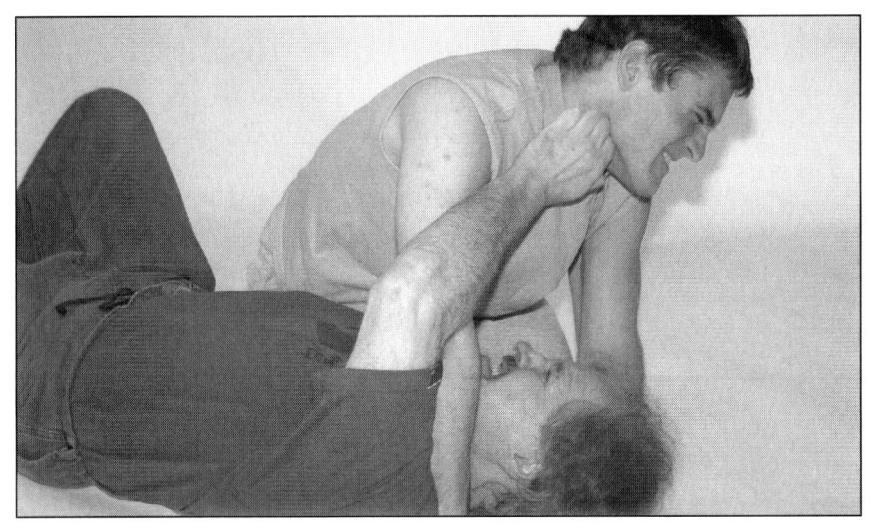

Figure 147

- Reach with whichever hand is free. (Fig. 146)
- Dig into his jaw hinge with your middle knuckles to effect pain and force him to release or at least weaken his grip on you. (Fig. 147)

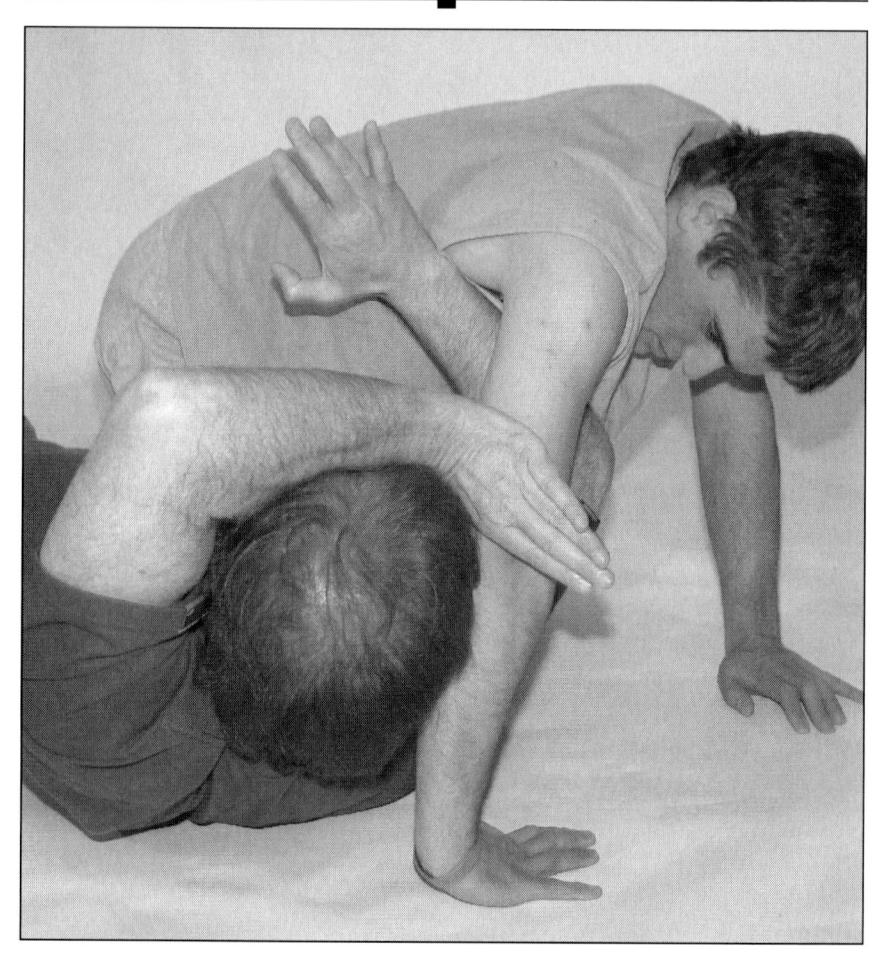

Figure 148

- Escape or maneuver into a counter hold. (Fig. 148)

Press to Force a Seated Person to Stand

A person refuses to get out of a chair and leave the premises.

- From behind, dig two or three fingers of each hand into his jaw hinges. (Fig. 149)
- Lift. (Fig. 150)

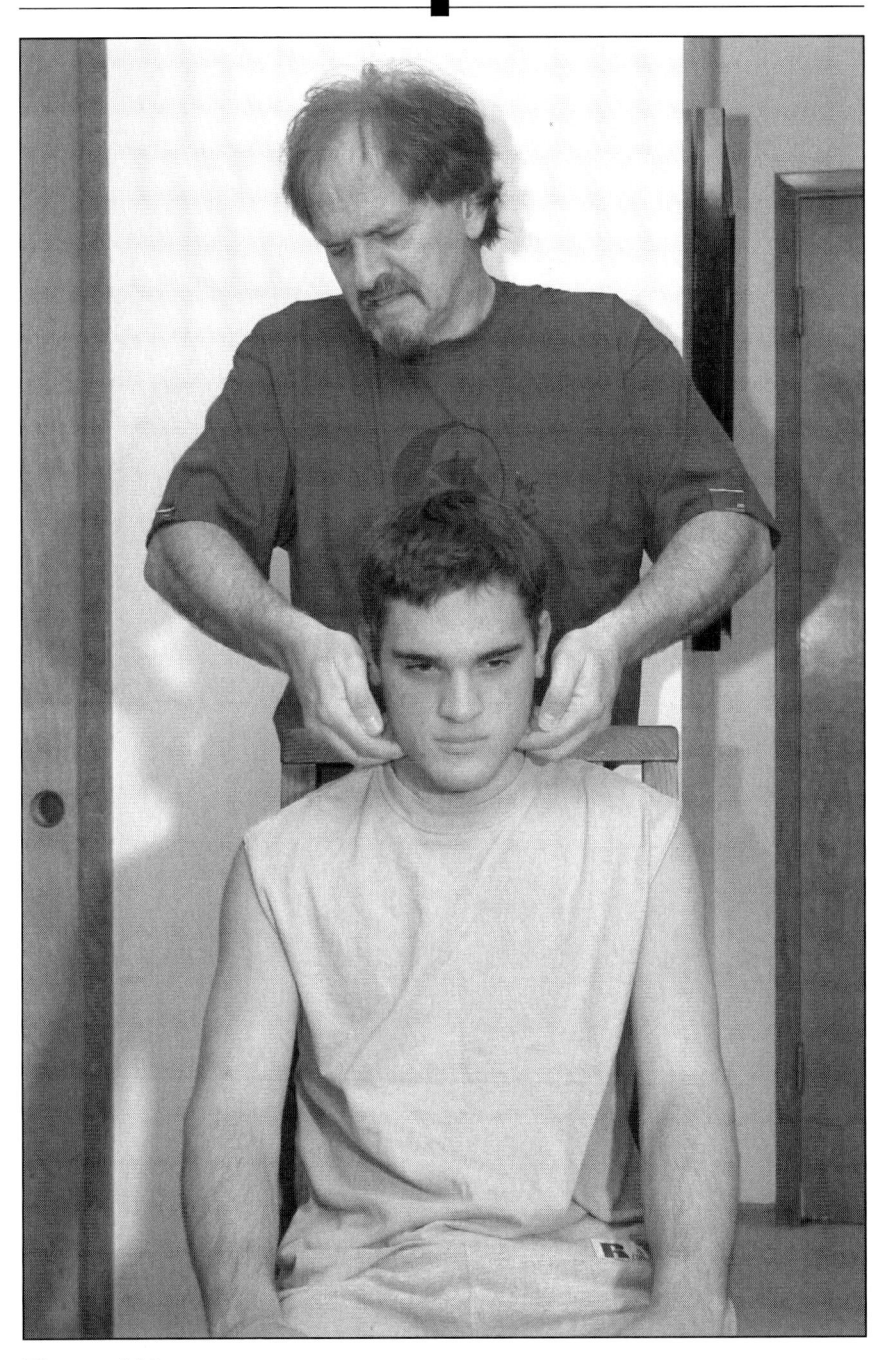

Figure 149

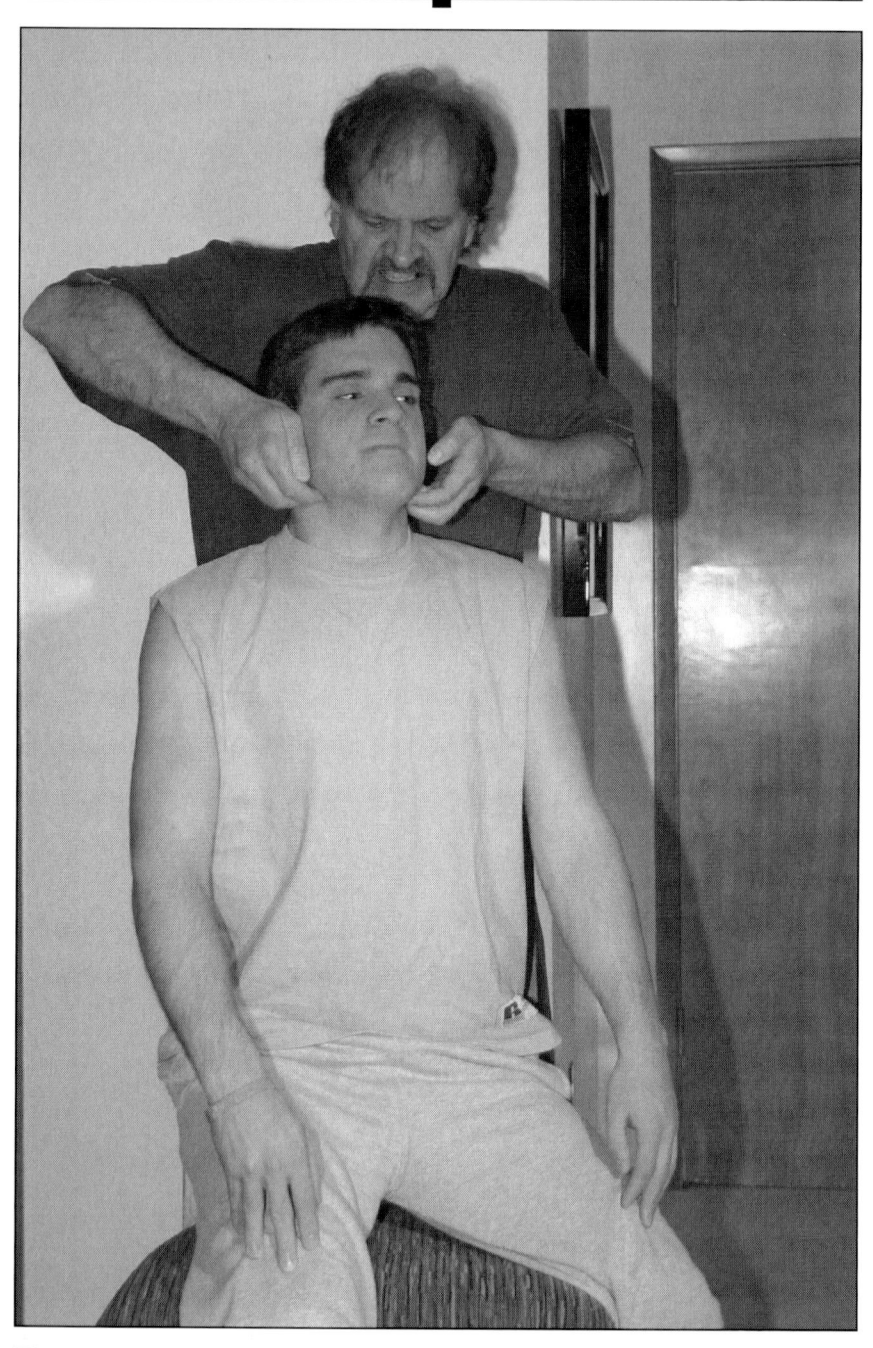

Figure 150

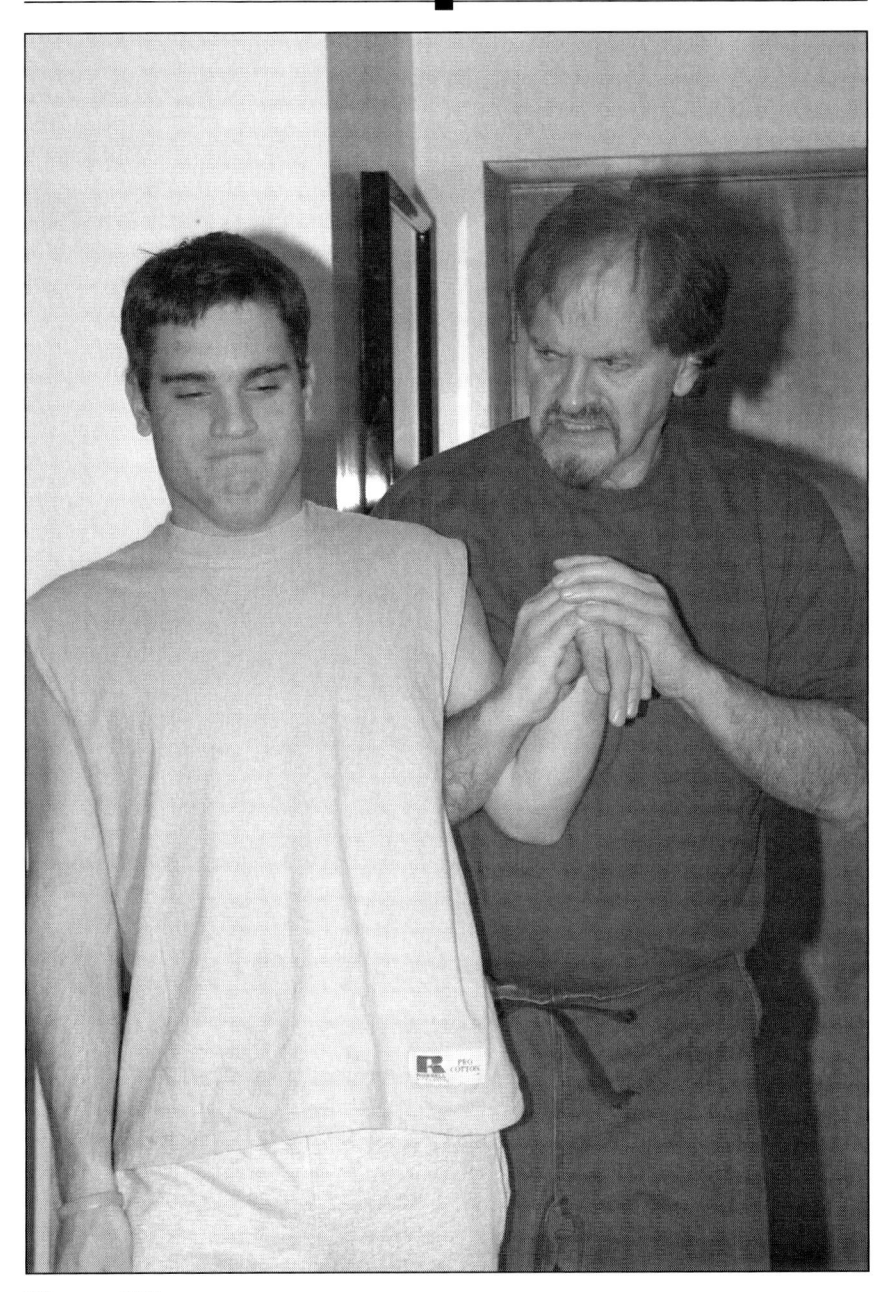

Figure 151

- Apply a restraint hold so you can escort him out. (Fig. 151)

EARS

The ear isn't as vulnerable to pressing, gouging, and ripping as are the eyes, nose, and other head targets, but that doesn't mean you won't get a reaction from your attacker when you target them. You will. Sometimes the reaction will be big, while other times it will be just enough to distract him for a second so you can apply a quick follow-up.

Armlock and Ear Press

You have taken your attacker down and you're controlling him with an armlock.

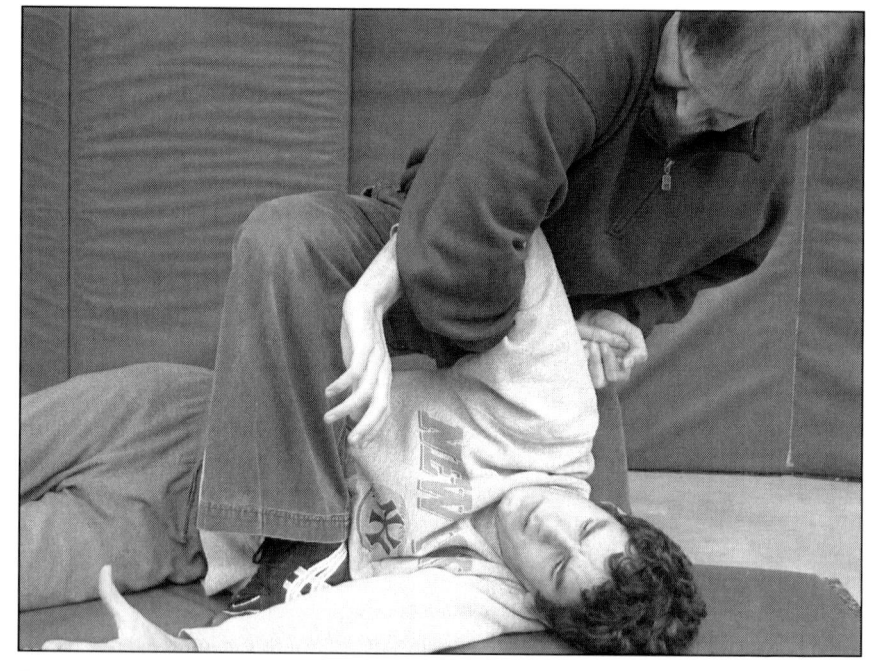

Figure 152

- For whatever reason, you're starting to lose the hold. (Fig. 152)
- Press your middle knuckle into his ear canal and twist it back and forth. (Fig. 153)
- The instant he reacts, re-grip your hold. (Fig. 154)

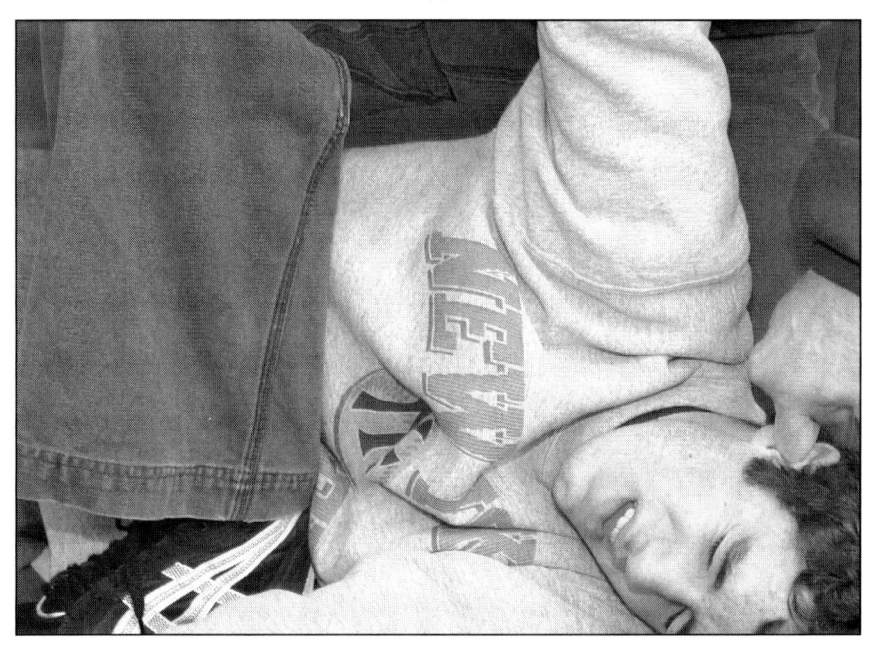

Figure 153

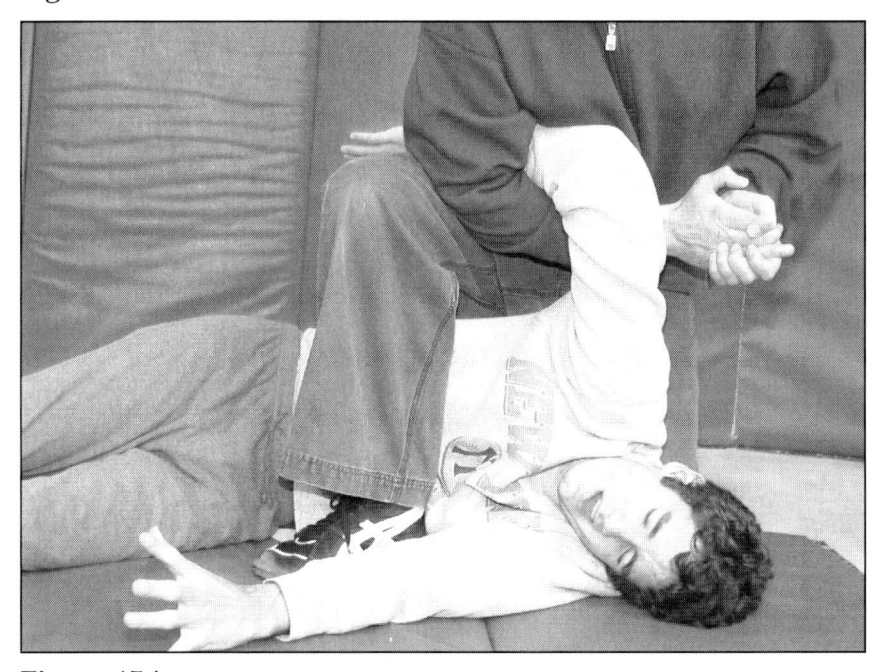

Figure 154

Attacker on Top

The attacker is trying to smother you with his weight.

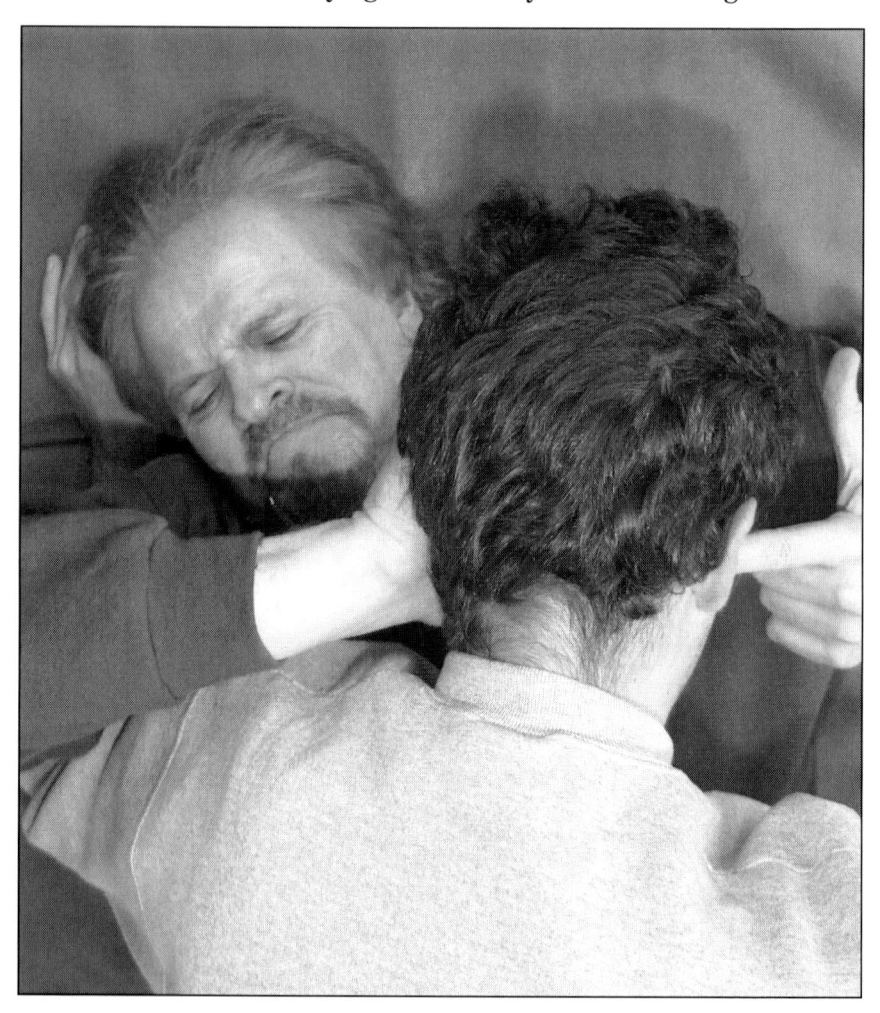

Figure 155

- Press your left index finger into his ear canal. Brace the opposite side of his head to force all the finger pressure into his ear. (Fig. 155)
- After five seconds of hard pressing, snap your bracing hand away so that he jerks toward the same direction. (Fig. 156)
- Simultaneously buck him off in that direction. (Fig. 157)

Head 105

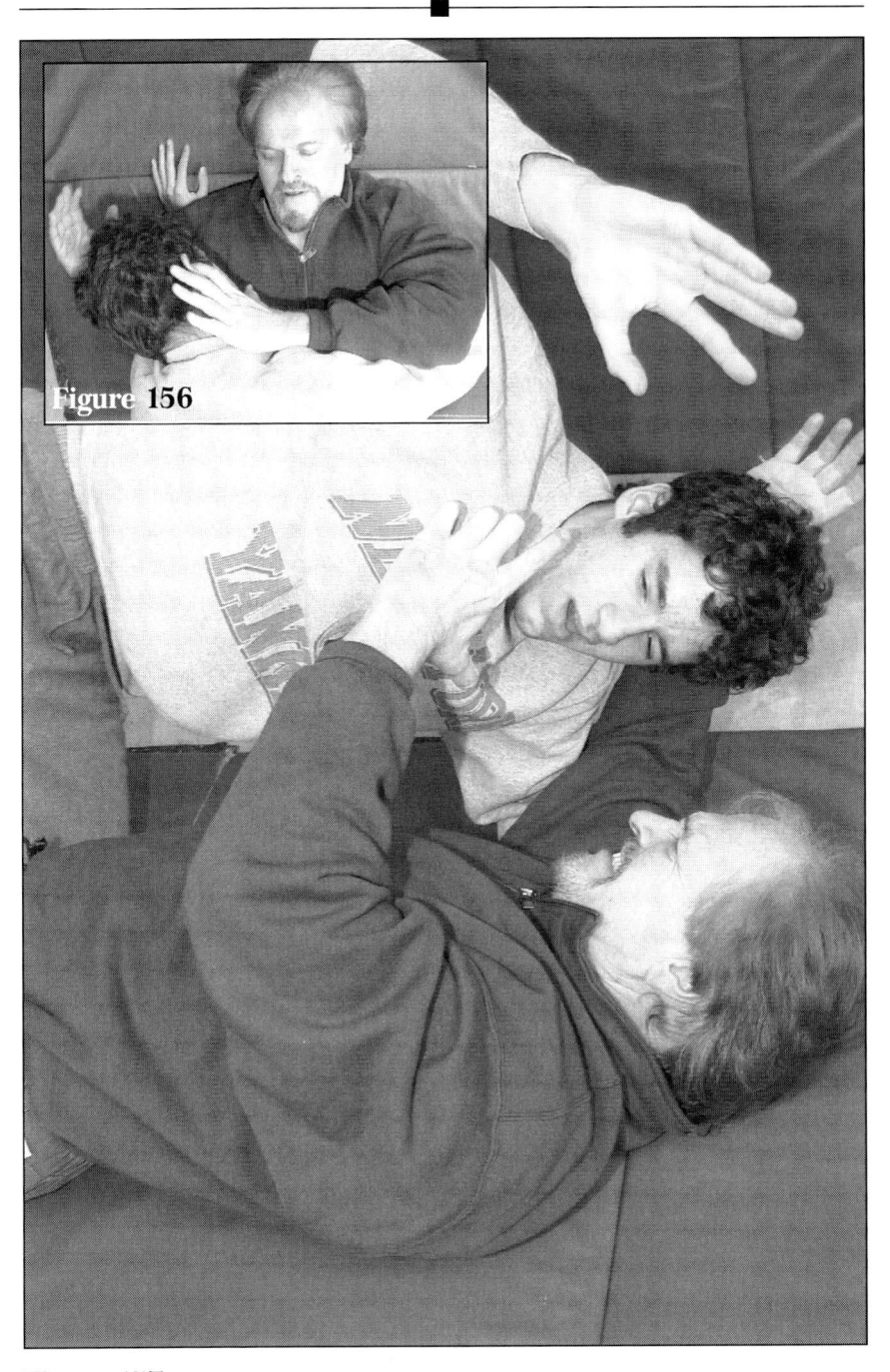

Figure 156

Figure 157

Attacker Grabs Your Shirt

Grabbing you this way is usually a setup
for a punch, so you must react quickly.

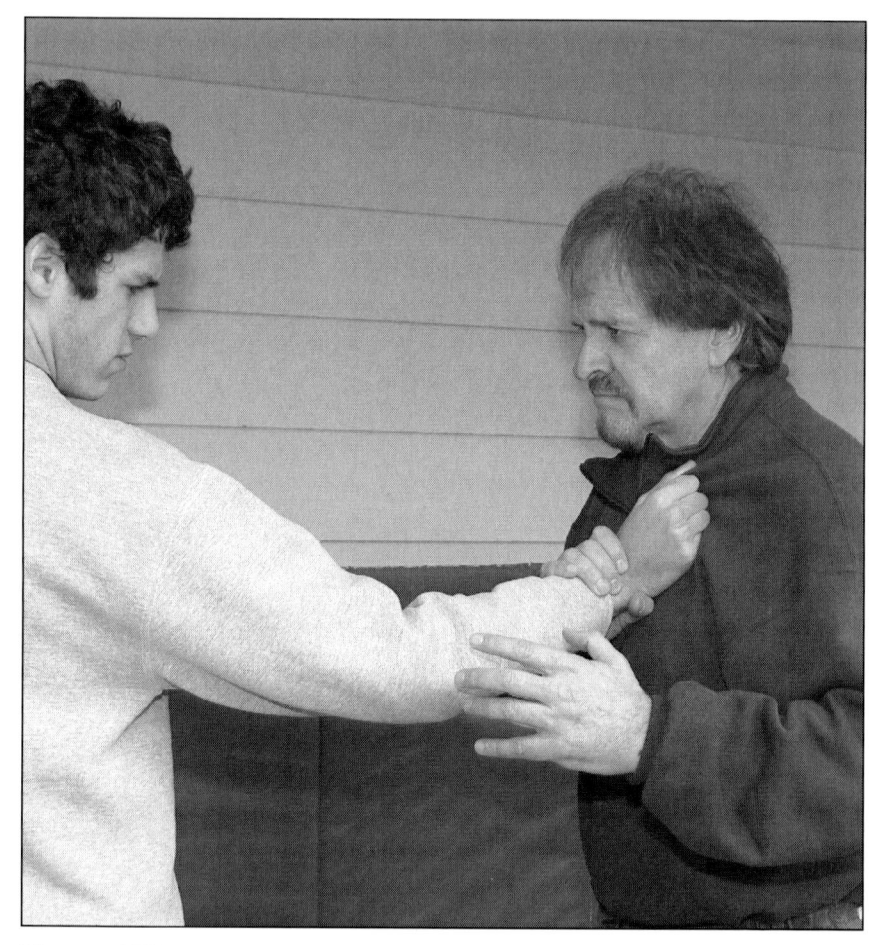

Figure 158

- Secure his wrist. (Fig. 158)
- Press your index finger or thumb into his ear canal. (Fig. 159)
- When he turns away from the pressure, strike his elbow with your forearm to shock the nerves in the joint. (Fig. 160)
- Palm his ear. (Fig. 161)

Head

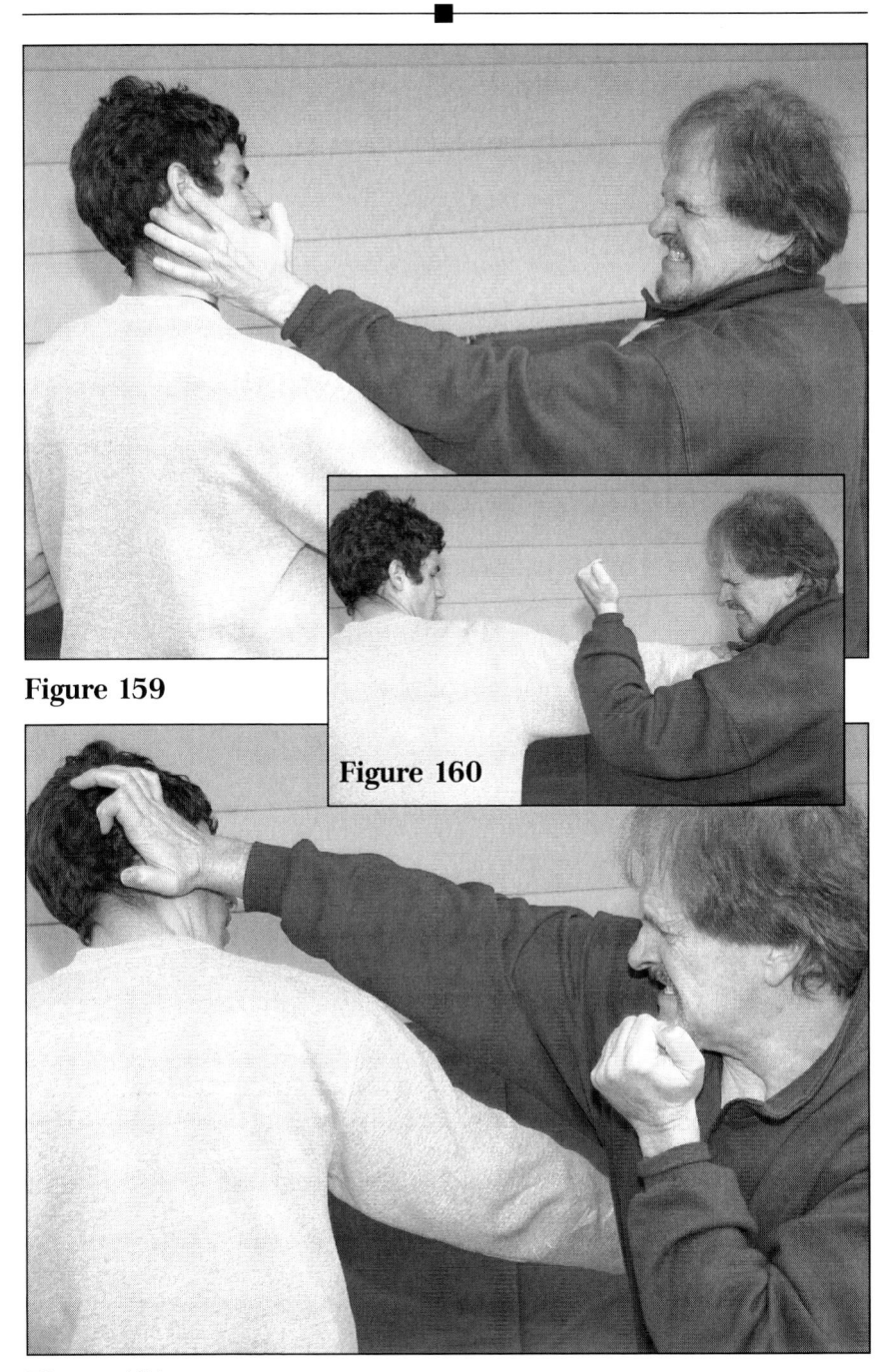

Figure 159

Figure 160

Figure 161

Attacker Resists Your Takedown

You're behind the attacker.

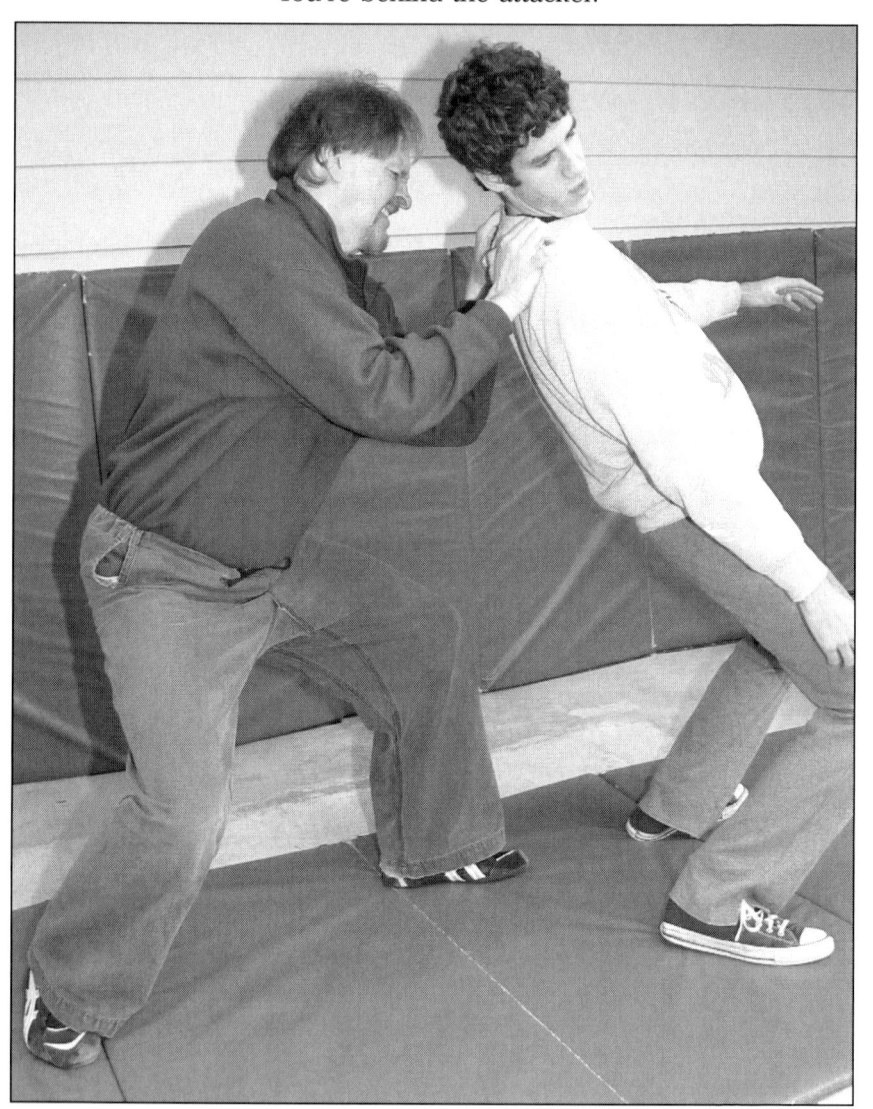

Figure 162

- Grab his shoulders and jerk. Make sure your elbows are pointing downward. (Fig. 162)

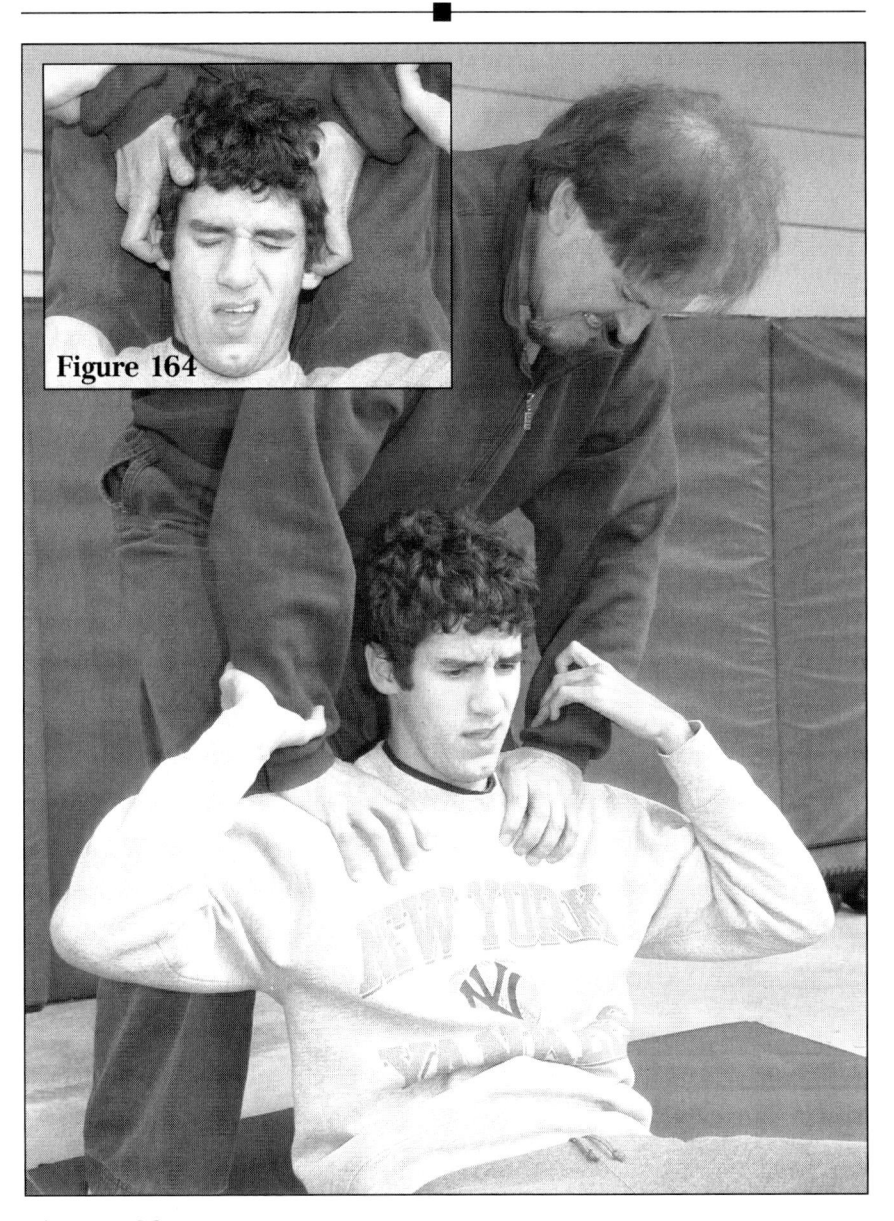

Figure 163

- As he lands on his rear, he reaches up and grabs your upper arms. (Fig. 163)
- Press both of your index fingers into his ear canals. (Fig. 164)

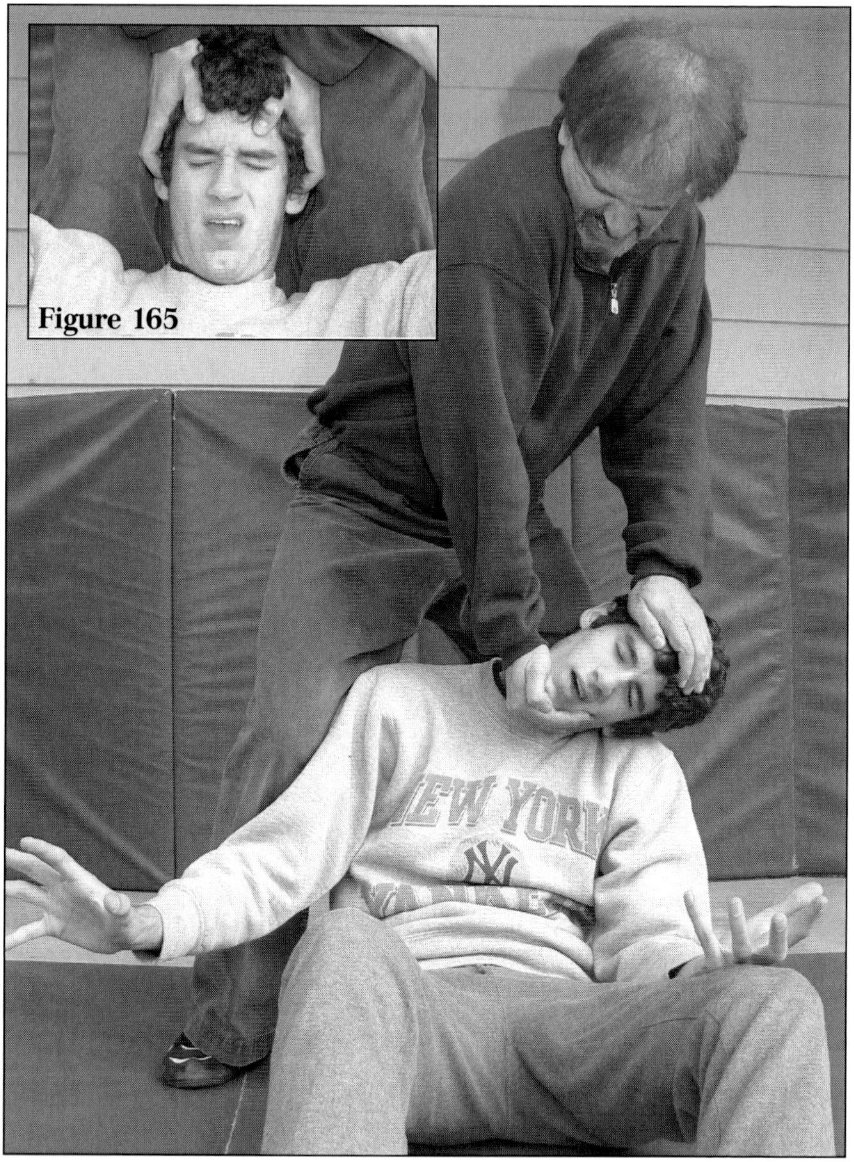

Figure 165

Figure 166

- Use the inside of your knees to press your fingers more deeply into his ears as you command him to let go of your arms. (Fig. 165)
- When he releases, quickly apply a neck crank or any other technique of your choice. (Fig. 166)

To Disengage from the Attacker

You're on top but not doing well.

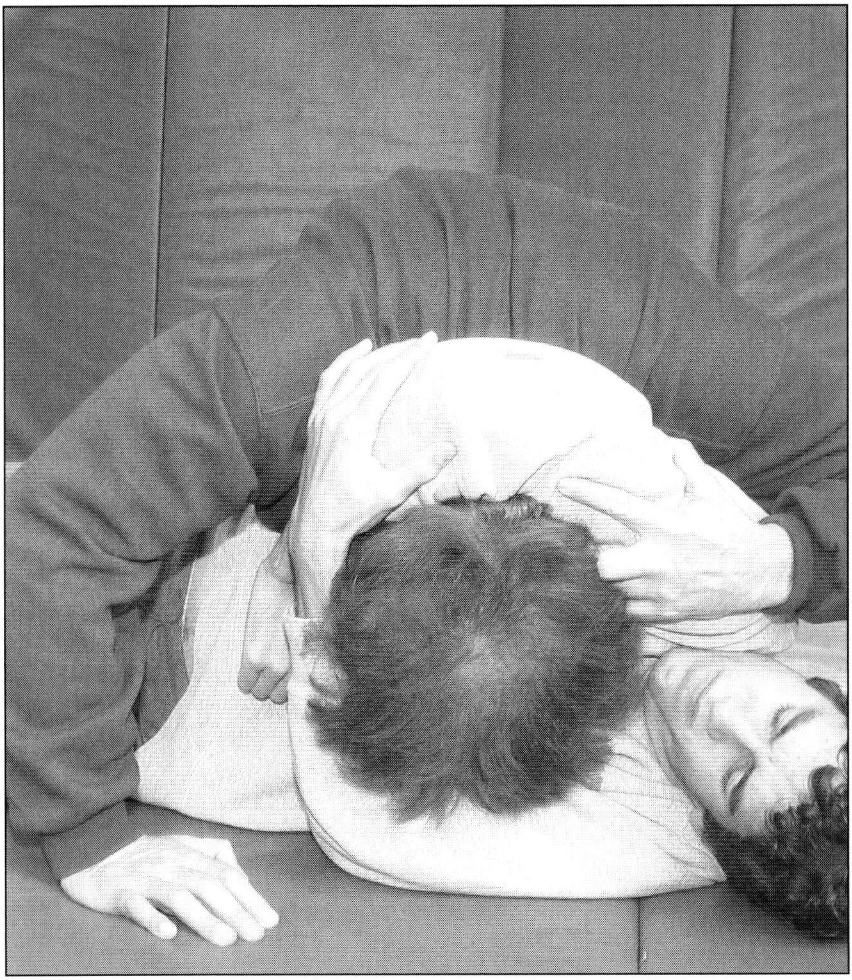

Figure 167

- You want to distract your attacker so you can get off of him. (Fig. 167)
- Press your left elbow into his right ear and begin to scoot off. (Fig. 168)
- Once you're off, you can scoot away, hit him, or try for another hold. (Fig. 169)

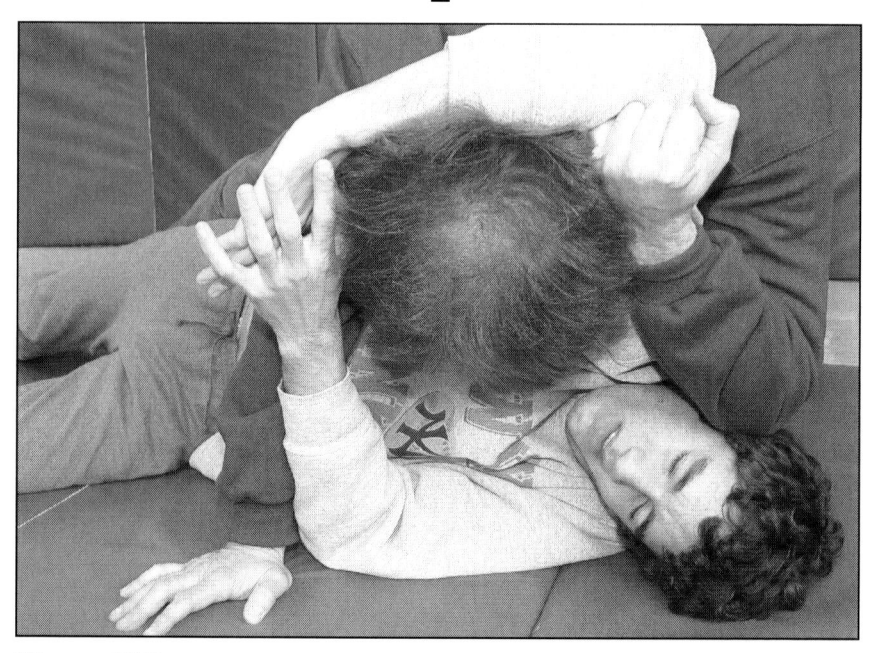

Figure 168

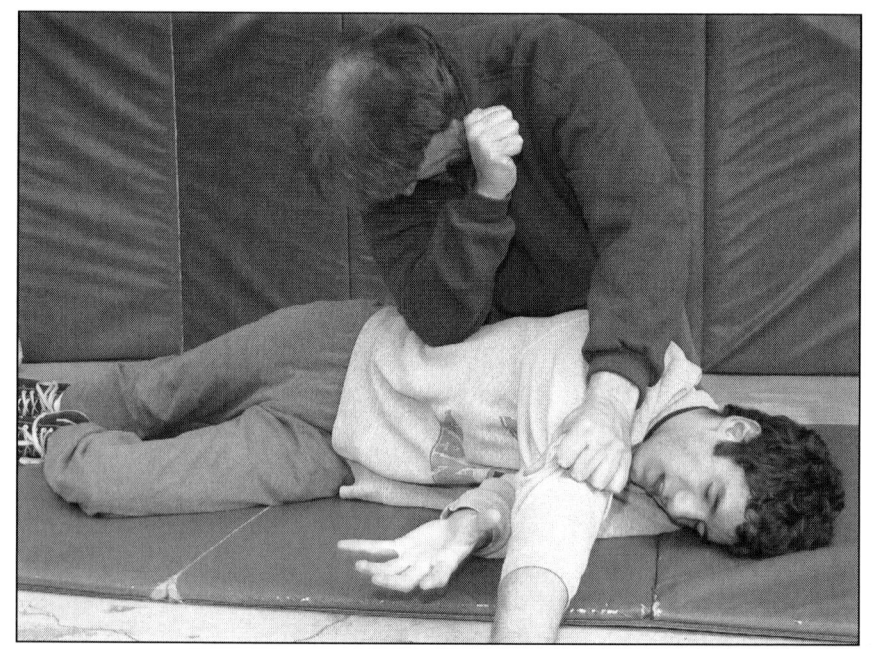

Figure 169

Head   113

Hook His Ear to Help Turn Him

Your attacker has stepped into your
space and is making threats to hurt you.

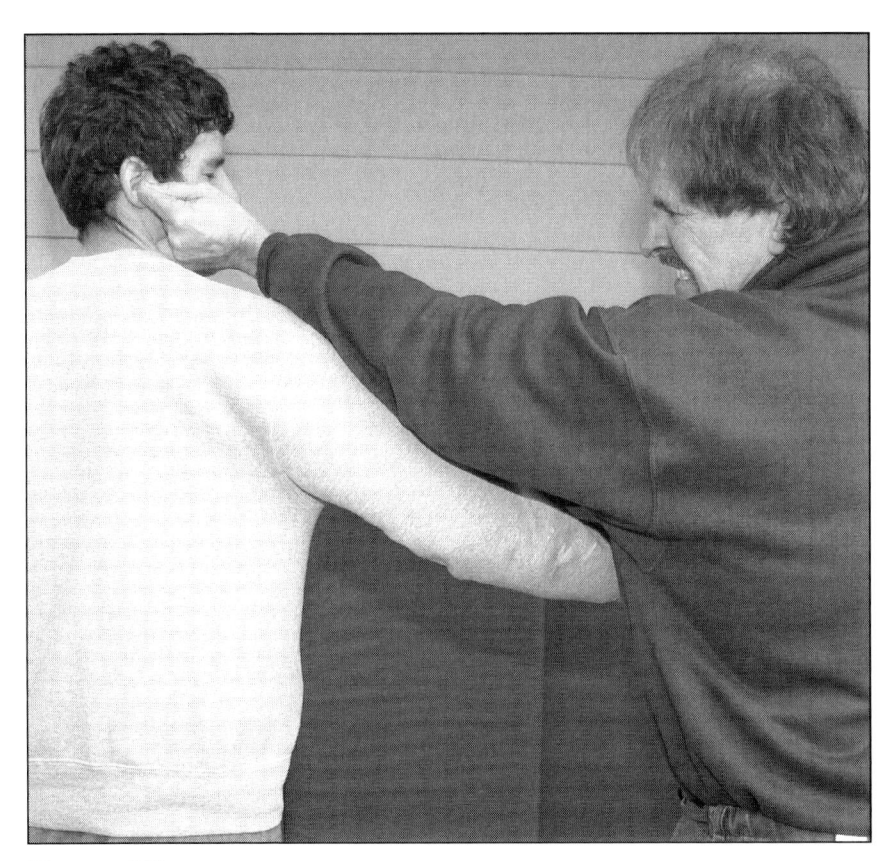

Figure 170

- Grab his closest upper arm and press the mantis finger of your other hand into his ear (think of it as a hook). Make these moves simultaneously or, depending on positioning, grab the arm first and then press the ear (or press the ear first and then grab the arm). (Fig. 170)
- Turn his body away by pulling his arm as your hook-like finger helps turn his head (this is an application of the principle, "where the head goes the body follows"). (Fig. 171)
- Once you're behind him, grapple or hit him. (Fig. 172)

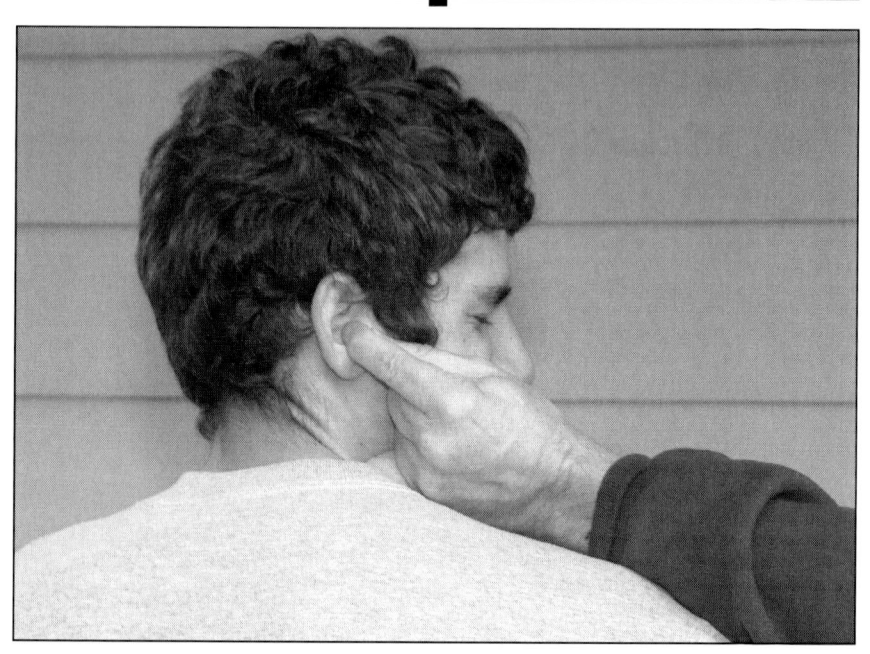

Figure 171

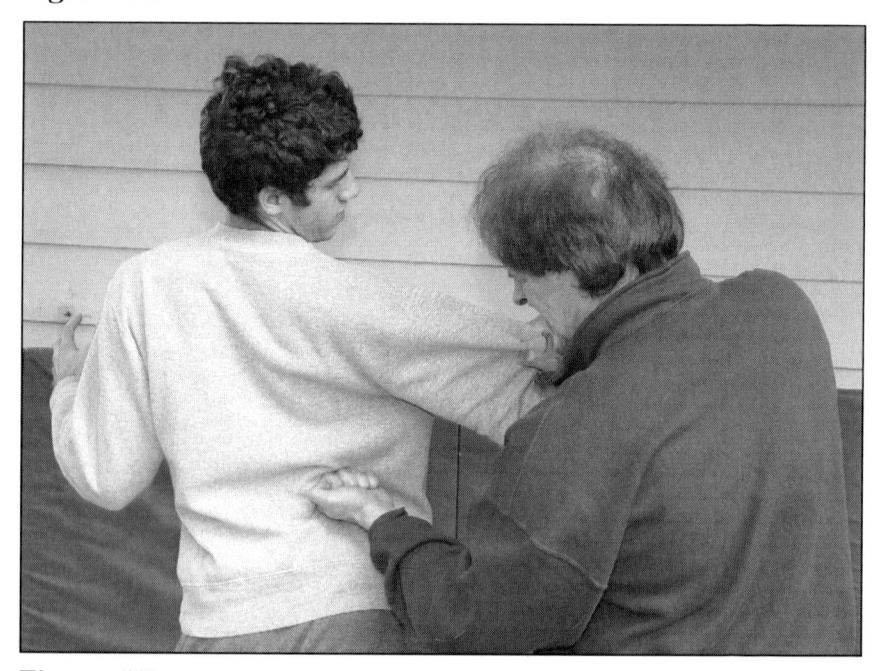

Figure 172

Ear Rip

Practice this on a live opponent or a mannequin-style bag. Your attacker throws a cross.

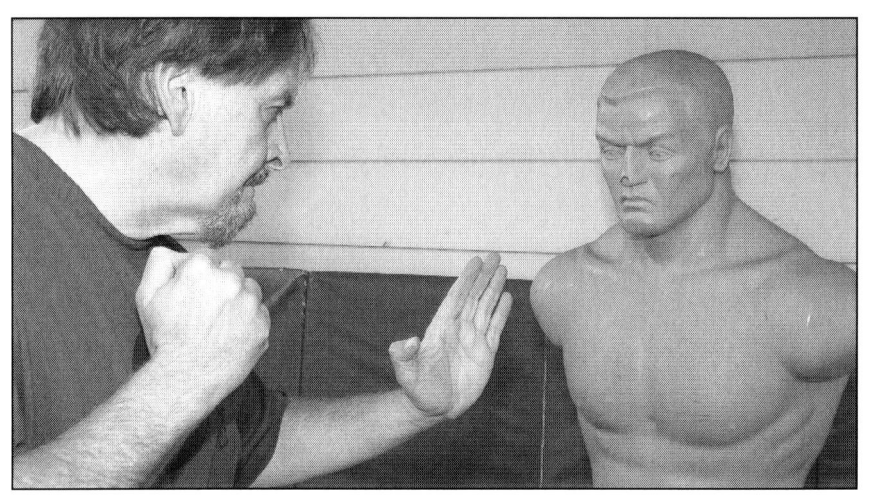

Figure 173

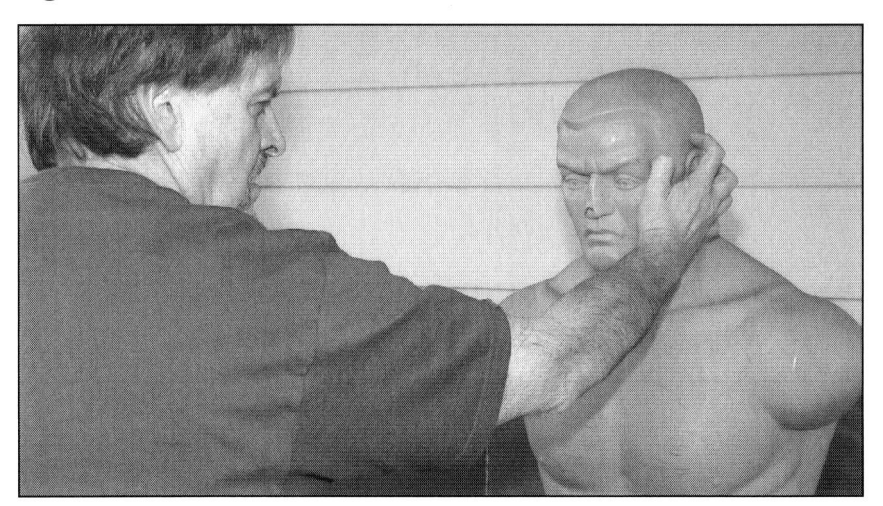

Figure 174

- Block it with a lead-hand sweep. (Fig. 173)
- Snap your rear, five-fingered claw hand out toward the side of his head. (Fig. 174)

Figure 175

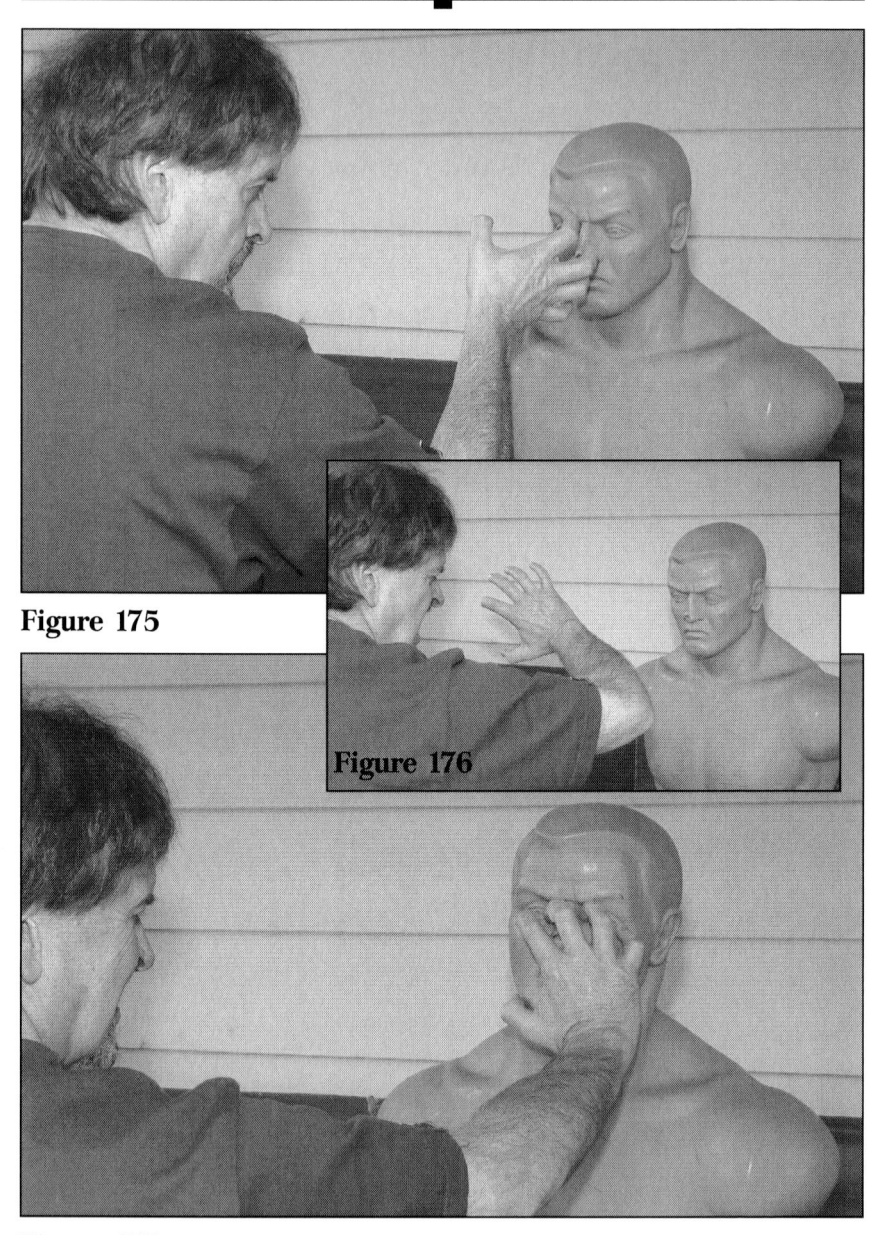

Figure 176

Figure 177

- Rip your claw hand across his ear and face. (Figs. 175, 176)
- This will likely snap his head to the side. Return your hand with a backfist or another ripping claw to his face. (Fig. 177)

Variation 1:

- Block as before, but this time grasp his ear in your five-fingered claw and rip it to the side. It's highly unlikely you will rip off his ear, but he will be looking at your hand through watery eyes to see if you have it. (Fig. 178)

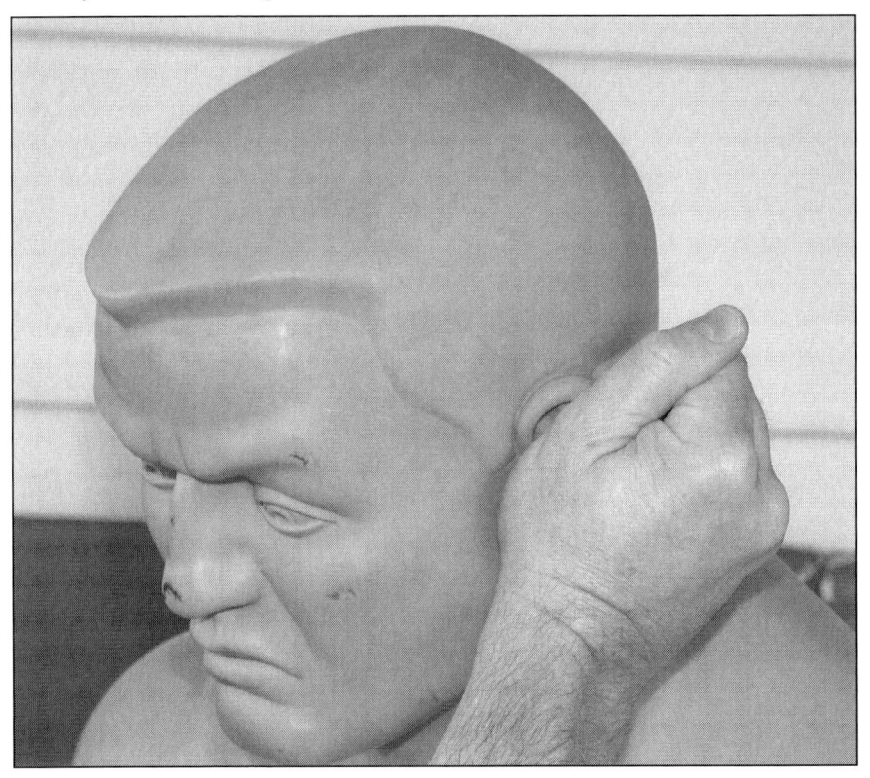

Figure 178

Variation 2:

- Block his punch with your sweep hand. (Fig. 179)
- Shoot your blocking hand to secure his shoulder as you step diagonally to the same side. (Fig. 180)
- As you execute the ear rip with your rear hand, push his shoulder slightly into the technique. This creates a brace effect, which makes the rip more intense. (Fig. 181)

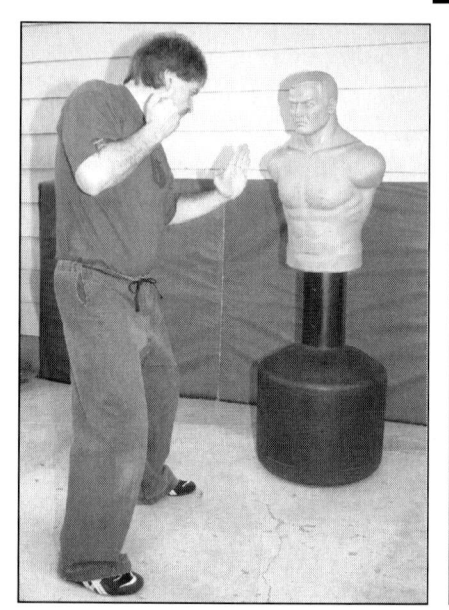

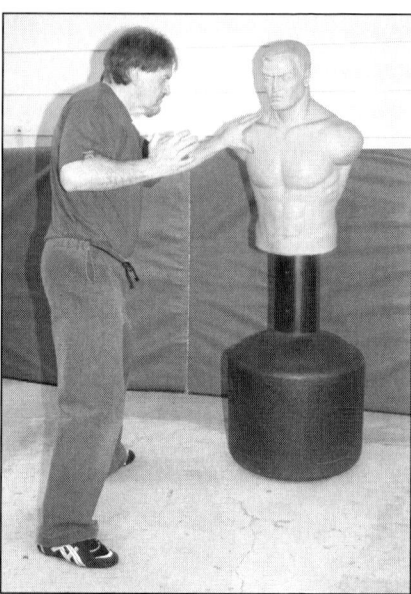

118   *The Brutal Art of Ripping, Poking, and Pressing Vital Targets*

Figure 179   **Figure 180**

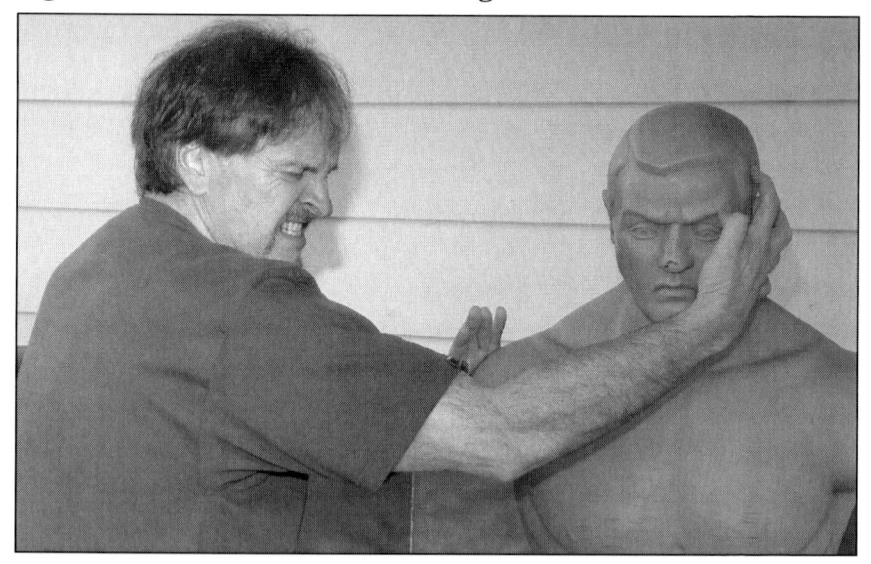

Figure 181

Variation:

- You can also brace the side of his head as you execute the rip. (Fig. 182)

Head   119

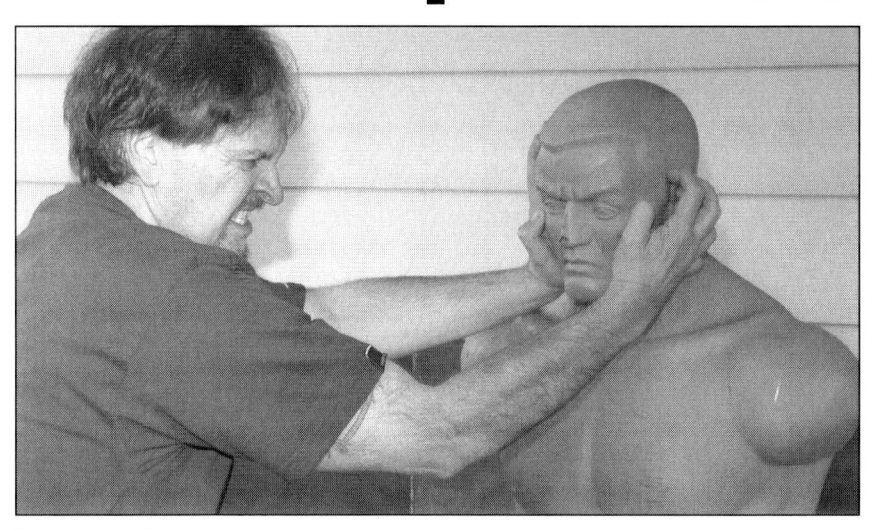

Figure 182

Mike Tyson His Ear

Your attacker has you in an arm-trapped bear hug. Practice on a mannequin-style bag when you don't have a partner with clean ears.

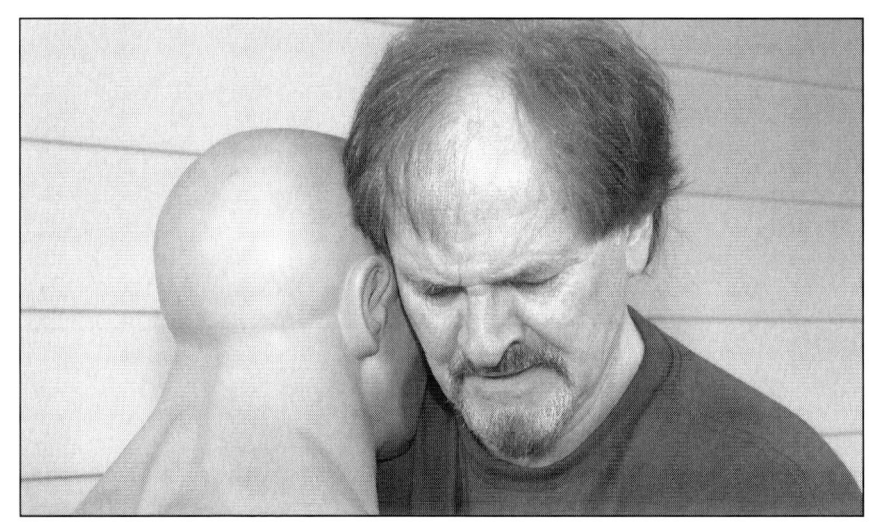

Figure 183
- Your head is next to his. (Fig. 183)

120   *The Brutal Art of Ripping, Poking, and Pressing Vital Targets*

- Chomp into his ear and do so with prejudice. Tear into his ear like a dog on a rabbit, jerking your head from side to side. (Fig. 184)
- Escape or follow with additional attacks. (Fig. 185)

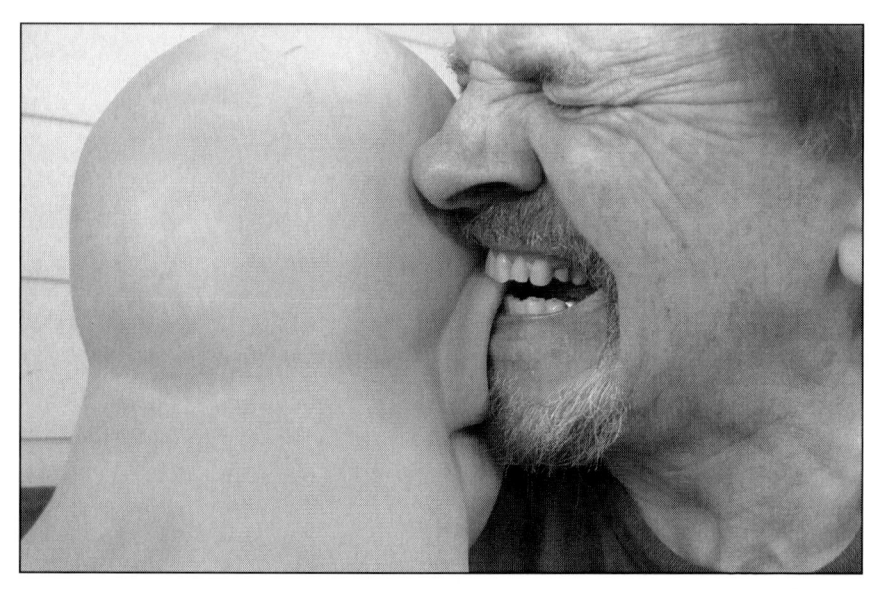

Figure 184

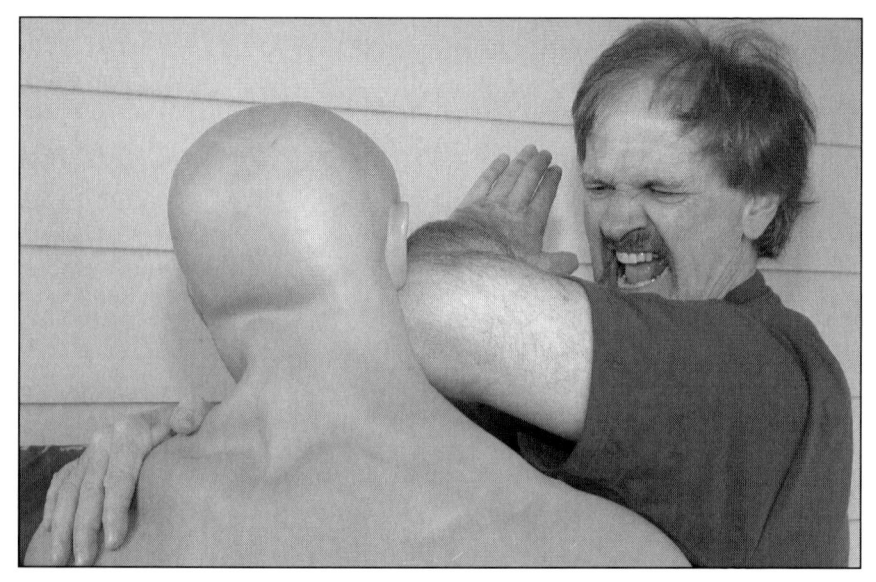

Figure 185

CHEEK

The face cheek—no matter if it's a fat face or a lean one—is ripe for pinching, pressing, twisting, and ripping. Because most people aren't comfortable with a stranger touching their face, let alone hurting it, they will pull away, which is exactly what you want so you can counter or escape.

Press to Turn Attacker's Head

The attacker is on top of you.

- He grips the front of your shirt. (Fig. 186)

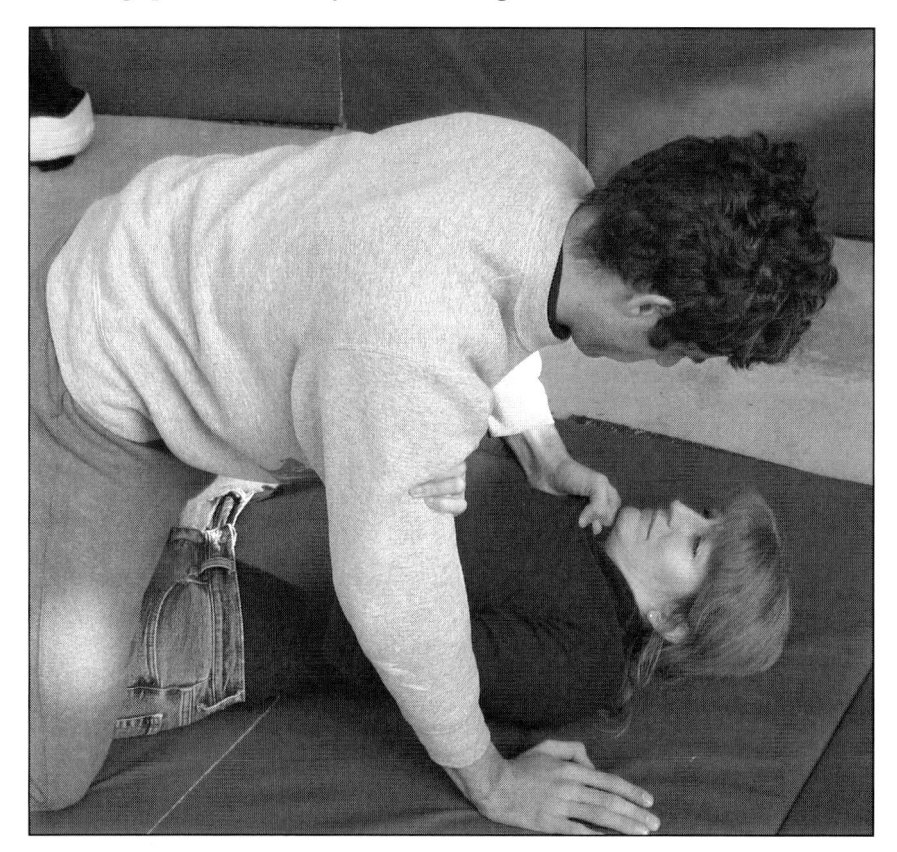

Figure 186

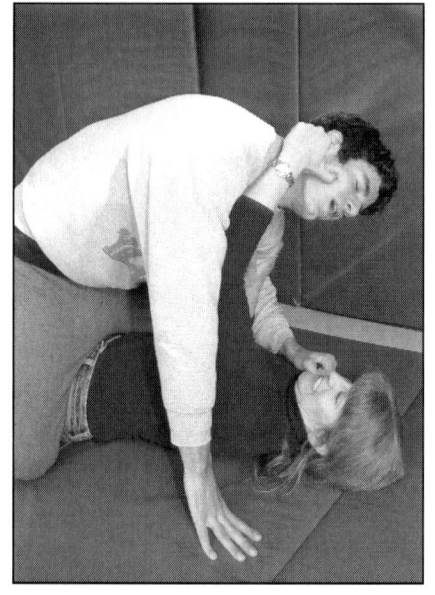

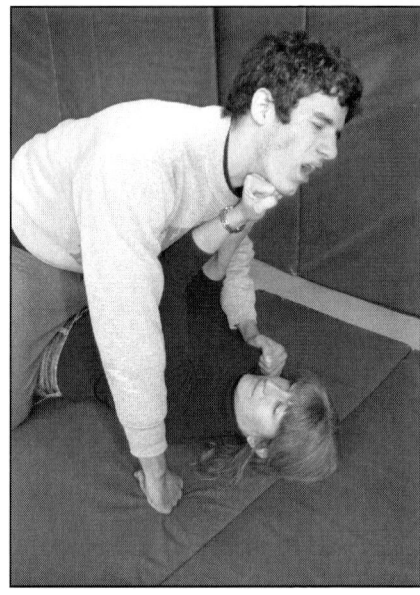

Figure 187

Figure 188

- Press your thumb into his cheek to expose his neck. (Fig. 187)
- Punch it. (Fig. 188)

Variation:

- If the situation allows, brace the other side of his face as you press with your thumb. (Fig. 189)

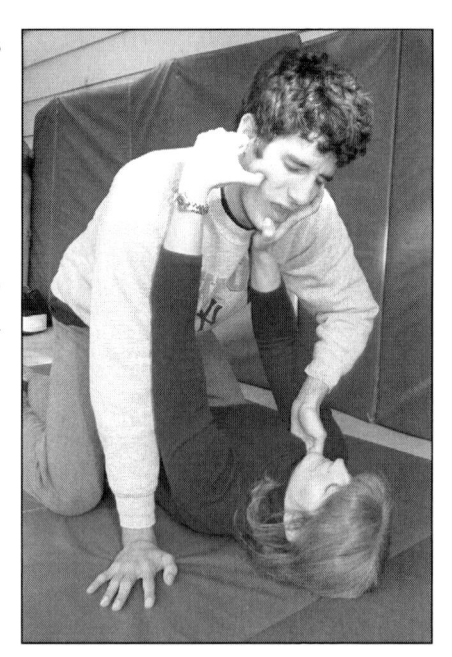

Figure 189

Cheek Press or Twist to Supplement Your arm Trap

You're applying a straight armlock with your knee on the attacker's head. For additional pain and restraint, apply a cheek technique.

- Press your knee into his cheekbone. The knee isn't as sharp as your elbow or thumb, but it still works well because of the sensitivity of the target. Your weight helps to restrain his head. (Fig. 190)

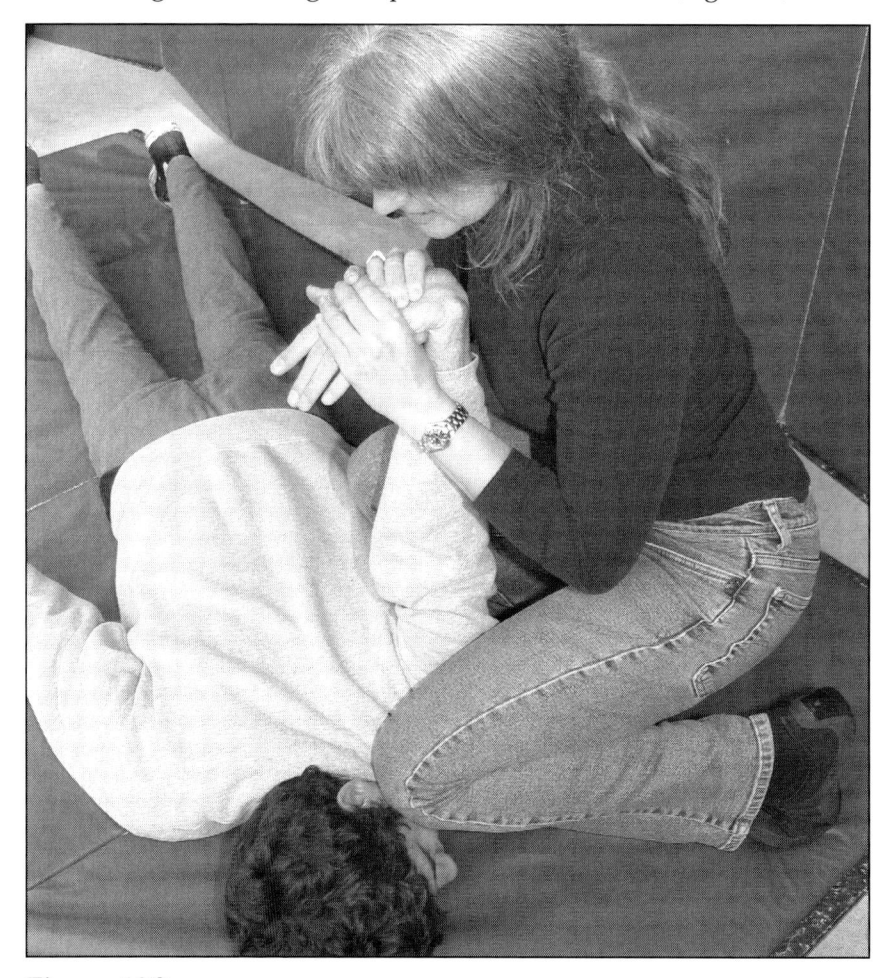

Figure 190

Variation 1:

- Place your knee on his shoulder and press your thumb or middle knuckle into his cheek cavity. (Fig. 191)

Variation 2:

- Pinch his cheek with your thumb and index finger and press the twisted flesh into his face. The floor acts as a brace. (Fig. 192)

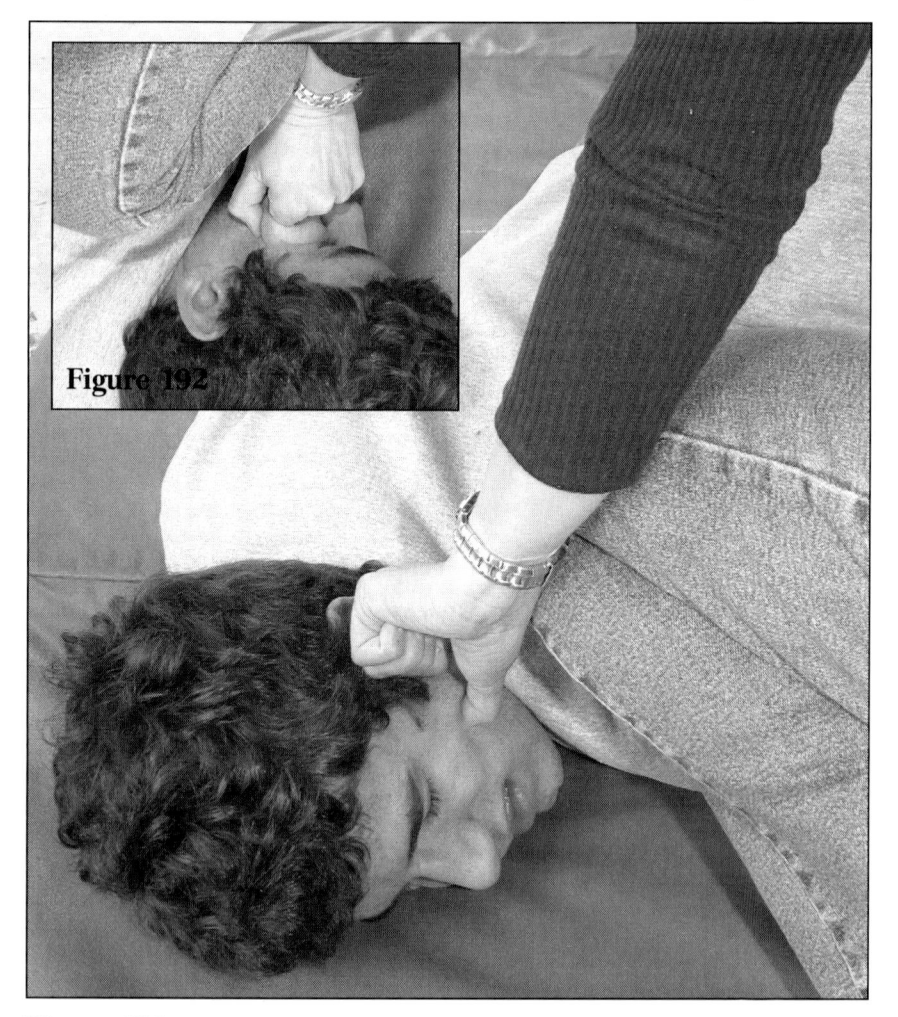

Figure 192

Figure 191

Cheek Press to Augment a Wristlock

You're on the ground on top of the attacker applying a wristlock.

- You begin to lose control of your attacker's trapped arm. (Fig. 193)
- To distract him, press the point of your elbow into his cheekbone. Dig it in and wiggle it as you work to better secure his arm. (Fig. 194)

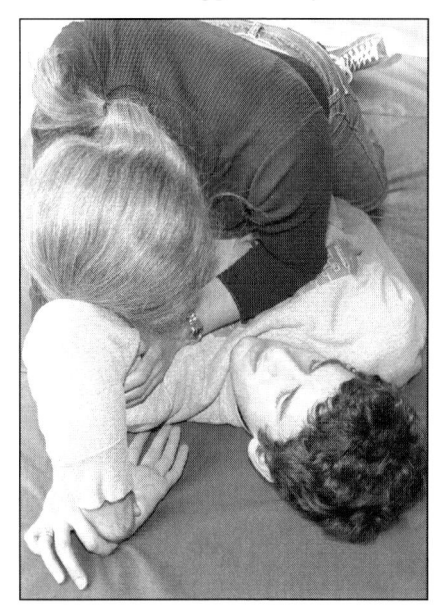

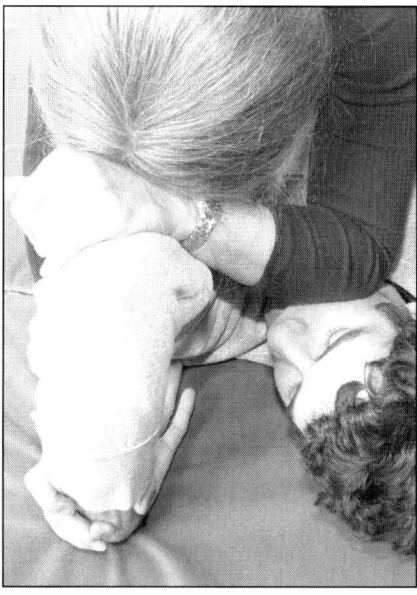

Figure 193   **Figure 194**

One night I was in the precinct house trying to write a report. I say "trying" because a drunk in the DUI room (a small room where motorists charged with driving under the influence are processed) was screaming, kicking, and generally acting like a fool. At least twice I heard banging, thumping, and cursing coming from the room as officers repeatedly wrestled him back into a chair.

Then it was quiet, but only for a minute or two before there was a sudden commotion of scraping chairs, an overturned table, shouting, doors hitting walls, and running feet. I learned later that the big prisoner had slammed into the officers like a bowling ball knocking down pins, smashed through the door, fled down the hall, and out an exterior door.

It took only about 10 seconds to get out into the parking lot, but already seven cops had piled onto the downed guy in a technique we used to call "pig pile." I circled the struggling mass looking in vain for a place to get in since the squad still hadn't controlled one of the man's flailing arms.

Then a window of opportunity opened through the blue mass of arms, legs, and torsos; it was a small two-second opening that led to the drunk's face. I thrust my hand into it and secured a piece of the man's cheek. I pinched and twisted it as if trying to remove a sample for a souvenir of our time together.

The man screamed like a bad actress in a horror movie, followed a moment later by all the tension going out of his arm. The other officers got control of him and a moment later the man was handcuffed.

Only one officer saw me do my little technique. I shook my head at him as I gave him a finger-to-my-lips hush sign, and then I walked back into the building.

Cheek Pinch or Rip

Remember when you were a kid and your Aunt Matilda would pinch a wad of your cheek, shake it back and forth, and tell you how precious you were? Remember how you wanted to return the favor? Well, now you can take it out on a hapless attacker.

Even a slight response to your technique will likely cause him distraction and open a window of opportunity for you to follow up.

You're clinching with an attacker who is pressing you against a wall.

- He has a secure grip on your right arm but your left hand, though restrained, is just close enough to reach his cheek. (Fig. 195)
- Use your left thumb and index finger to pinch and twist his cheek as hard as you can. He might react by jerking his head away or by closing his eyes and grimacing against the pain, or he might not react at all because he's too pumped with adrenaline to feel it. But it doesn't matter as long as his brain is diverted. Since a person can think of only one thing at a time, his thought process will momentarily focus on his face, not on the grip he has on your arms. (Fig. 196)

Head

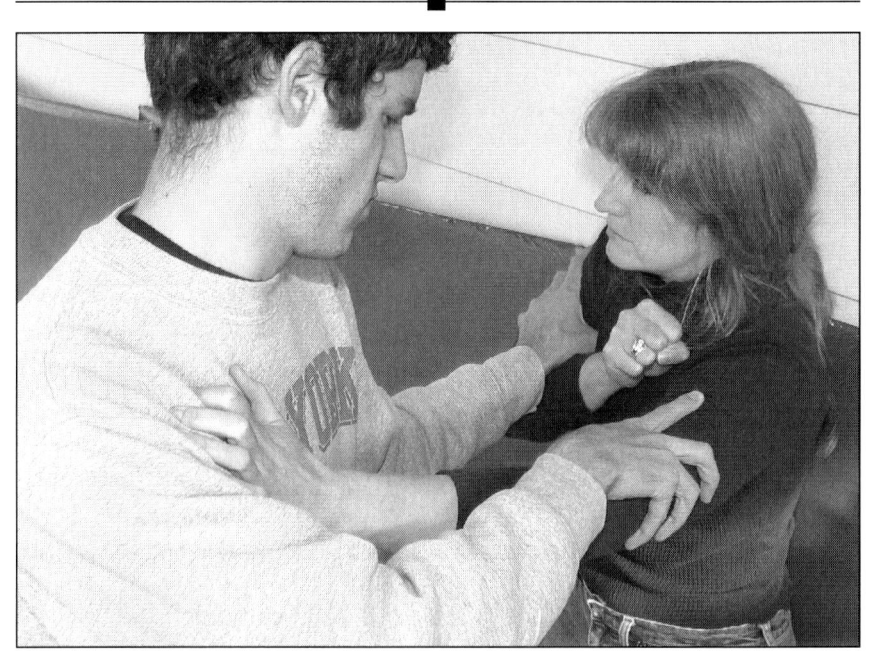

Figure 195

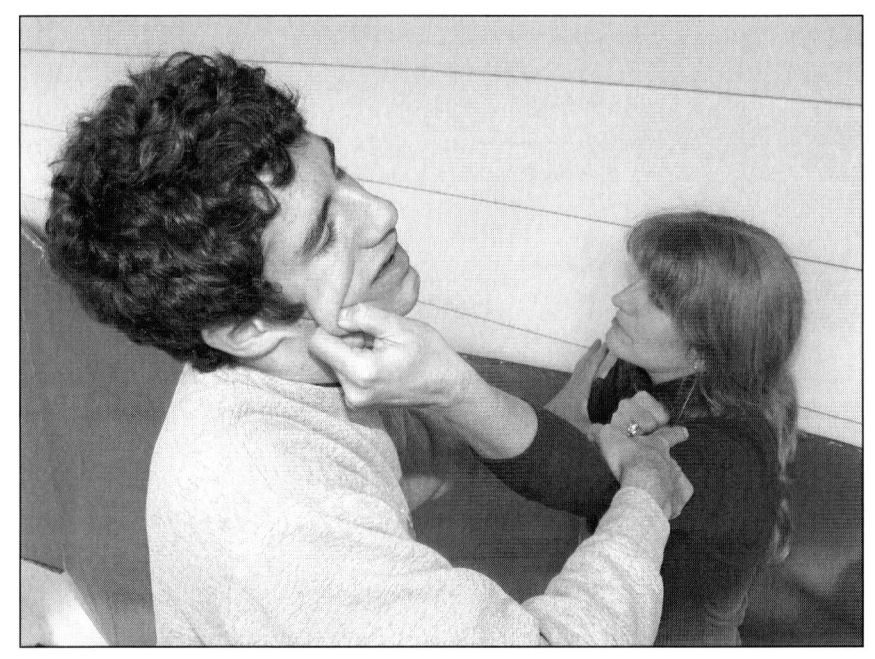

Figure 196

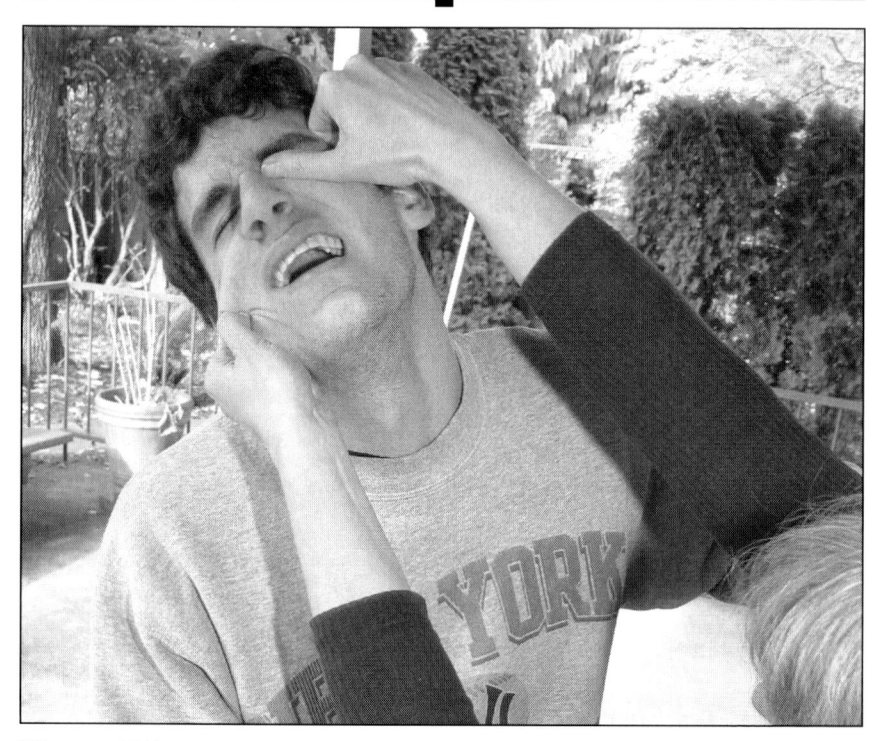

Figure 197

- Let's say he reacts by tightening his grip on your pinching arm but relaxes his grip on your right. Instantly ram your right thumb into his eye. (Fig. 197)

THROAT AND NECK

Anytime you apply a choke hold, you press the throat. Even carotid holds, where pressure is applied against one or both sides of the neck, affect the front of the throat to some degree. This section isn't about chokes but about pressing, twisting, and ripping techniques that cause pain to the neck area. Still, some might inadvertently choke the attacker or restrict his carotid arteries, both of which can cause serious injury, unconsciousness, and even death. So, while the primary function of the following techniques is to effect enough agony to get your attacker to stop his aggression toward you, you're ultimately responsible for any vulnerable target that is affected. Be justified.

Head 129

Standing Larynx Press

An attacker approached from your front.

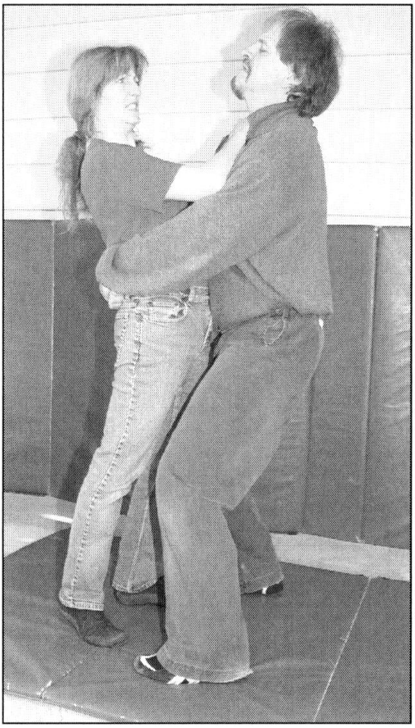

Figure 198

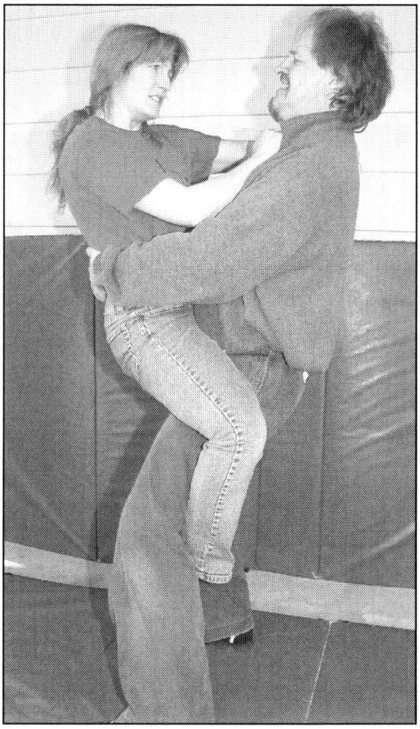

Figure 199

- He grabs you in an arms-free bear hug. (Fig. 198)
- Jump up and straddle his legs, your calves behind his knees. (Fig. 199)
- Press the side of your right wrist into his throat (turn your hand so that your wrist protrudes outward) and push it with your left hand. (Fig. 200)
- Force him to release his hug by pulling on the back of his knees with your claves and pressing your wrist deeply into his throat. (Fig. 201)

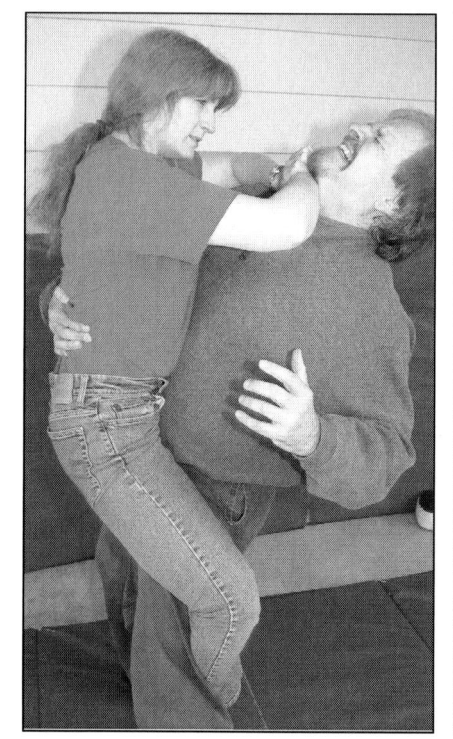

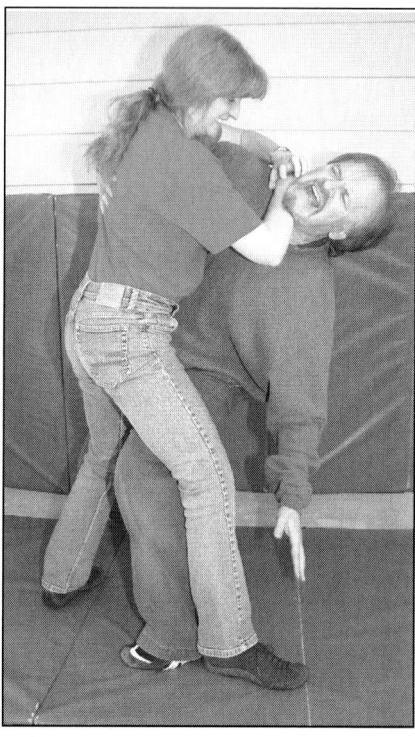

Figure 200   **Figure 201**

Shin-on-Throat Press

I used this technique three or four times when I was a cop. It has the potential for causing internal damage or death, so be justified to use it.

You're thrashing about on the floor with an armed attacker. At one point you're lying perpendicular across him as you restrain his right weapon arm.

- Trap his left arm by leaning on it and place your right shin across his throat. If he turns his head before you can pin it completely, it's okay because your shin will still hurt him, though not as acutely as when your leg is on the front of his throat. (Fig. 202)
- As you to press his throat, apply pressure to the armlock as you order him to release the weapon. If he complies, reward him by

easing off his throat a little, but don't move your shin away. If he doesn't release it, or does but suddenly gets combative again, apply more weight to the throat press and more pressure on the armlock. If he reaches for the weapon, slam your shin in hard. (Fig. 203)

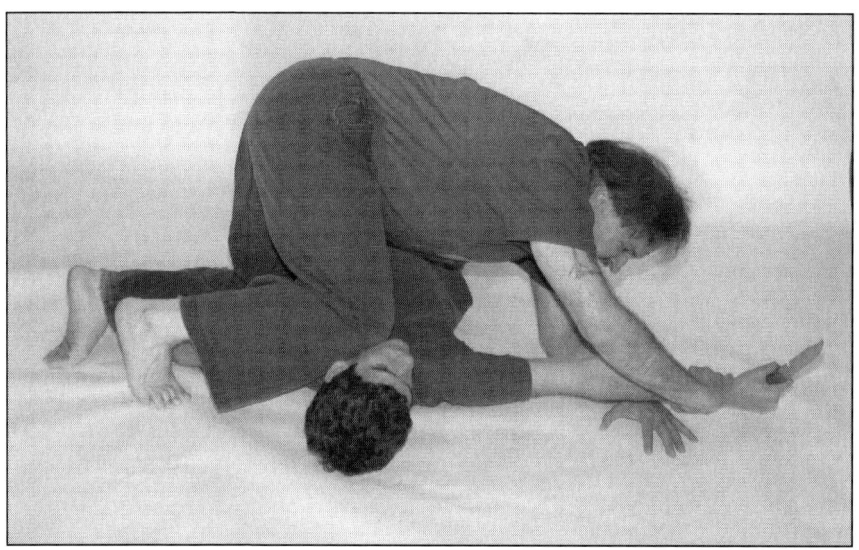

Figure 202

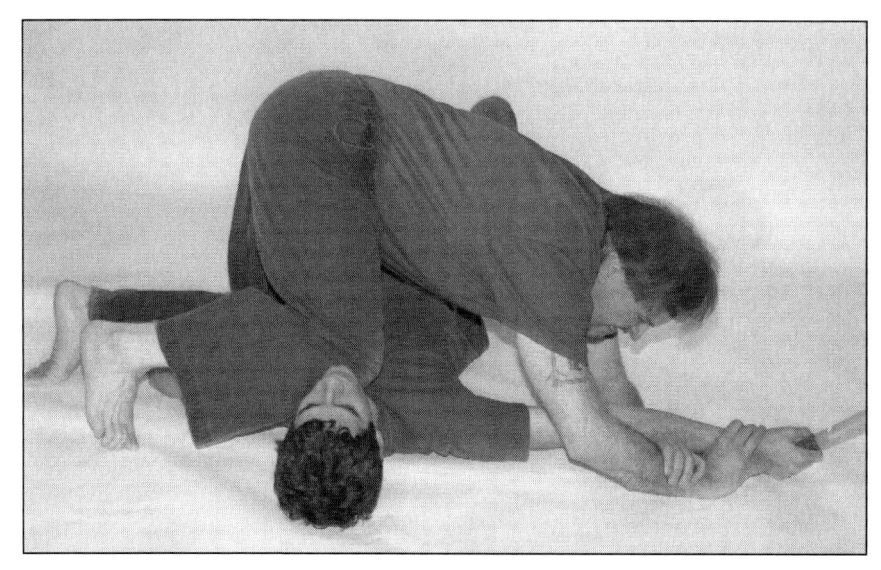

Figure 203

A word on squeezing the throat. Throat squeezing techniques hurt, they cause panic, and they give direction (usually away from your squeeze). Now, if you have a grip that can tear up street asphalt, or your attacker has an especially tender throat, there is a good chance you might cause serious internal damage. Be careful with this one, and be justified to use such severe force.

Squeeze to Release Headlock

The attacker has you in a headlock.

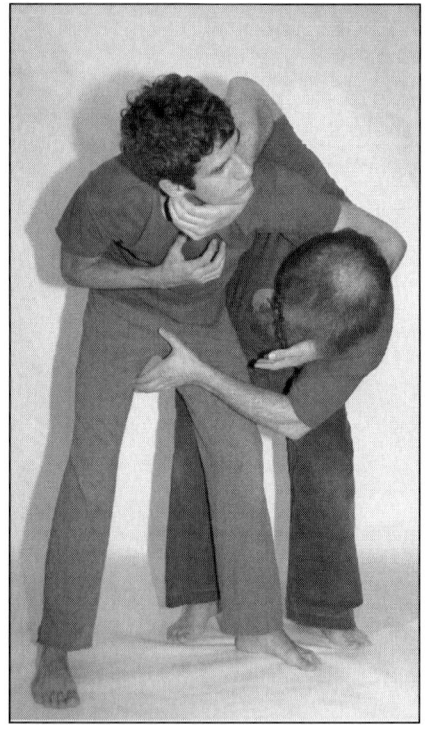

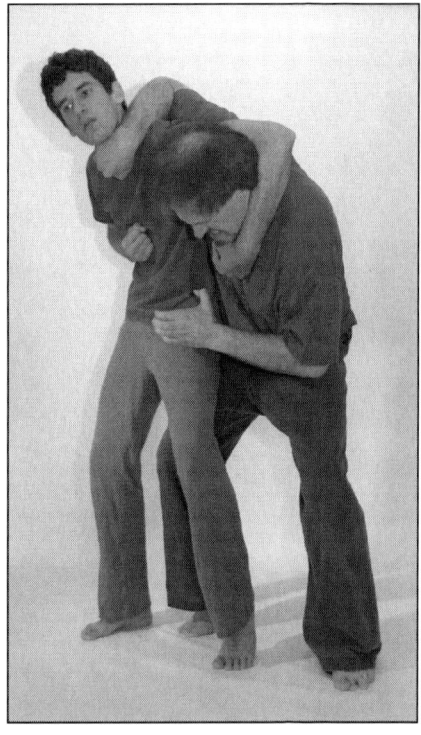

Figure 204

Figure 205

- Reach up and squeeze the front of his throat as you simultaneously slap his groin. Most people will snap their heads back and lean away. That is exactly what you want. (Fig. 204)
- Bump your hip into the back of his. (Fig. 205)

Head

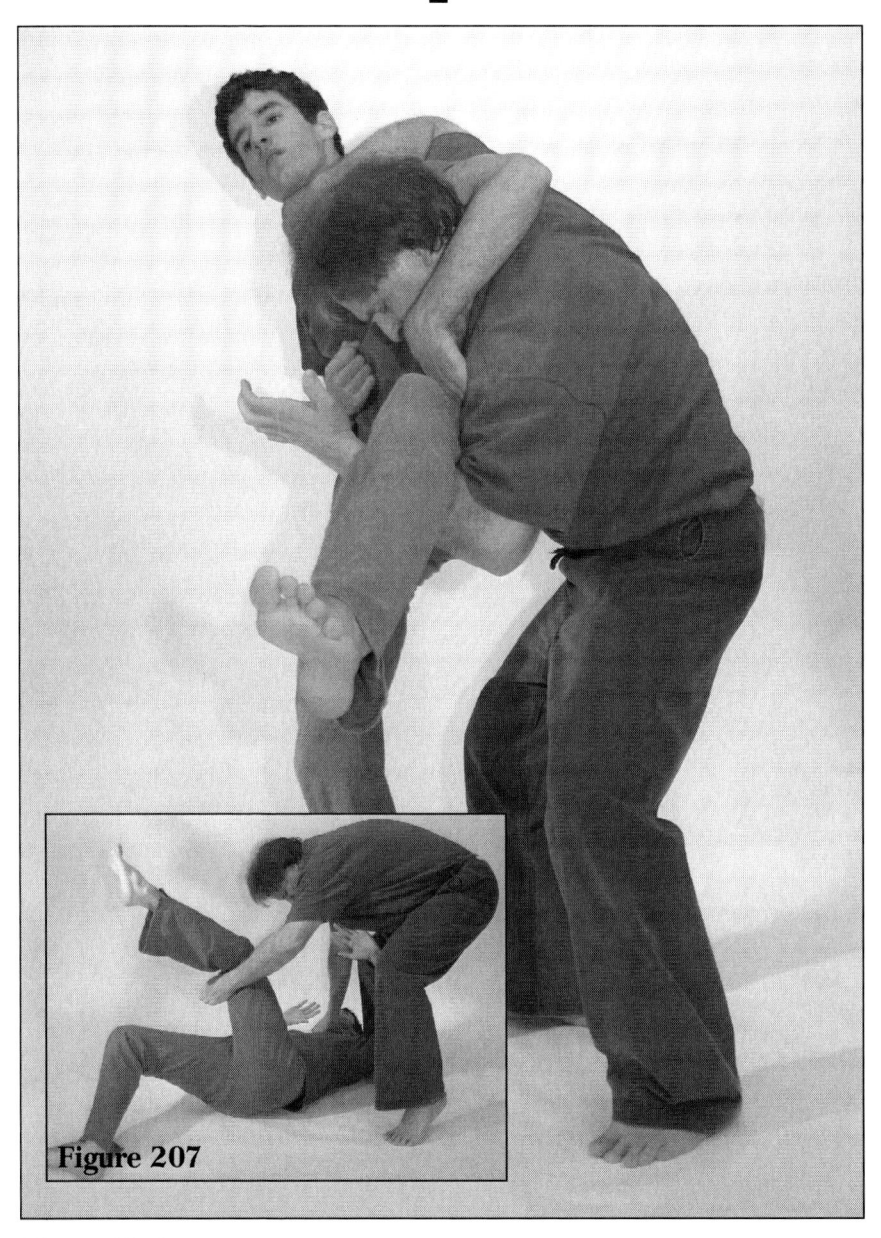

Figure 206

Figure 207

- Lift his closest leg as you continue to squeeze his throat. (Fig. 206)
- Dump him onto his back. (Fig. 207)

A Long Squeeze

I used this on the street a few times as a cop, back before times changed and we were commanded to handle rapists, killers, and arsonists more kindly and gently.

The attacker throws an arcing haymaker at you.

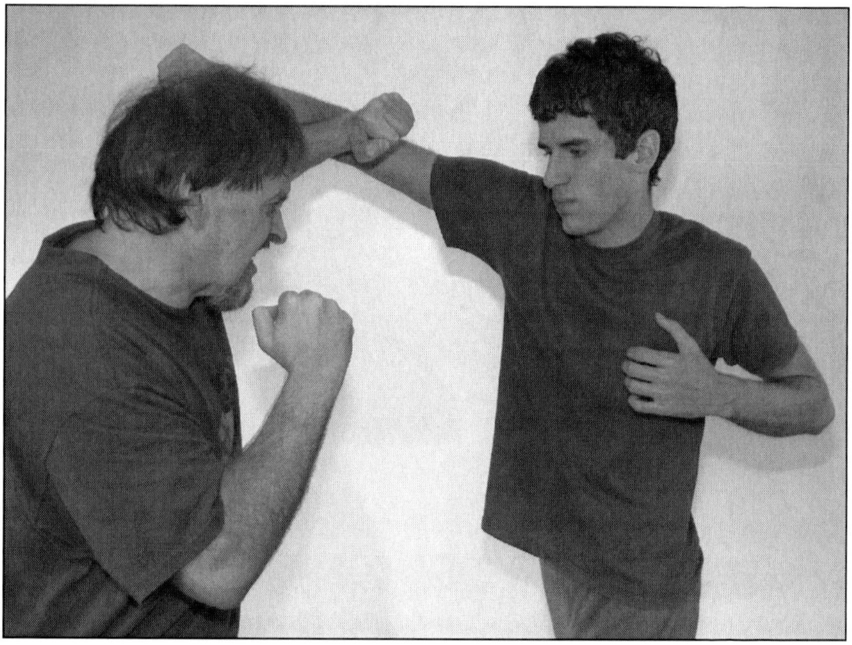

Figure 208

- Make yourself solid and block. (Fig. 208)
- Wrap your blocking arm around his attacking arm and thrust your other hand in to squeeze his throat. (Fig. 209)
- Drive with your legs and force the attacker backwards into a wall. Hold him against the wall for a second so that he can feel all the wonders of the throat squeeze. (Fig. 210)
- Simultaneously do three actions: pull his trapped arm inward, keep squeezing as you push his throat, and pivot your body to the left. (Fig. 211)
- Take him to the ground and keep squeezing as you press your hand into his throat. (Fig. 212)

Head

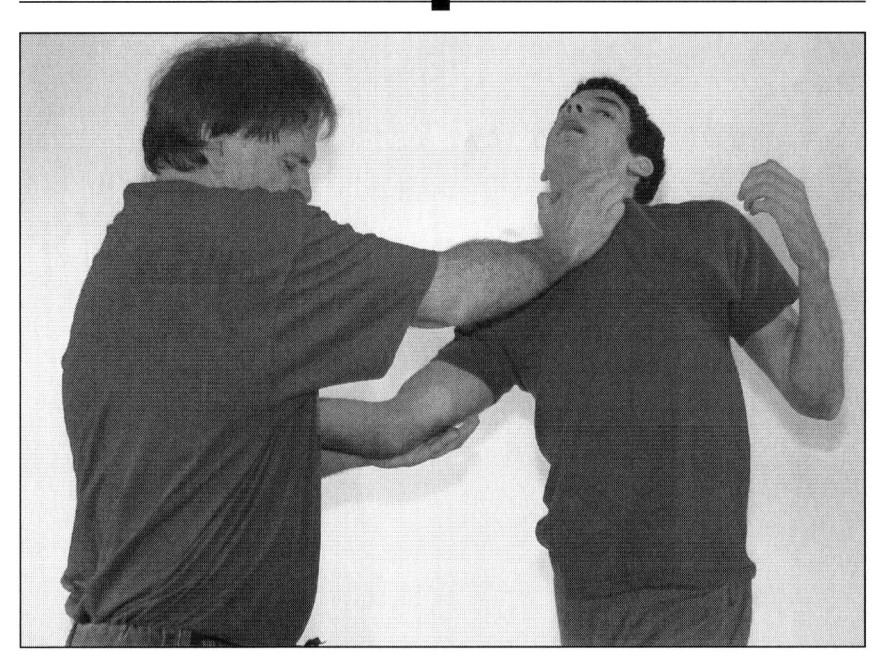

Figure 209

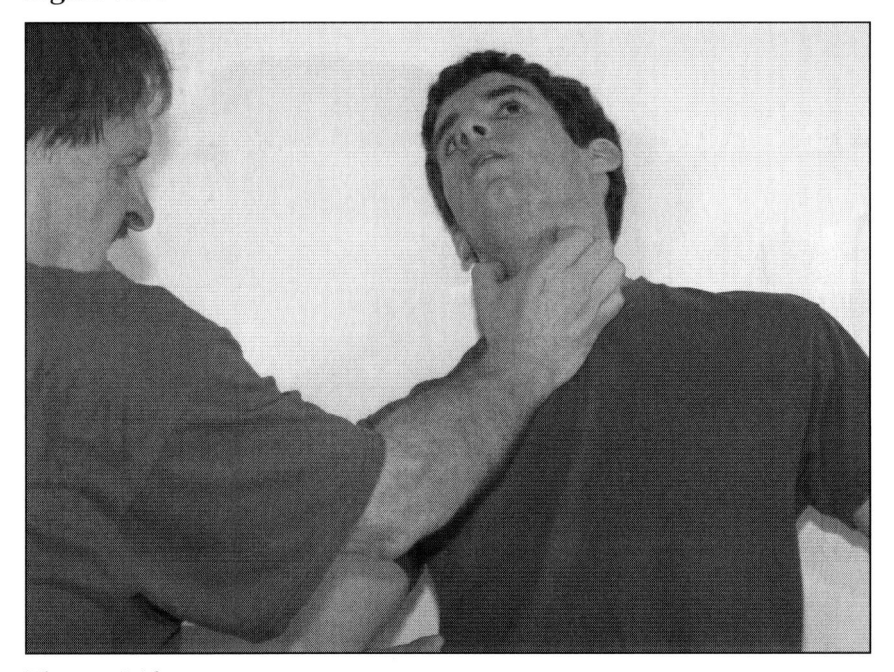

Figure 210

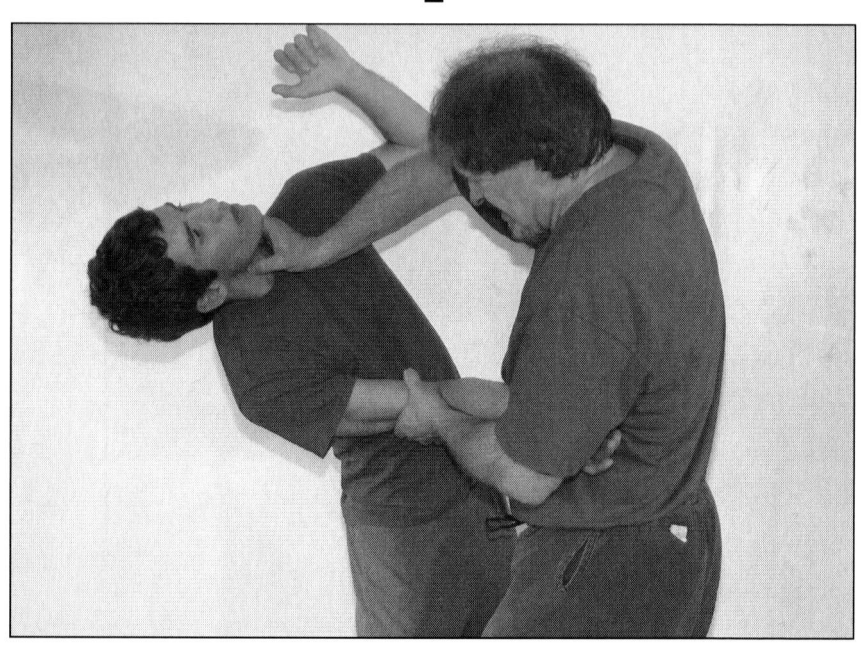

Figure 211

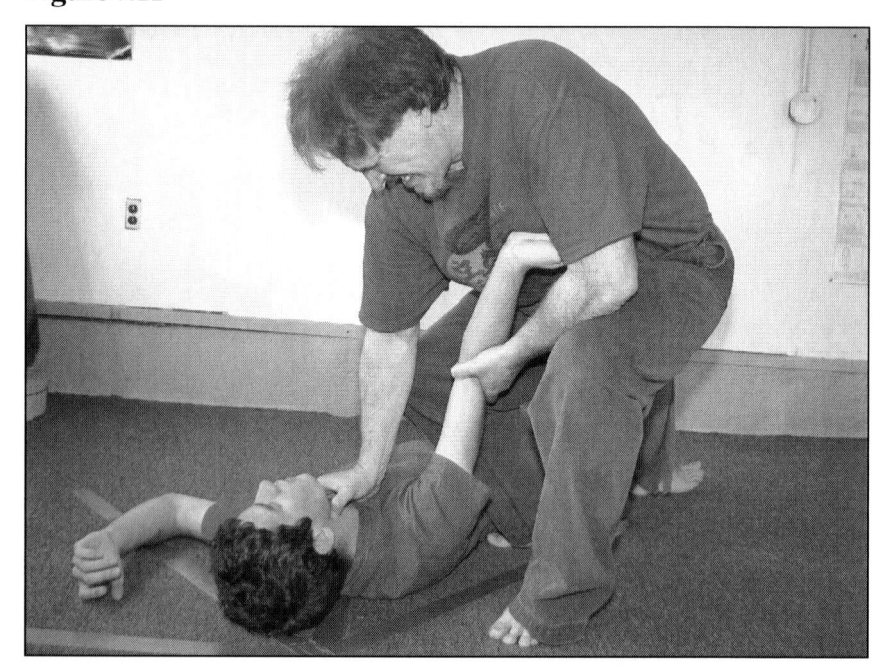

Figure 212

Throat Rip

Whether you actually rip anything with this technique depends on your power, the vulnerability of the recipient's throat, and how you're both positioned. At the least, you will give your attacker some shock and awe. At the most you will cause internal and possibly fatal damage. As always, be justified to use this level of force.

Let's look at three kinds of rips in response to an attack with a bottle (not shown).

Against a haymaker attack:

- Block with both arms. (Fig. 213)

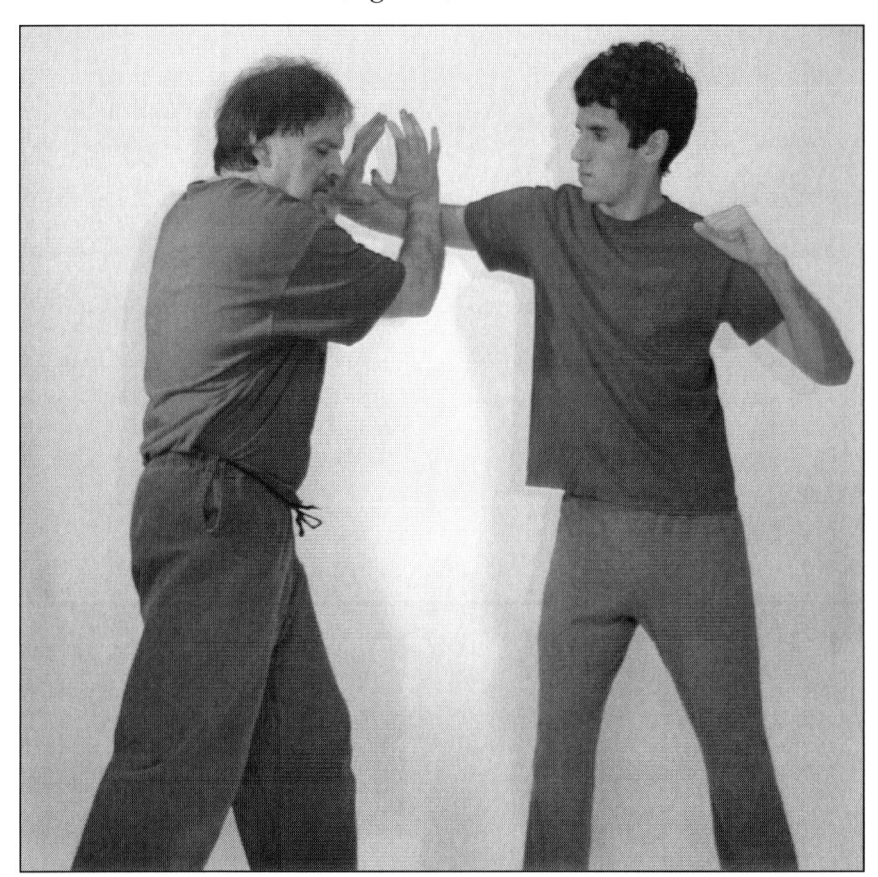

Figure 213

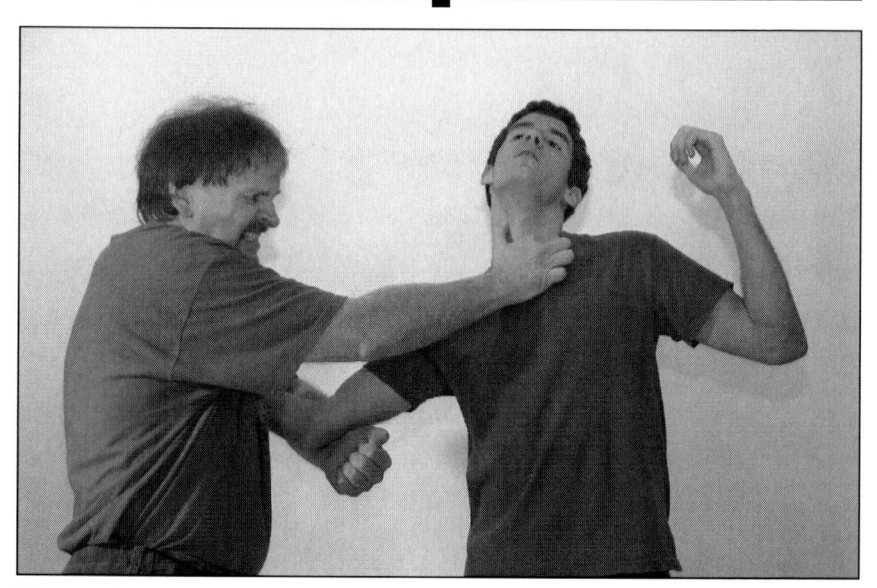

Figure 214

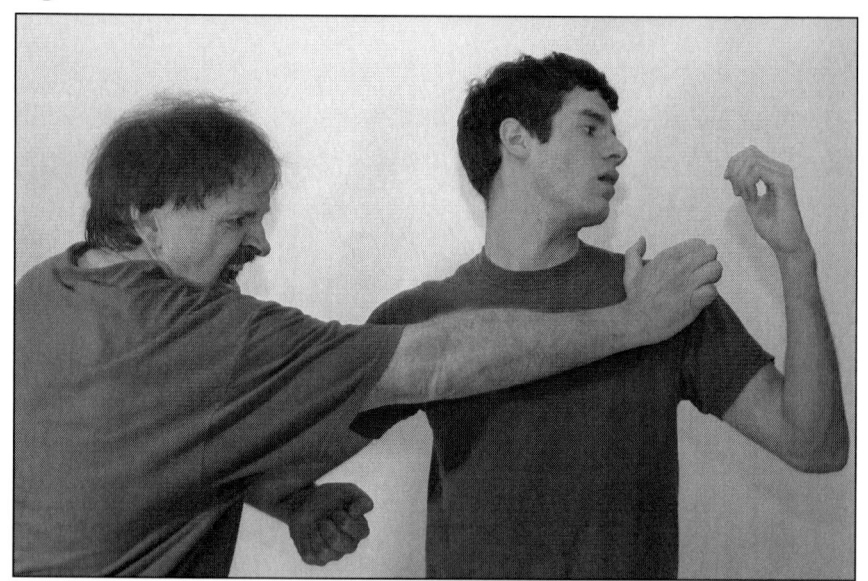

Figure 215

- Wrap the attacker's arm in a lock and jab your thumb into the side of his Adam's apple. (Fig. 214)
- Rip your thumb and his apple away from you. (Fig. 215)

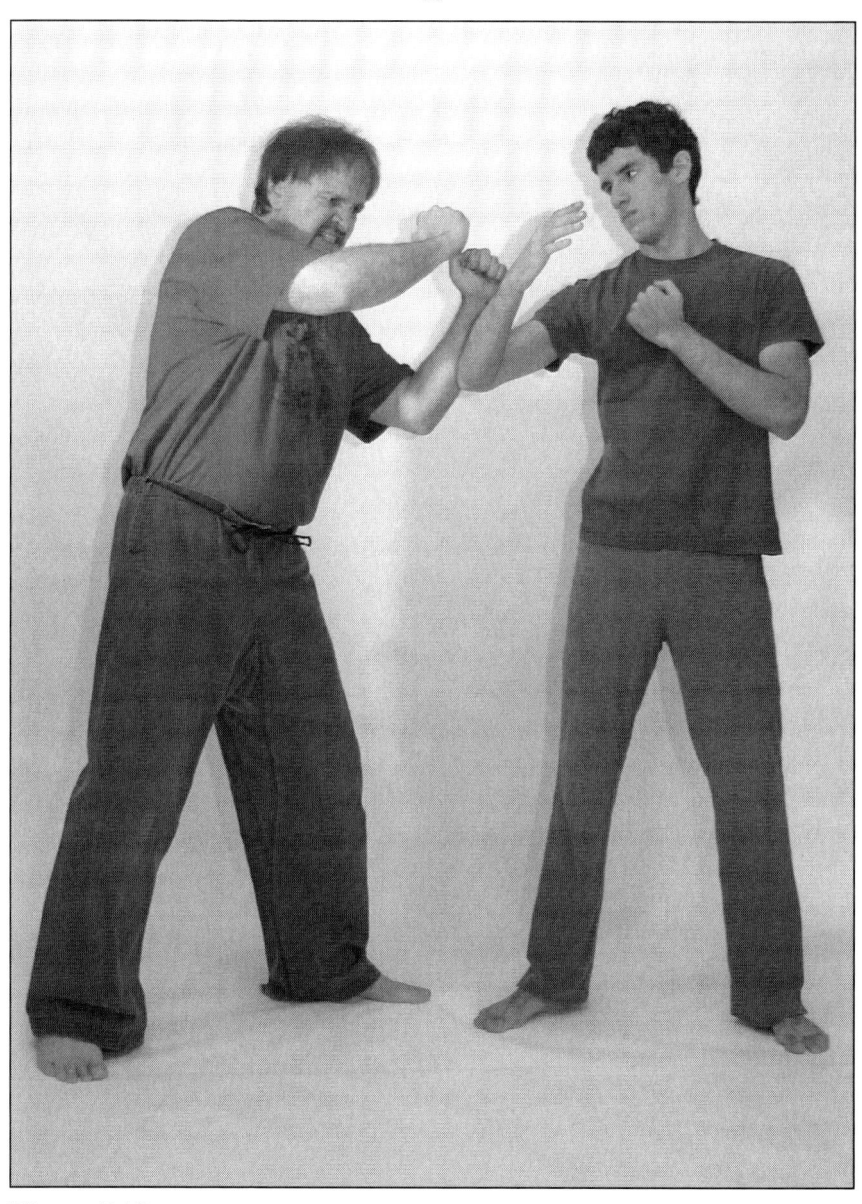

Figure 216

Against a backhand attack:

- Block with both arms. (Fig. 216)

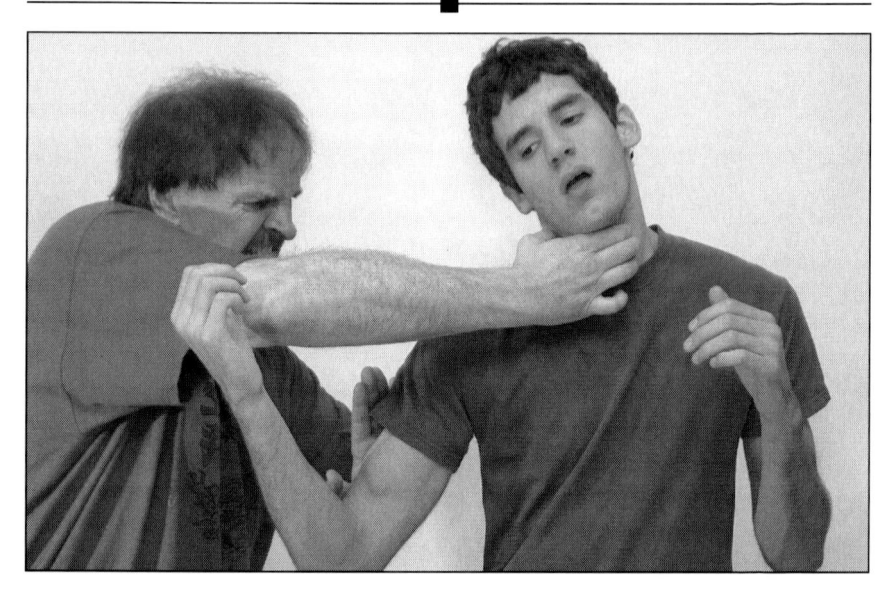

Figure 217

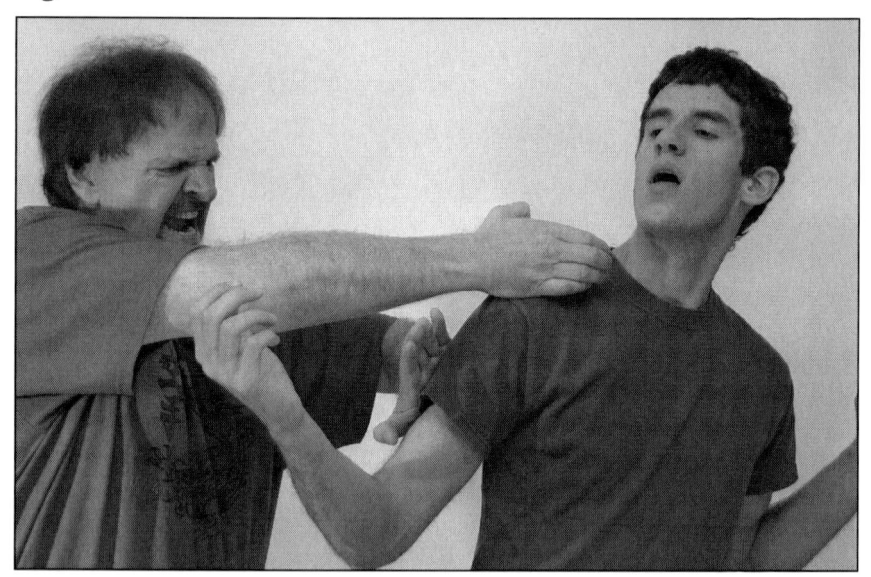

Figure 218

- Keep pressing his upper arm to turn him slightly and then ram your four fingers in the far side of his throat. (Fig. 217)
- Push his arm so his body turns away as you simultaneously pull his throat in a ripping motion toward you. (Fig. 218)

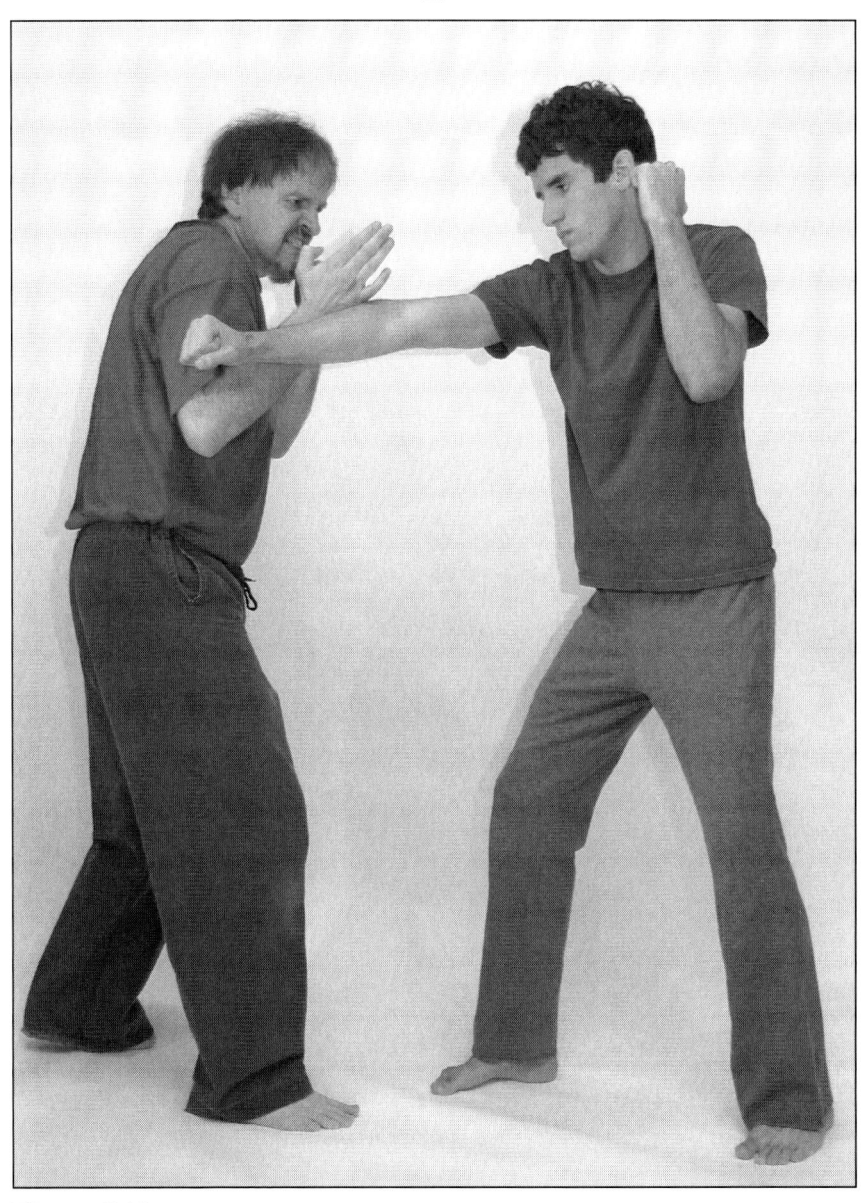

Figure 219

Against a straight thrust attack:

- Backhand block his thrust. (Fig. 219)

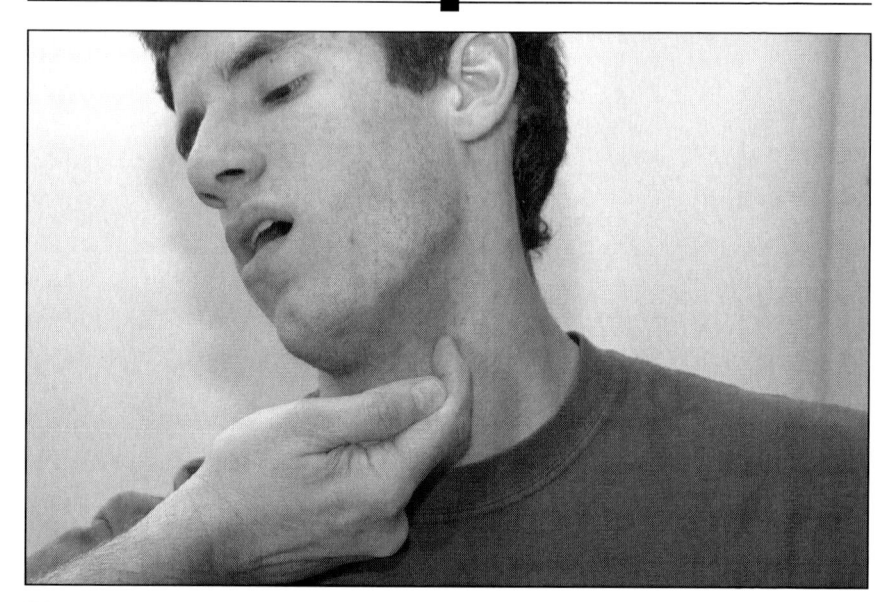

Figure 220

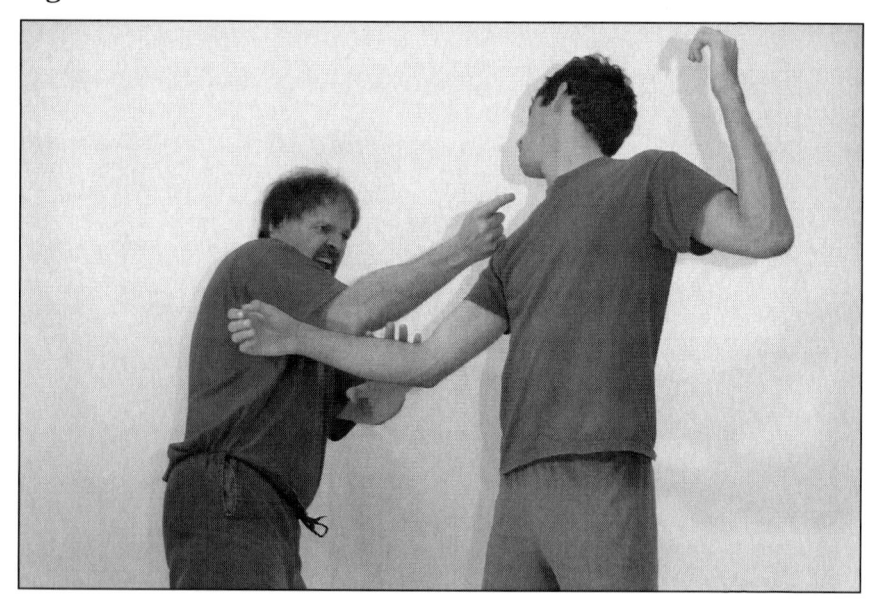

Figure 221

- Shoot your mantis finger against the far side of his throat. (Fig. 220)
- Rip it toward you as you drop to the side. (Fig. 221)

Neck Press with Fist

There are three possibilities with this press, depending on how your attacker is lying and where you push on his neck.

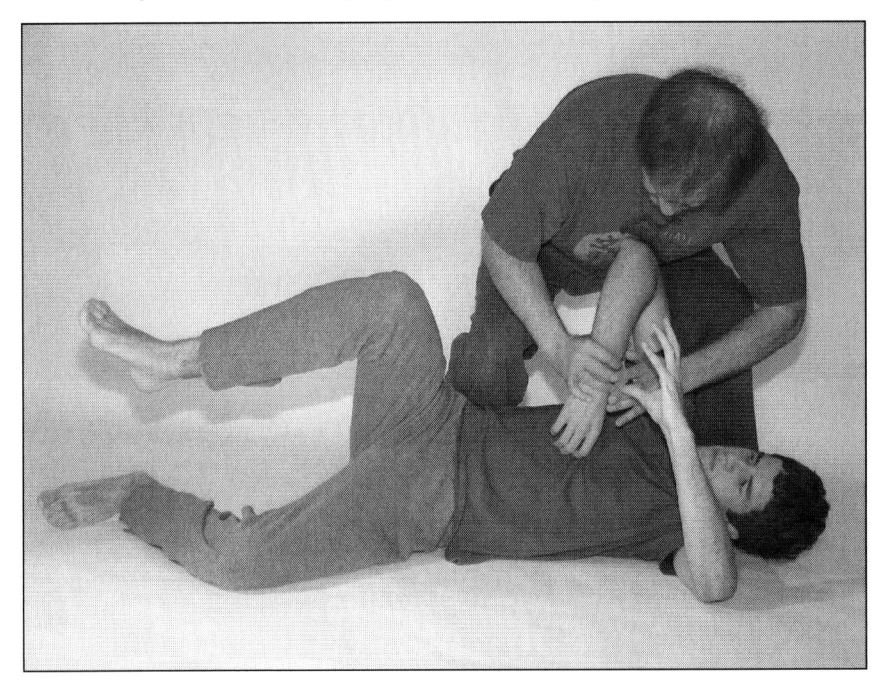

Figure 222

- You've taken your attacker down but, as you try to apply an armlock, he thrashes about so that you are about to lose your hold. (Fig. 222)
- Place your fist into his neck. If he is lying face up, press into the front of his throat (Fig. 223). If he is on his side, press your fist into his carotid artery below his ear. If his head is braced by the floor and your press is directly into his artery, he will likely lose consciousness. (Fig. 224) (See the warning on p. 150.)

  You can also position your hand so that it presses into his carotid artery while at the same time it presses into the nerve below his jaw hinge. (Fig. 225) (Again, see the warning.)

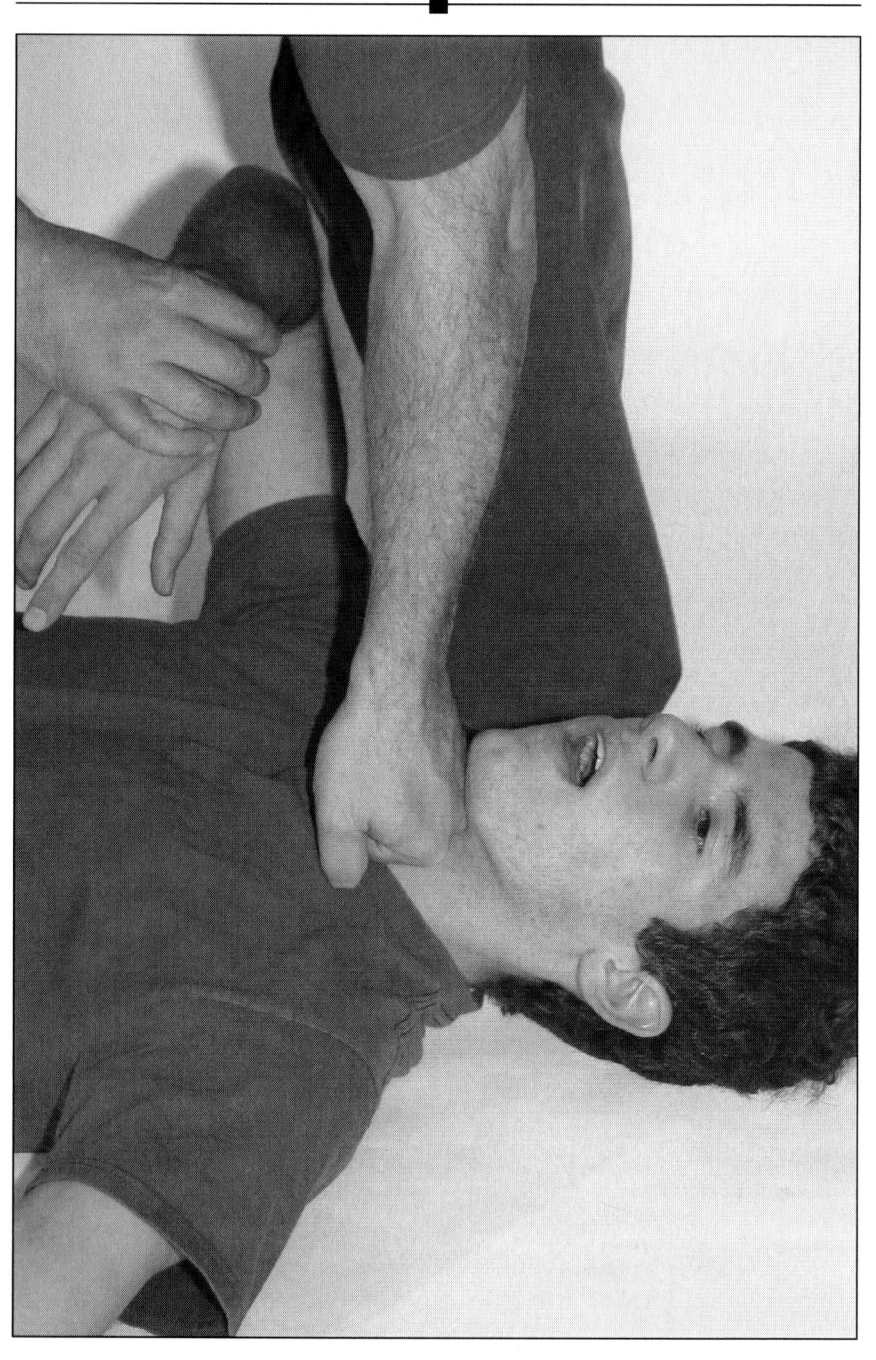

Figure 223

Head

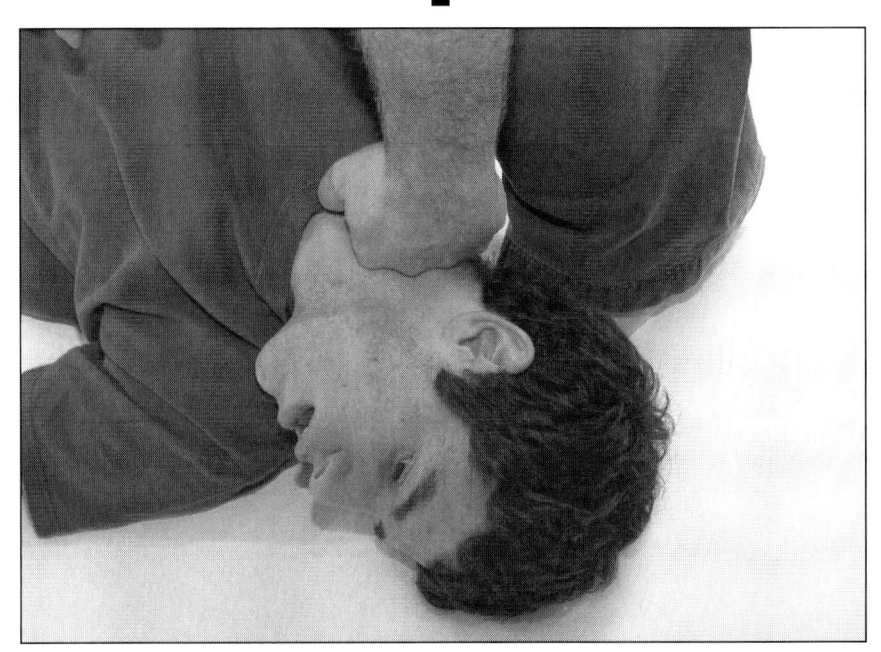

Figure 224

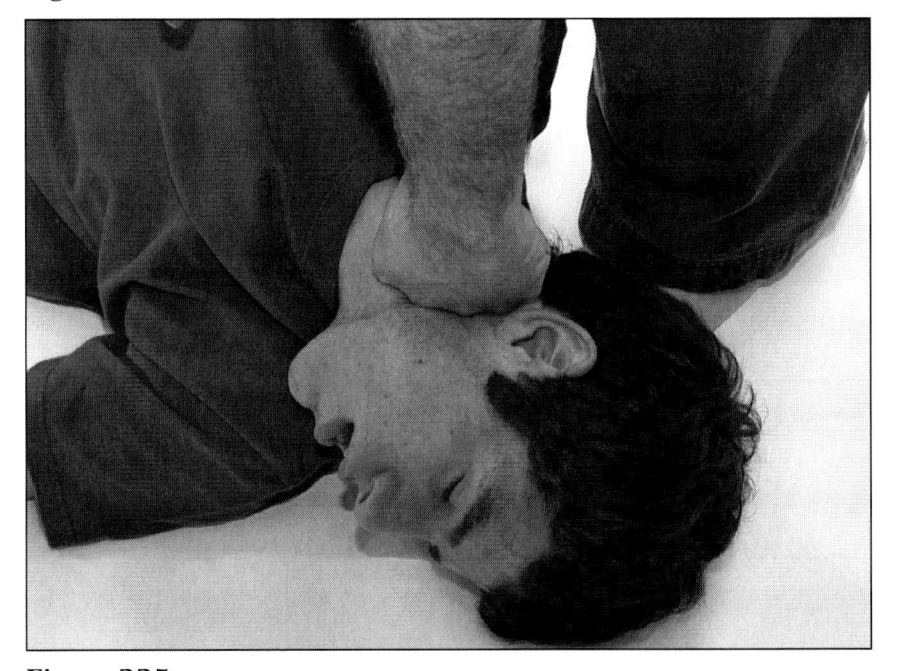

Figure 225

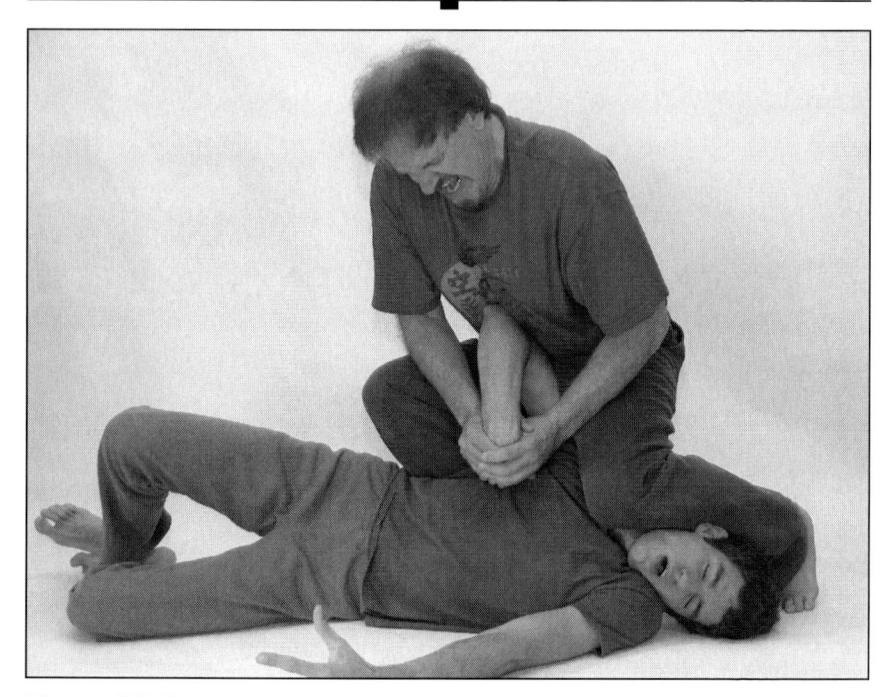

Figure 226

- The neck pain or loss of consciousness will distract him from squirming and kicking, and thus provide you with a couple of seconds to apply a better hold or to roll him over onto his stomach. (Fig. 226)

Throat Press with Fist and Chest

This one makes it hard for onlookers to see what you're doing, though they wonder why your attacker is flopping about like a beached fish.

Your attacker shoves you.

- Block it. (Fig. 227)
- Grab his shoulders and jerk him toward the ground face first, your elbows pointing downward. Be careful that you don't bang heads. (Fig. 228)
- Splay your legs out behind you as you go down. (Fig. 229)
- Quickly slip your hands under his throat. Place one hand palm down on the floor and your other fisted hand on top of it. (Fig. 230)

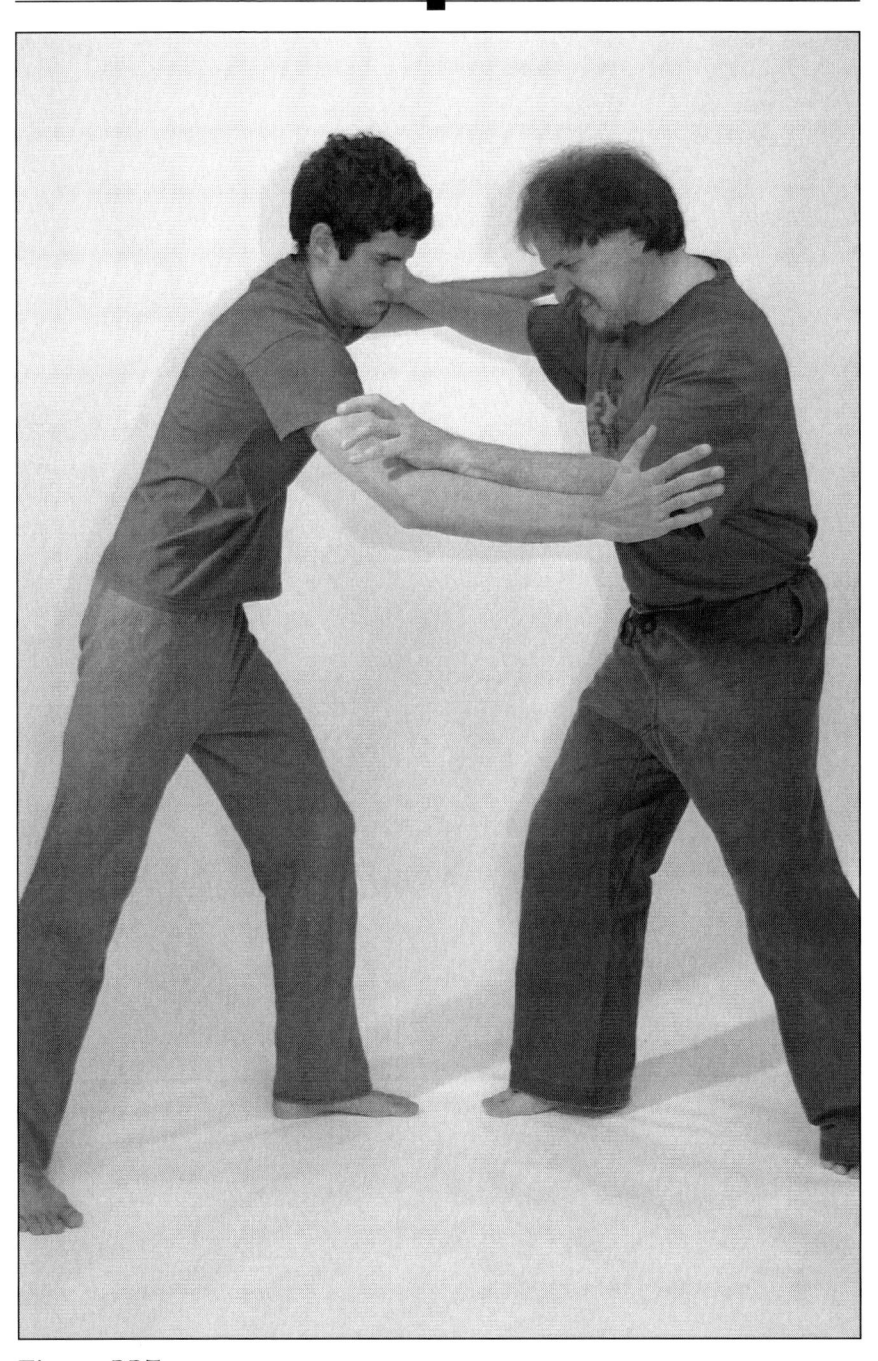

Figure 227

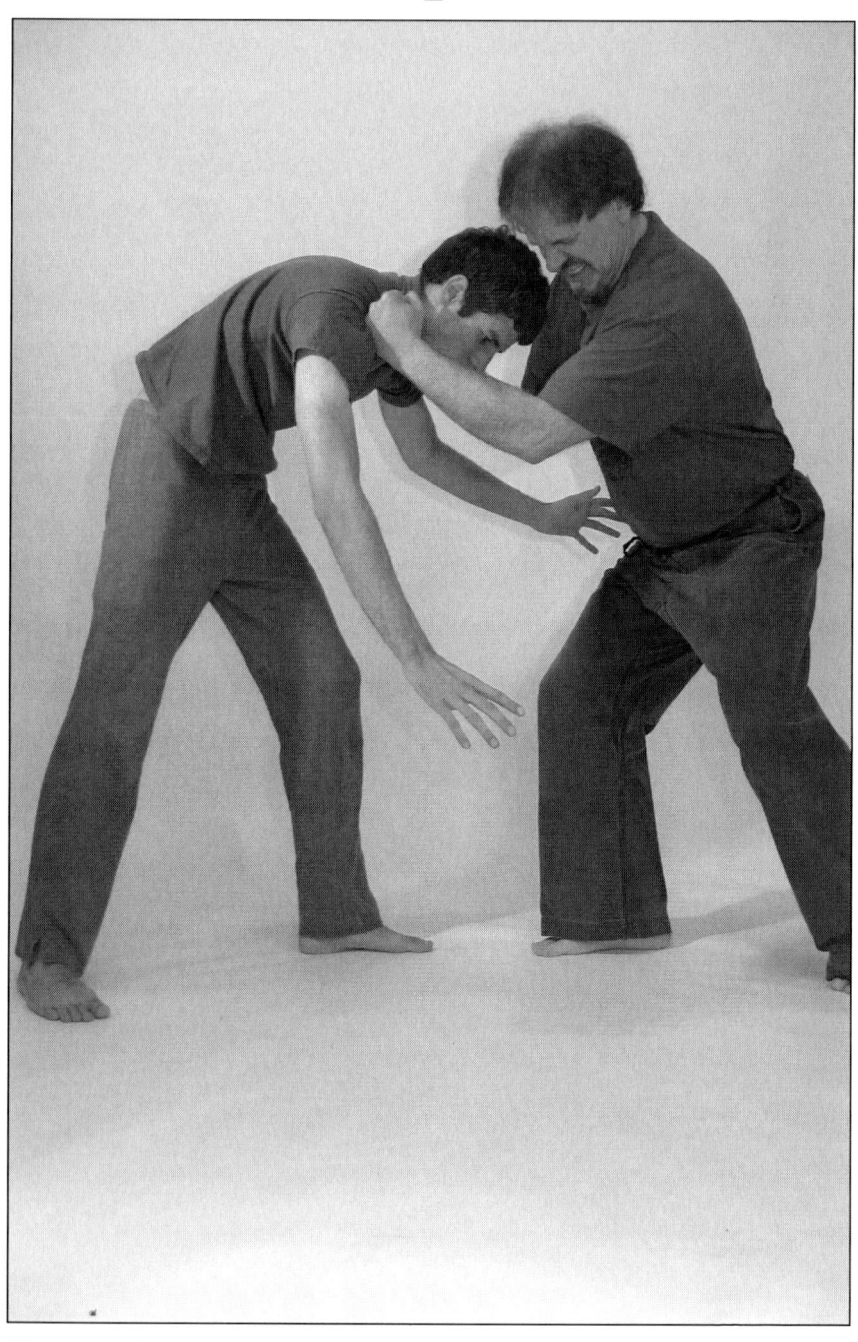

Figure 228

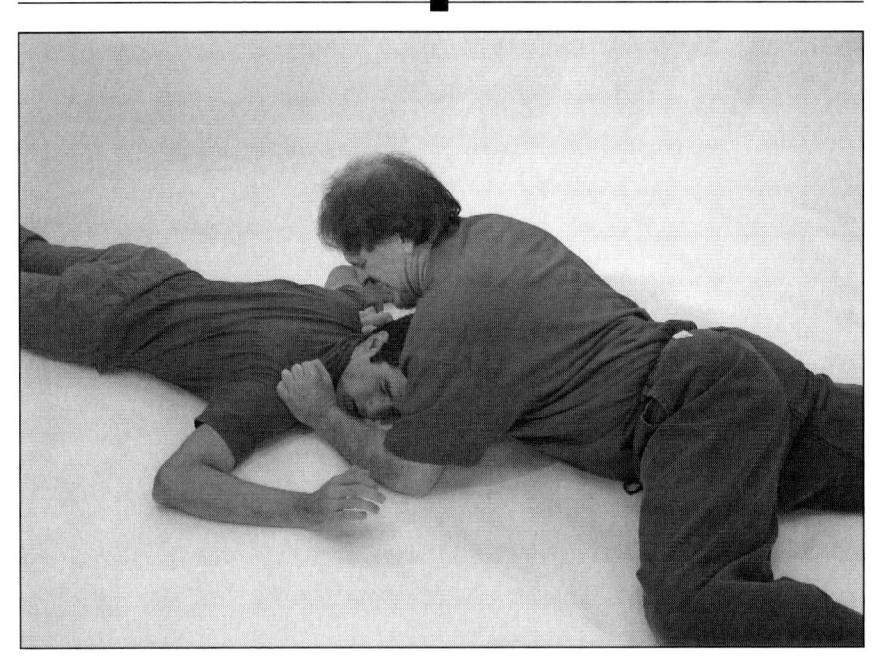

Figure 229

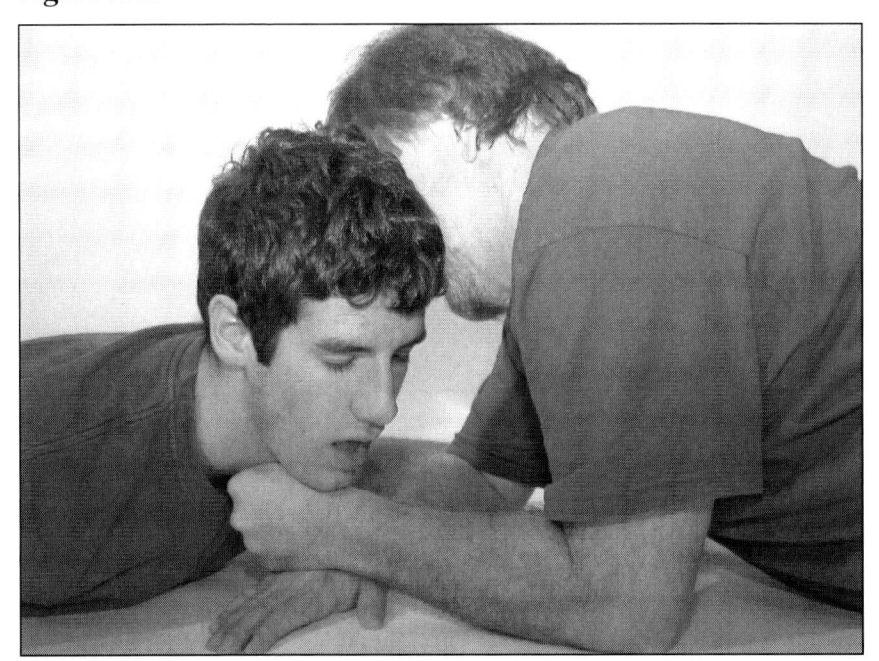

Figure 230

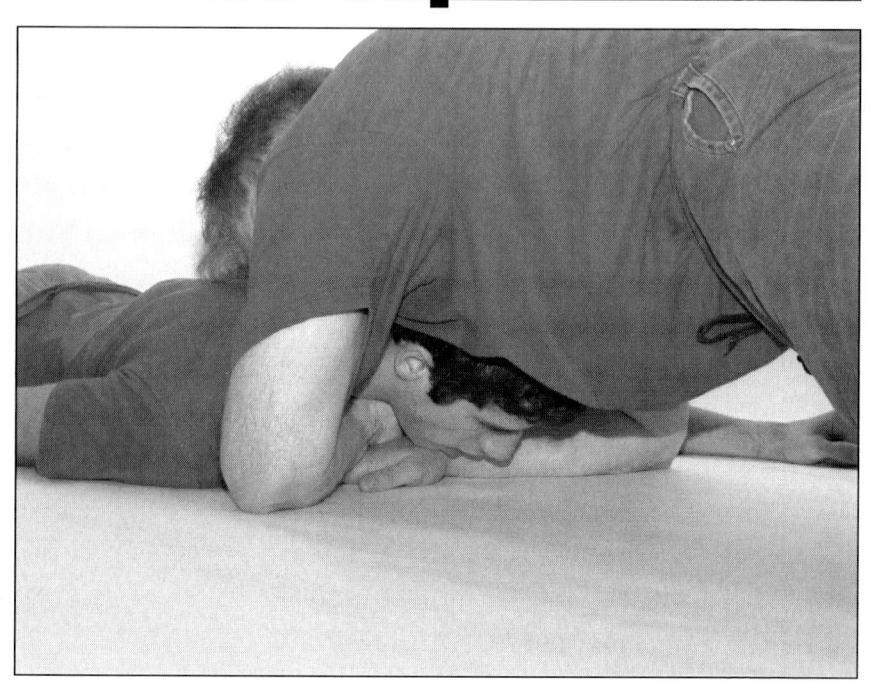

Figure 231

- Scoot yourself forward so that your chest and upper body weight presses down on the back of his head, forcing his throat down onto your fist. I'm holding my body off the floor so you can see the technique, but in actuality you want to lie on the floor to place as much weight as you can on top of his head. If you maintain this hold for a few seconds you might cause injury or unconsciousness. (Fig. 231)

Warning: Should he lose consciousness from pressure on the carotid artery, immediately release the hold and apply a restraint hold of some kind. Continuing to restrict blood to the brain can cause brain damage and even death.

HEAD OR FACE

Let's finish this section with a few techniques that impact the head and face in general.

Face Rip

Here are three ways to execute a face rip using the five-fingered claw.

Your attacker launches a haymaker punch.

- Block the punch. (Fig. 232)

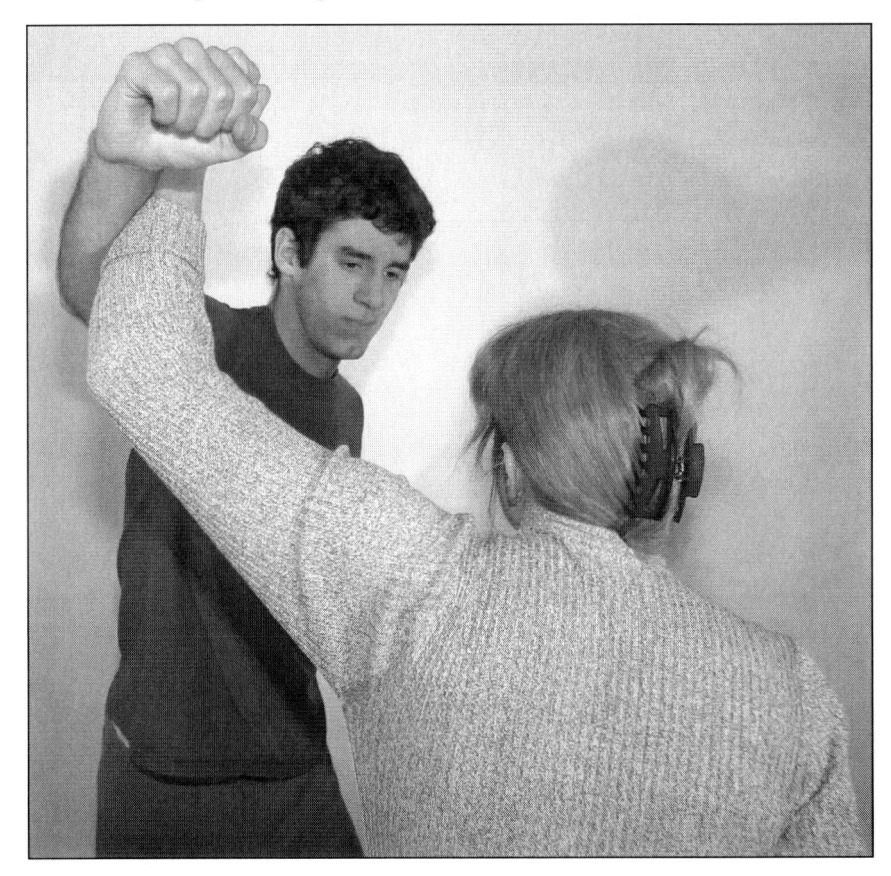

Figure 232

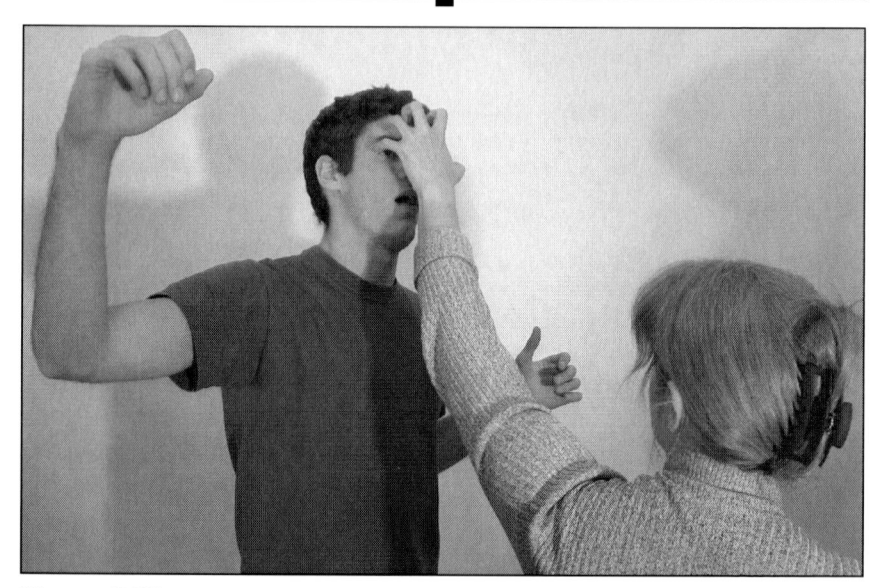

Figure 233

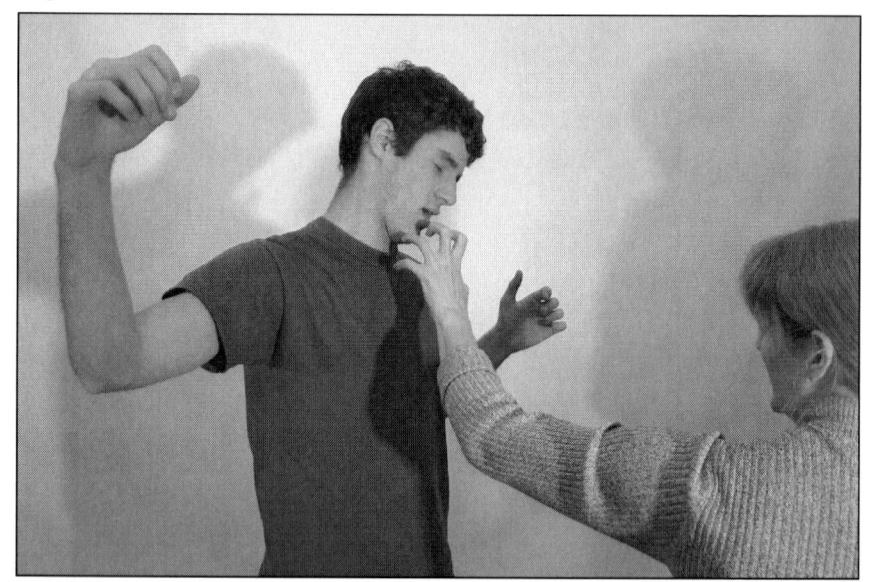

Figure 234

- Use the blocking arm to whip your claw hand straight down his face, from his forehead . . . (Fig. 232)
- . . . to his chin. (Fig. 234)

Head

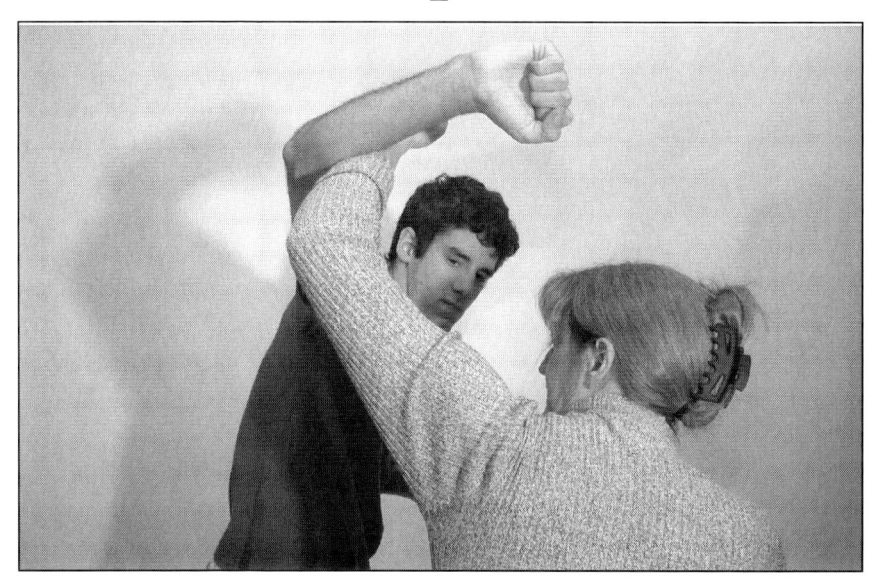

Figure 235

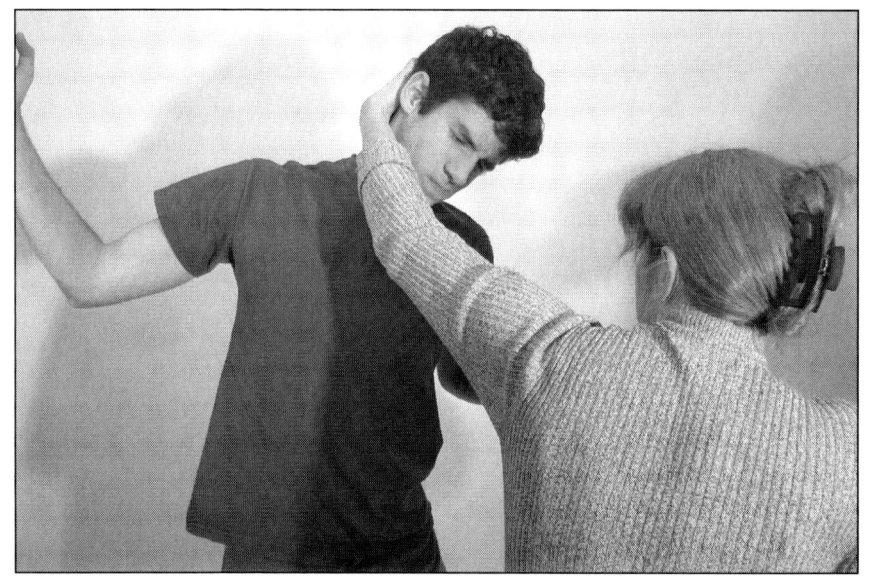

Figure 236

Your attacker launches a haymaker.

- Block. (Fig. 235)
- Step in and use the same hand to brace the back of his head. (Fig. 236)

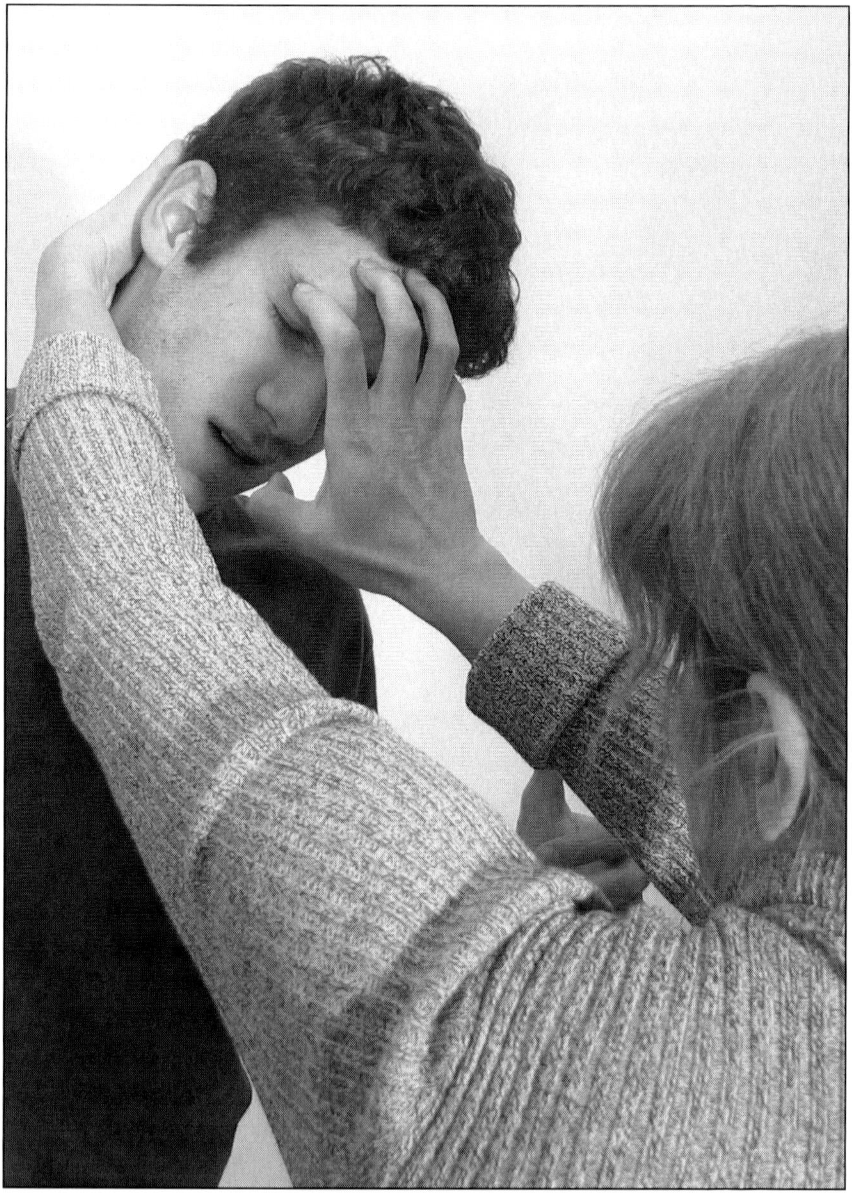

Figure 237

- Rip down his face with your other hand using a five-fingered claw. (Fig. 237)

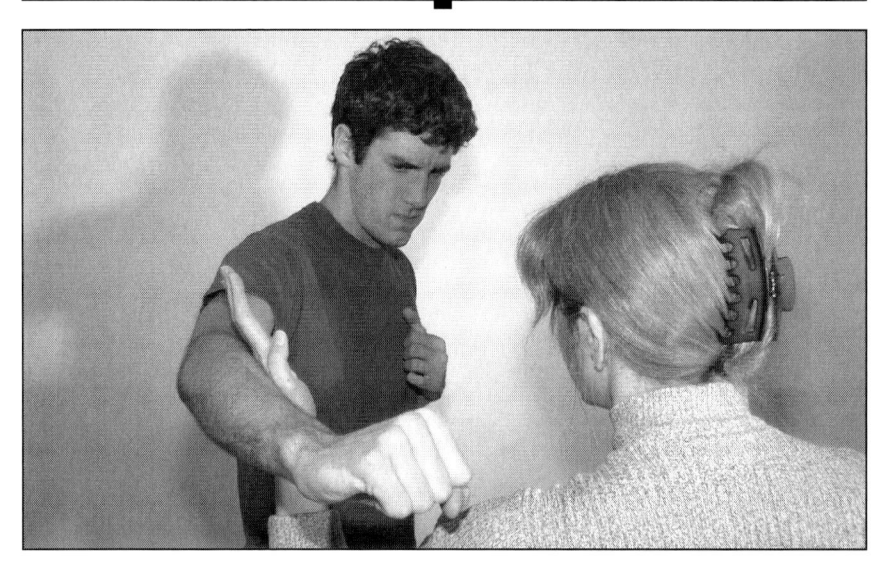

Figure 238

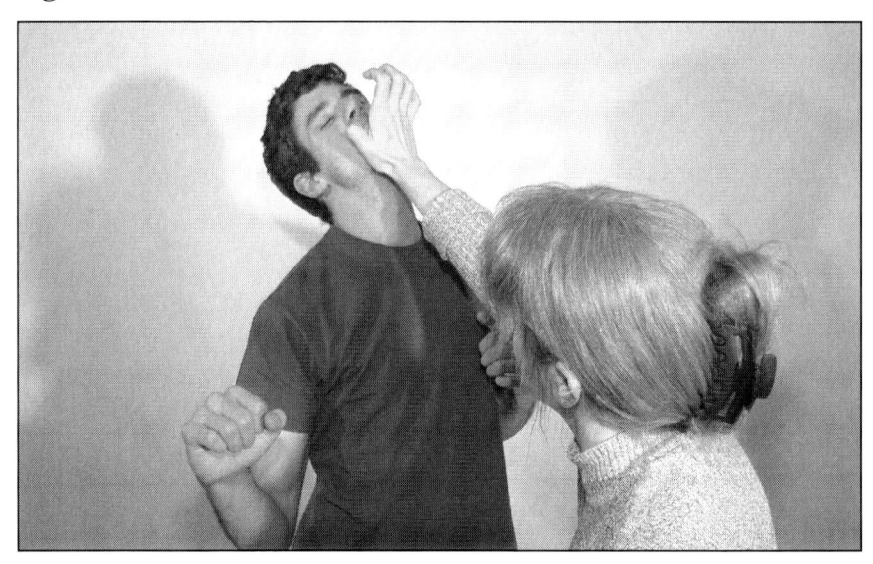

Figure 239

Your attacker throws a straight cross at your face.

- Backhand block. (Fig. 238)
- Slam your other hand into his chin with a palm-heel to push his face upward. (Fig. 239)

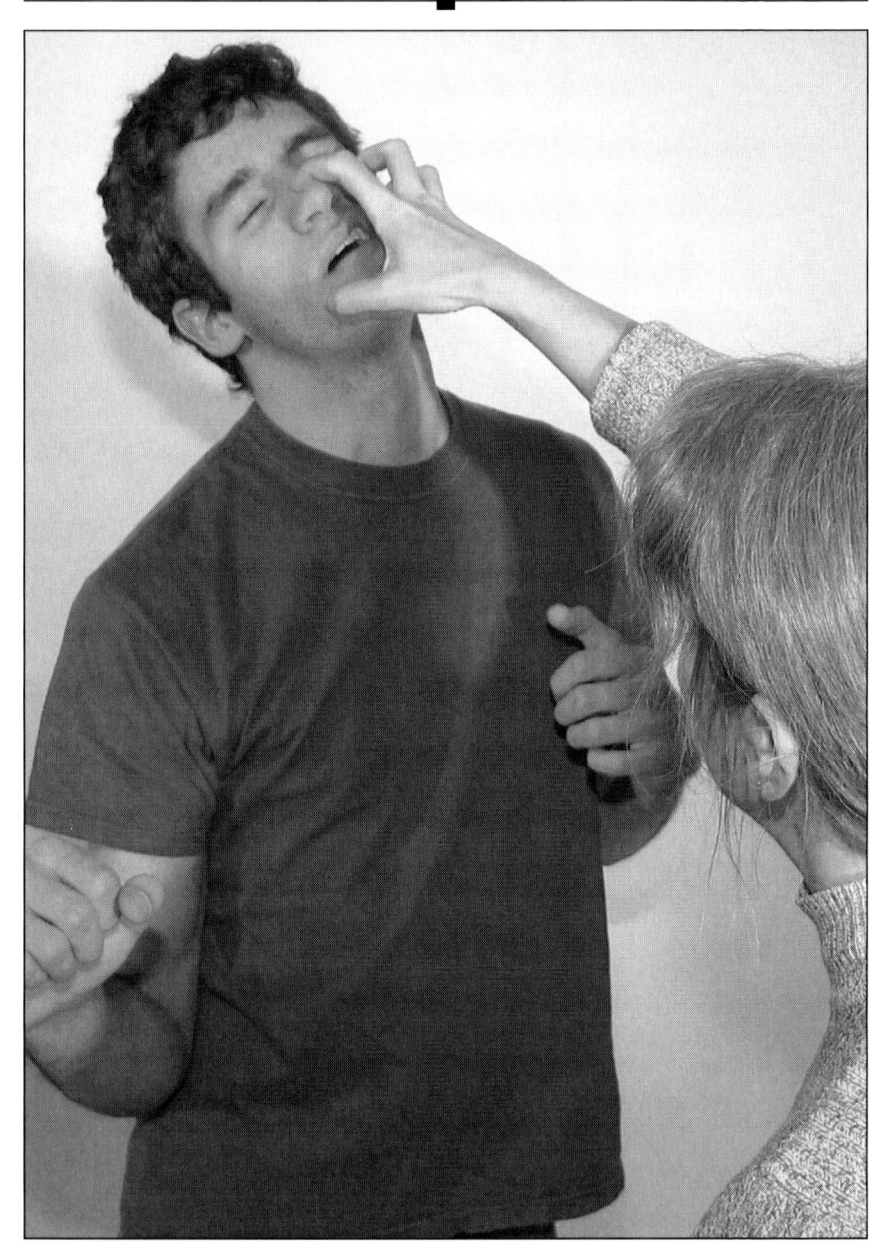

Figure 240

- Rip down his face with the same hand. (Fig. 240)

Head

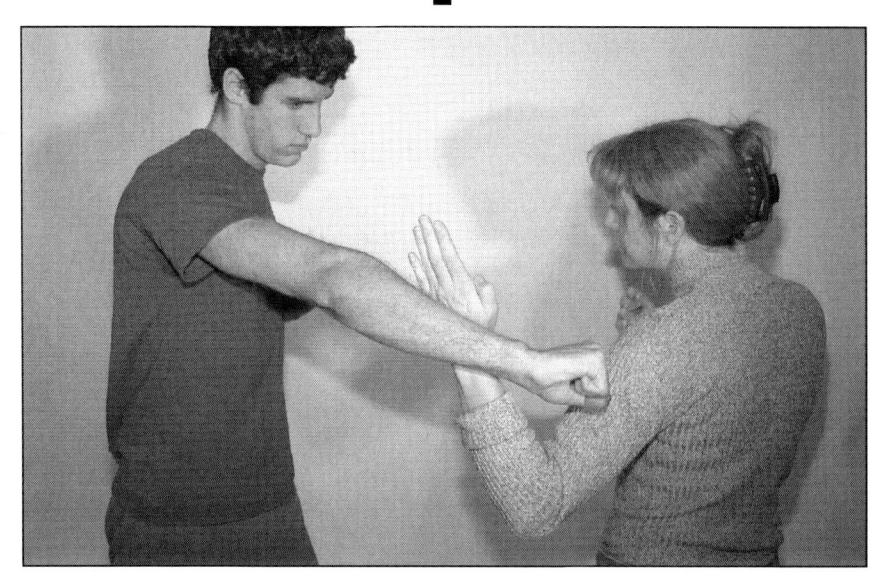

Figure 241

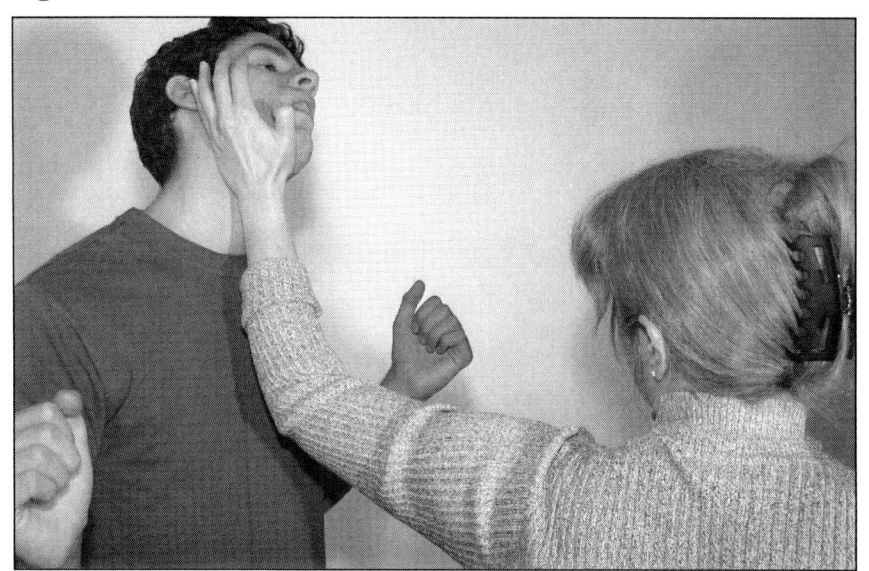

Figure 242

Your attacker throws a right cross.

- Block. (Fig. 241)
- Palm his chin. (Fig. 242)

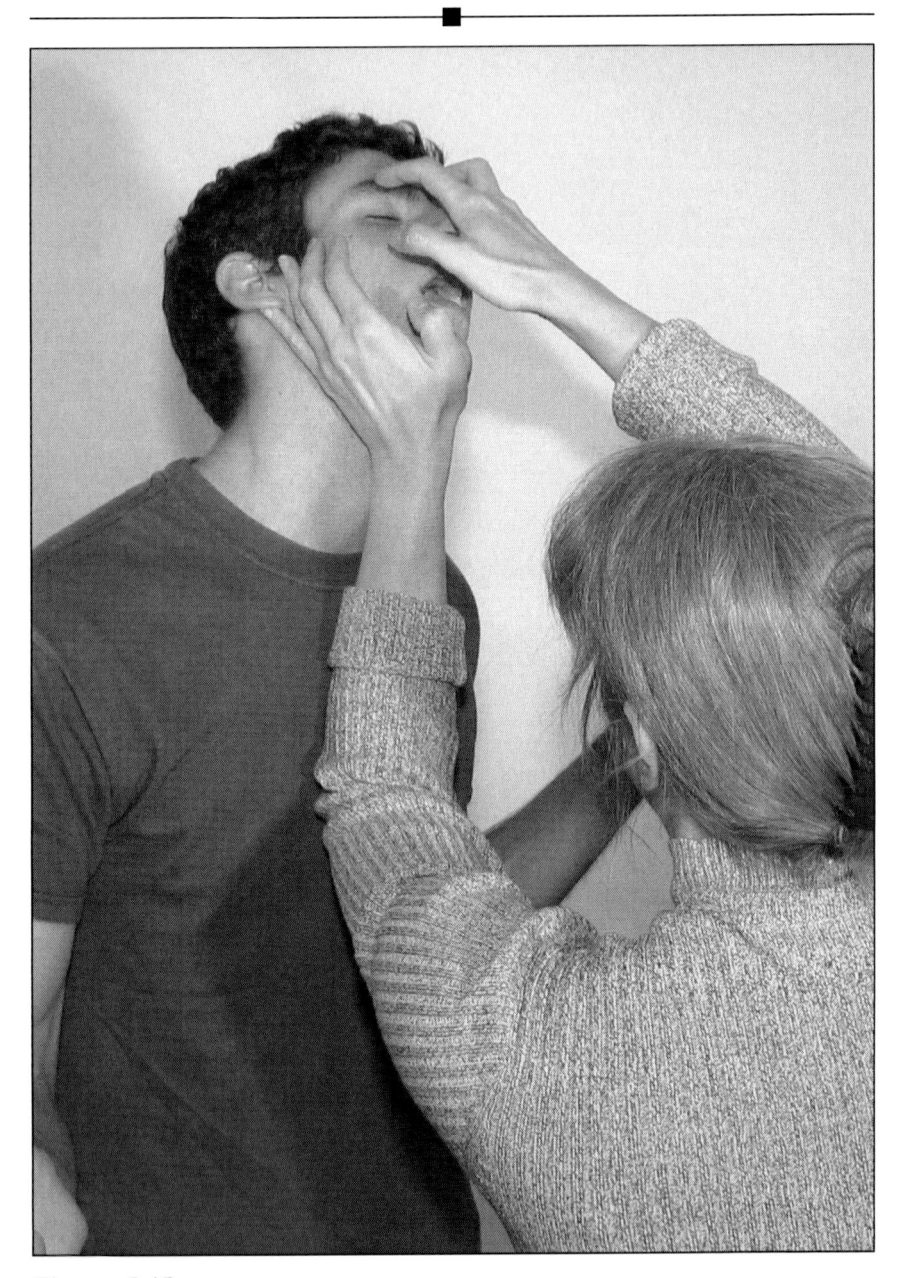

Figure 243

- Leave your palm in place to act as a brace as you rip across his face with your other hand. (Fig. 243)

3
Arms and Shoulders

"Slowly pull out your empty left hand. Do it slowly. If there is a weapon in your hand I will take out your eye. Any part of that you don't understand?"

The arms and shoulders aren't as target-rich as the head, but there are several vulnerable places that can be attacked with a variety of weapons. Few of these will end the fight, but they are good weapons to distract, break your attacker's focus, startle, and move him in a given direction.

Standing Inside Upper Arm Rip

This technique delivers surprise and shearing pain.

- An attacker grabs the front of your shirt and starts to utter a threat. (Fig. 244)
- Before he can get it out, reach across and pinch/grab the skin on the inside of his arm with a four-fingers-to-palm grip. Keep your elbow high to keep from getting struck with his other hand. (Fig. 245)
- Twist the flesh toward you as if turning a faucet handle. (Fig. 246)
- Pull his arm to the inside a little as you simultaneously step to the outside. (Fig. 247)
- Counter with a palm to his ear. (Fig. 248)

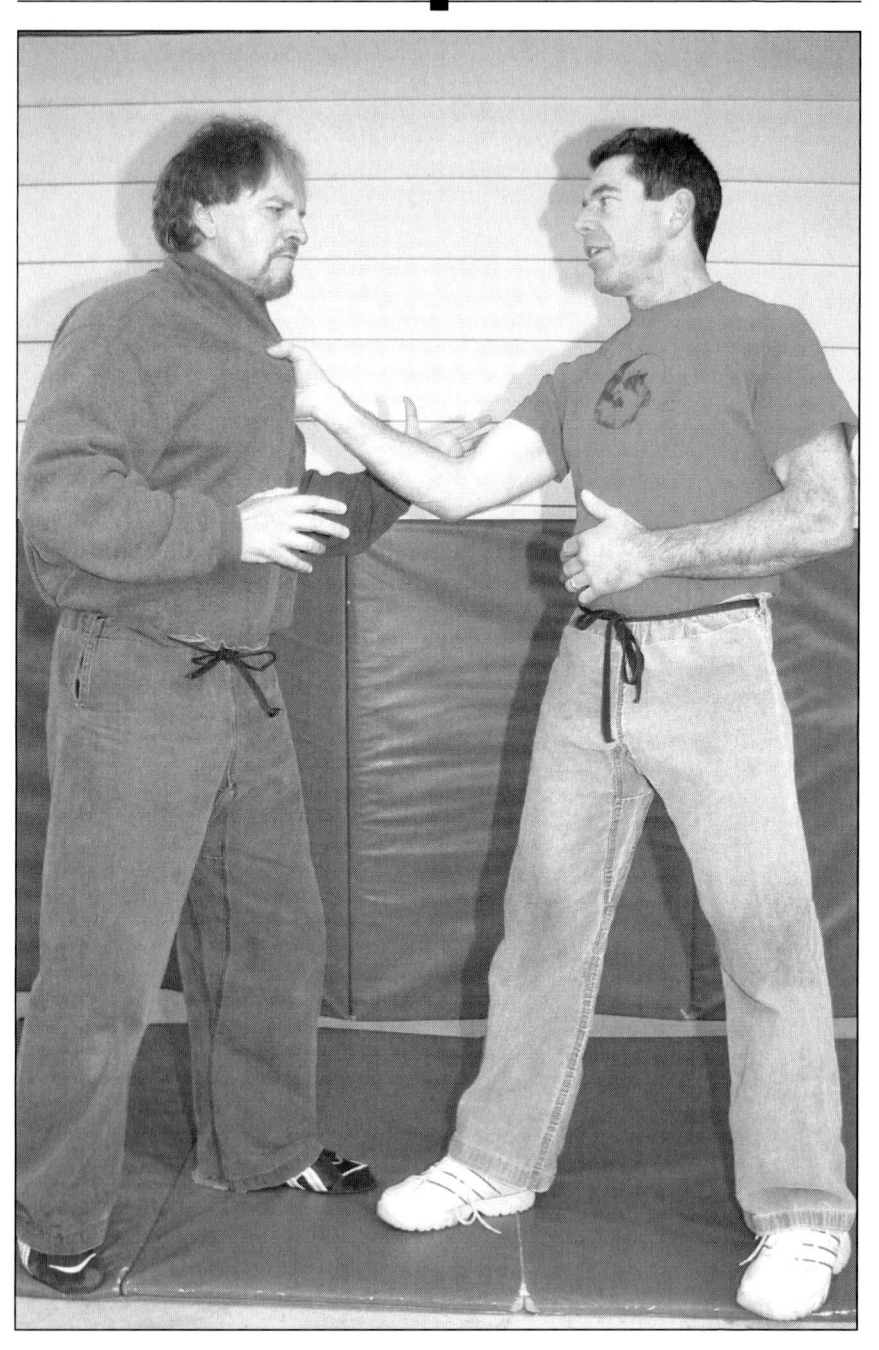

Figure 244

Arms and Shoulders 161

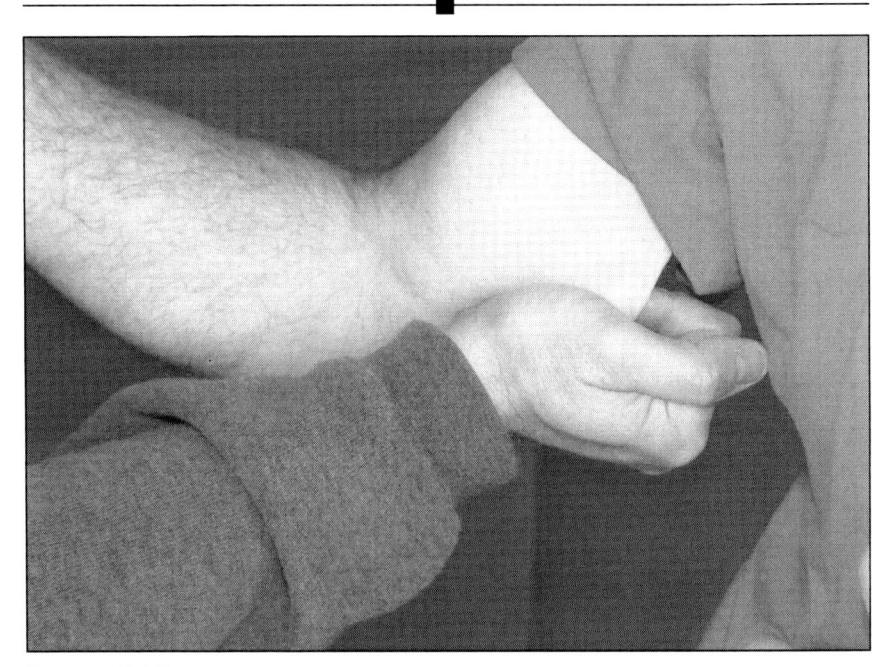

Figure 245

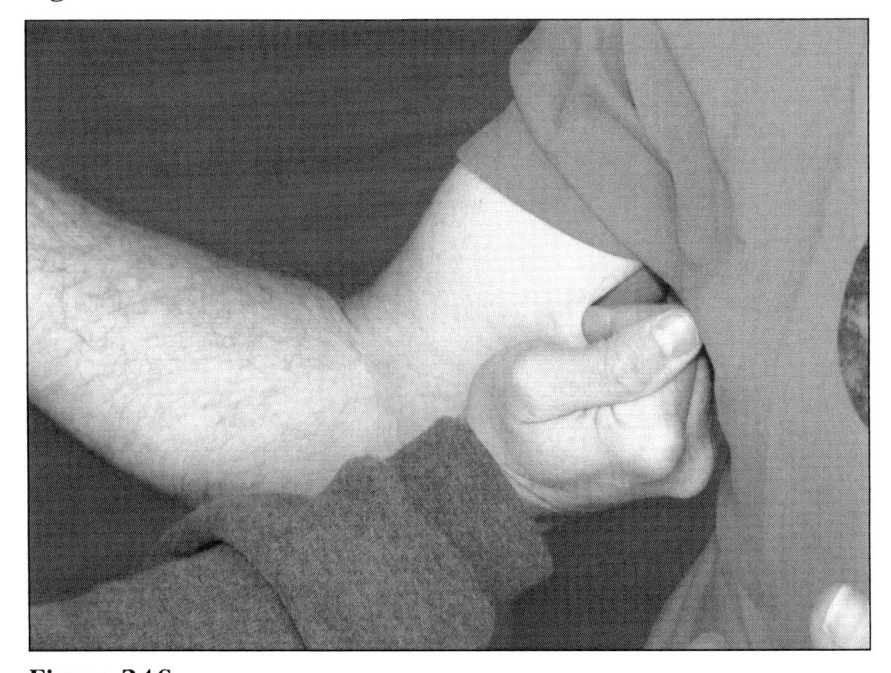

Figure 246

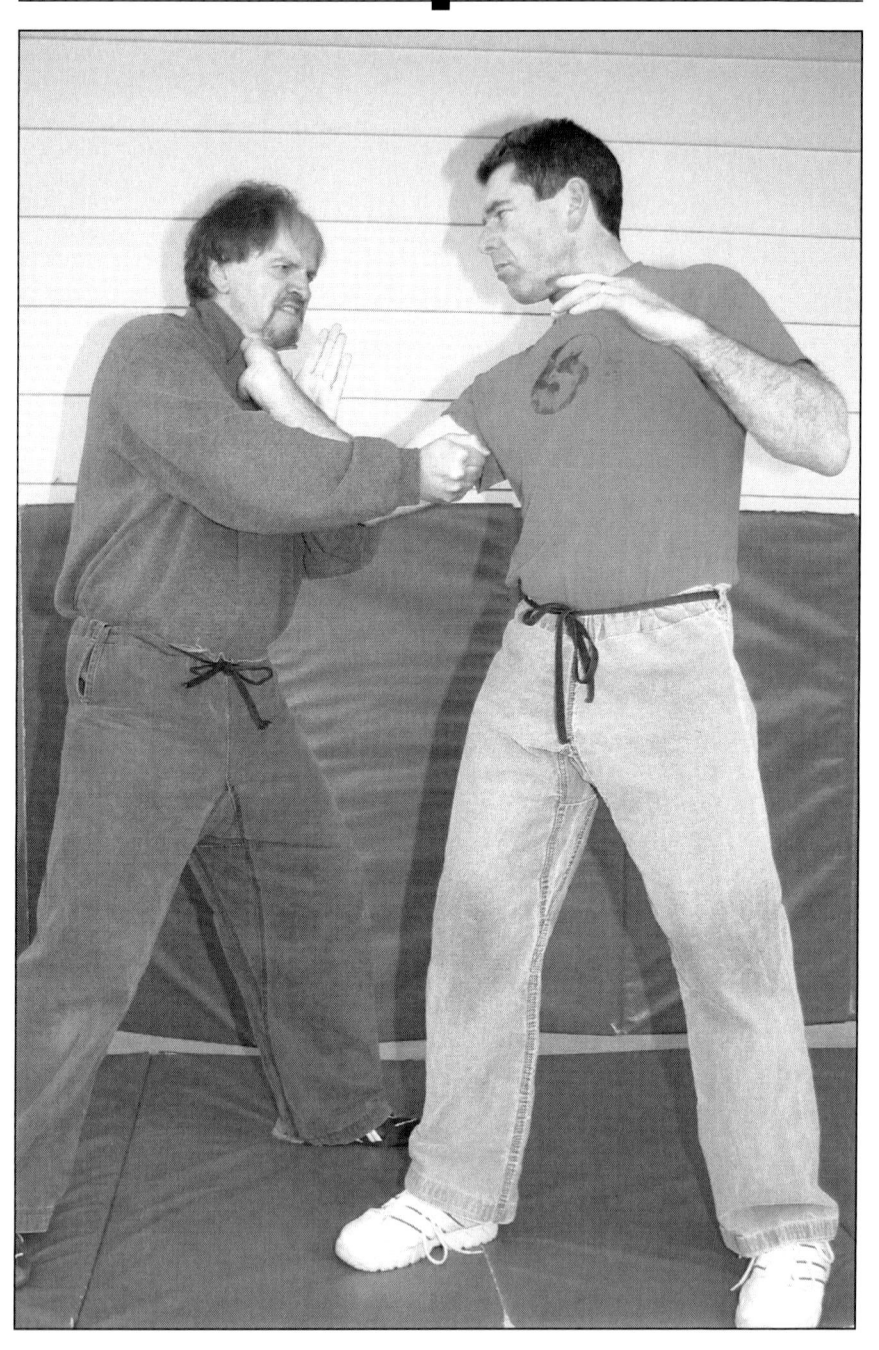

Figure 247

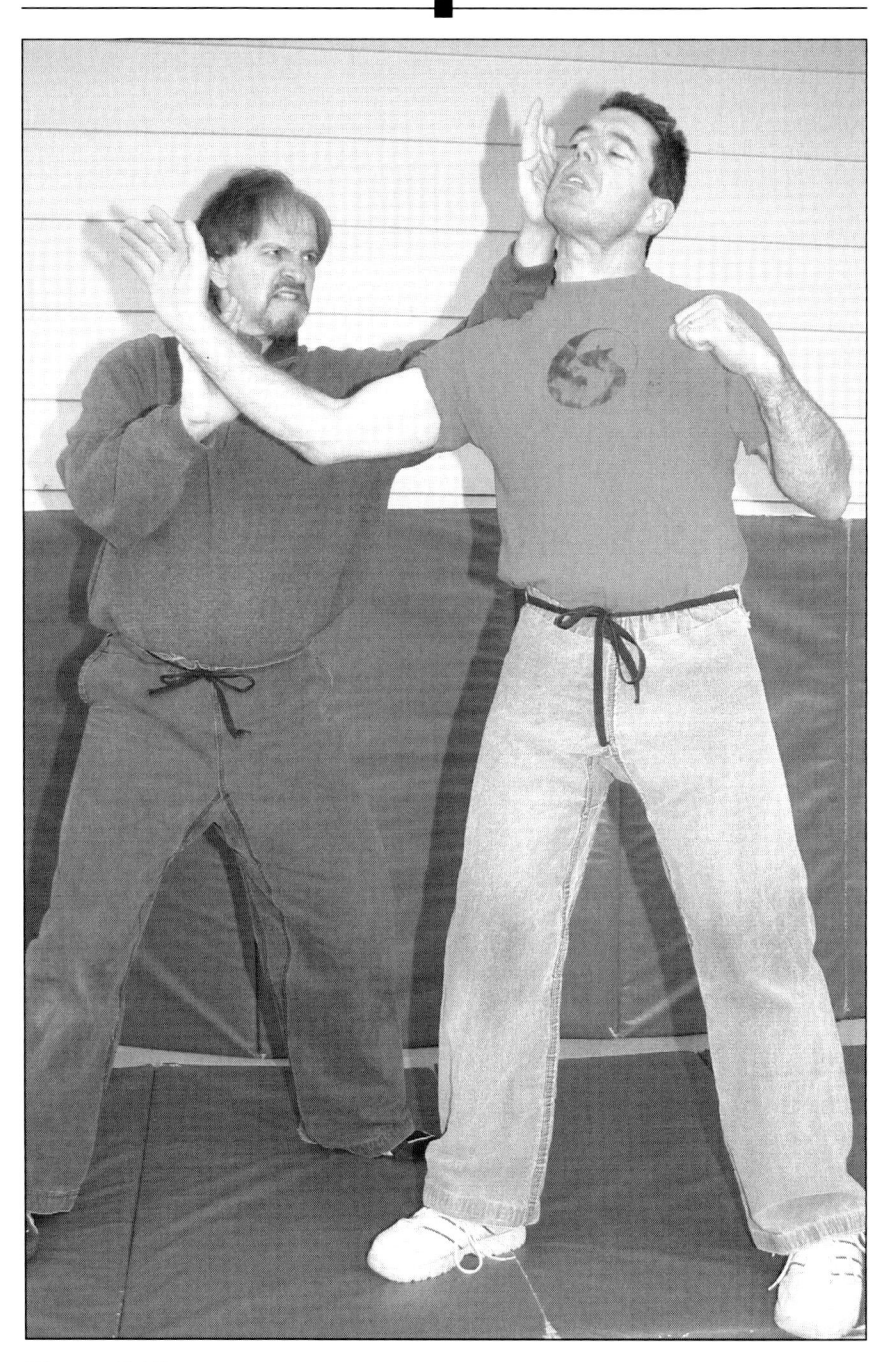

Figure 248

On the Floor Inside Upper Arm Rip

Unlike in training, when you dump a real attacker on the ground, he will likely grab a part of your body or clothing. Here is one solution:

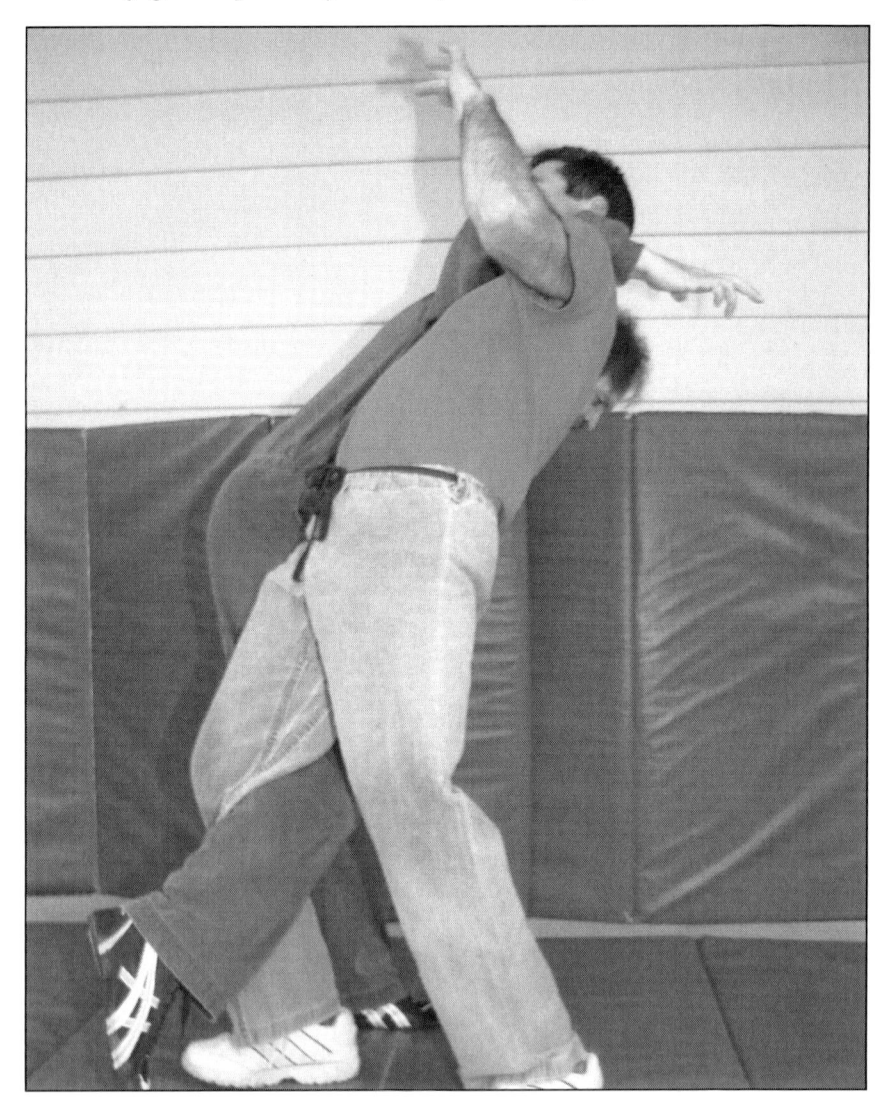

Figure 249

- Right after you execute a takedown on your attacker . . . (Fig. 249)

Arms and Shoulders

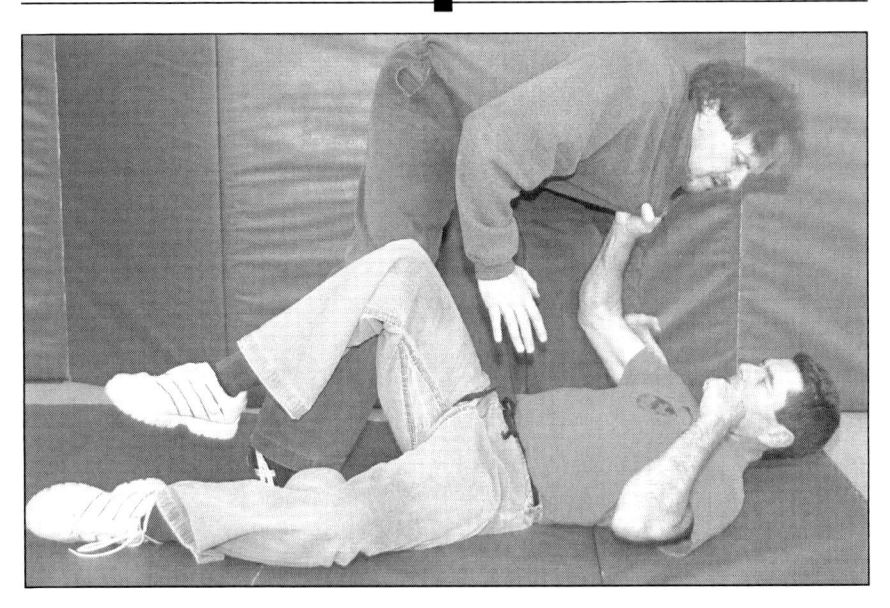

Figure 250

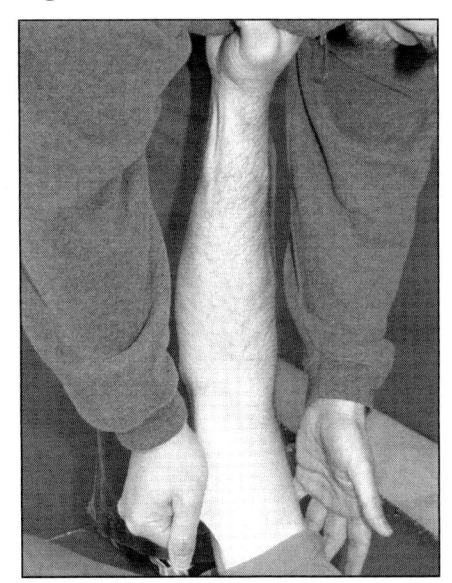

Figure 251

- . . . he grabs the front of your shirt as he lands. (Fig. 250)
- Instantly, grab the tender flesh on the inside of his arm, pinch with a four-fingers-to-palm grip . . . (Fig. 251)

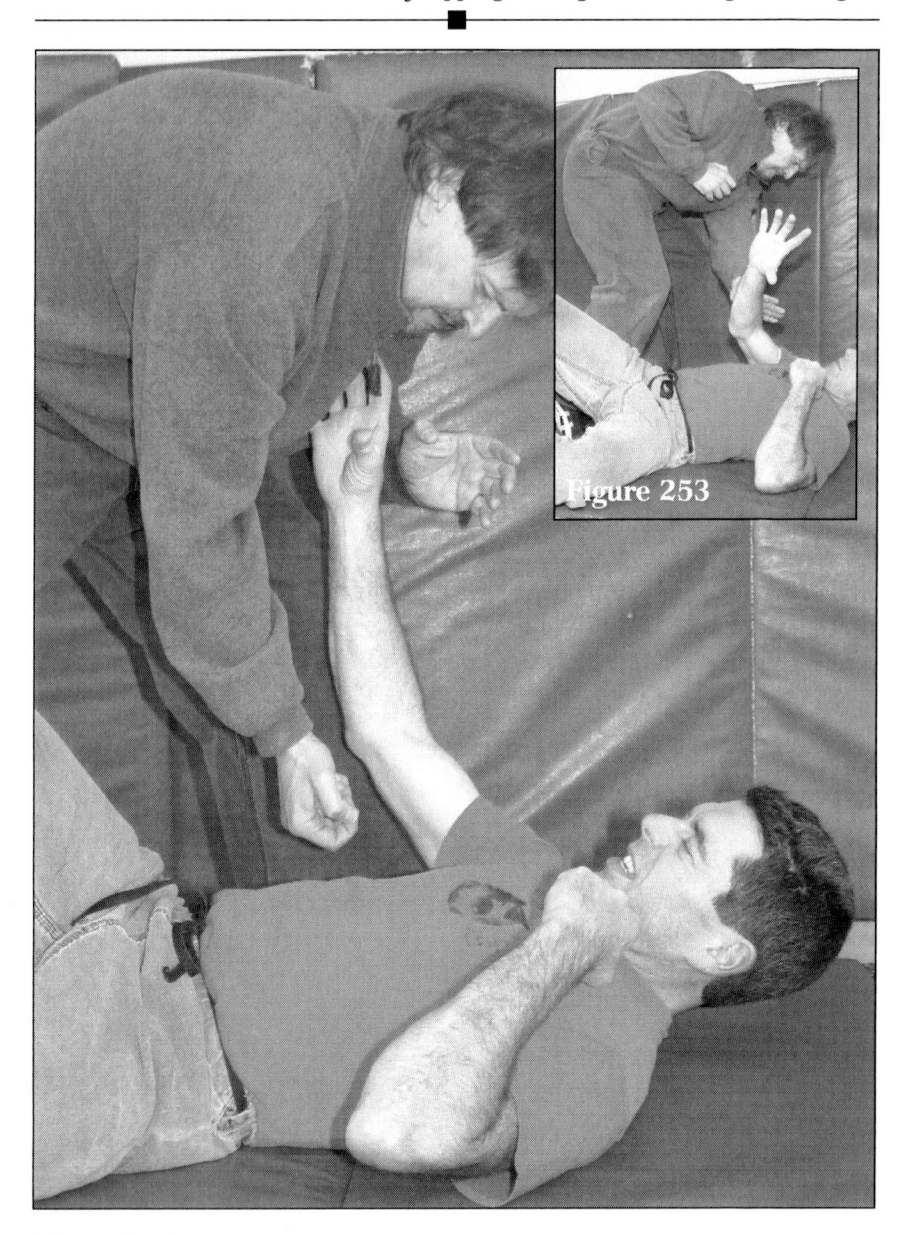

Figure 252

- . . . and rip by rotating your hand and yanking it away. (Fig. 252)
- As he releases his grip, use your other hand to knock his away so that you can either flee or apply a restraint hold. (Fig. 253)

Arms and Shoulders 167

Prone Triceps Squeeze

    This is a good technique that hurts and gives direction.
- You're taking the attacker down with an arm bar, but he lands on all fours instead of his belly. (Fig. 254)
- Keep hold of his wrist and use your other hand to pinch his upper triceps near his armpit with the four-fingers-to-palm squeeze. (Fig. 255)
- Twist with prejudice as you simultaneously press his arm into the floor. (Fig. 256)

Variation:

- You can also pinch and press just above the elbow joint at the ulnar leverage point. The skin here isn't as sensitive as it is near his armpit, but adding the press to the pinch usually flattens the arm. (Fig. 257)

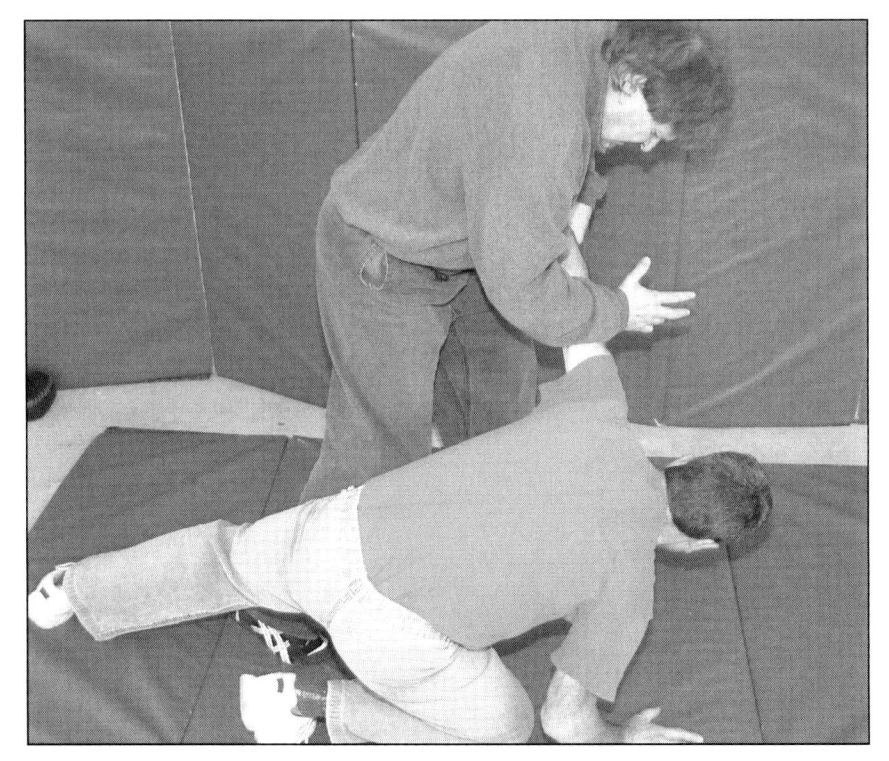

Figure 254

Figure 256

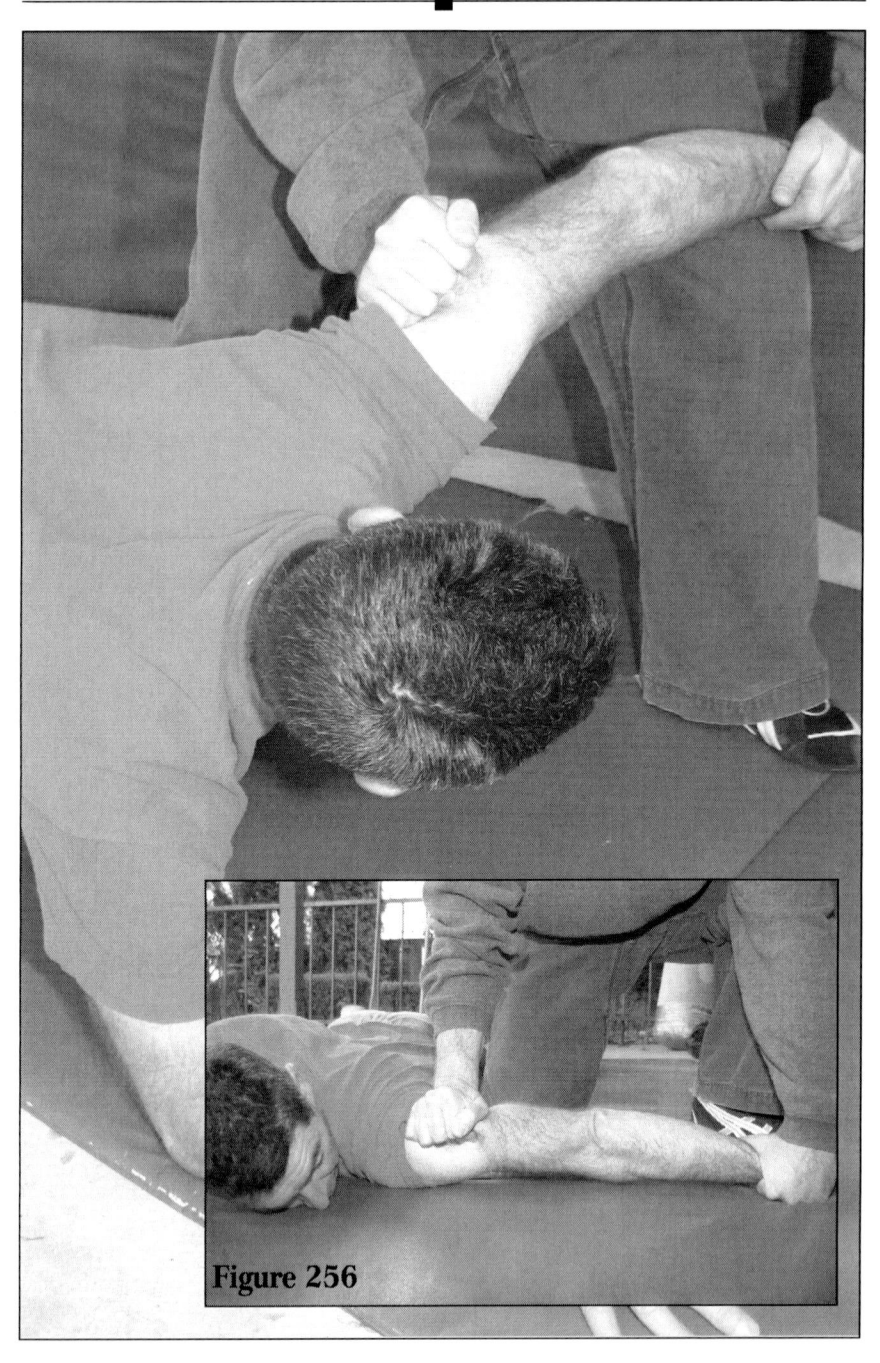

Figure 255

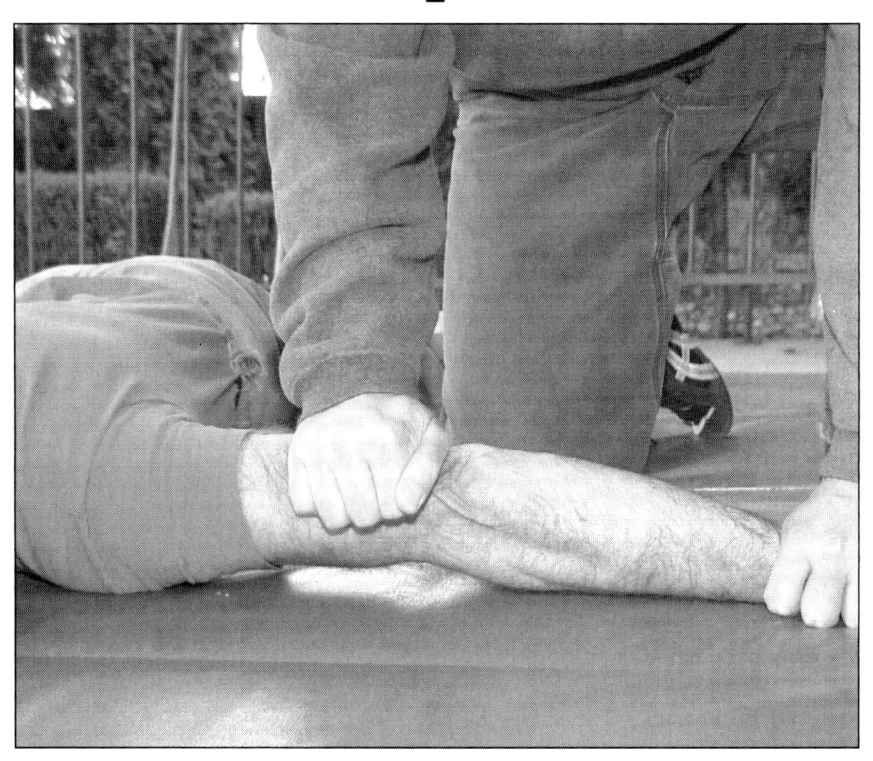

Figure 257

Chair Extract with Triceps Squeeze

This is a quick and effective way to get a person out of a chair and onto the floor. Pull his hair to assist.

- Your attacker balks at getting out of a chair. (Fig. 258)
- Approach from the side. Grab a handful of his hair close to the roots with one hand and pinch his triceps muscle with your other. (Fig. 259)
- Tuck the elbow of the hand that is pulling his hair and squeeze and pull his triceps to bend him forward. (Fig. 260)
- Force him to the floor (Fig. 261)
- Apply a control hold. (Fig. 262)

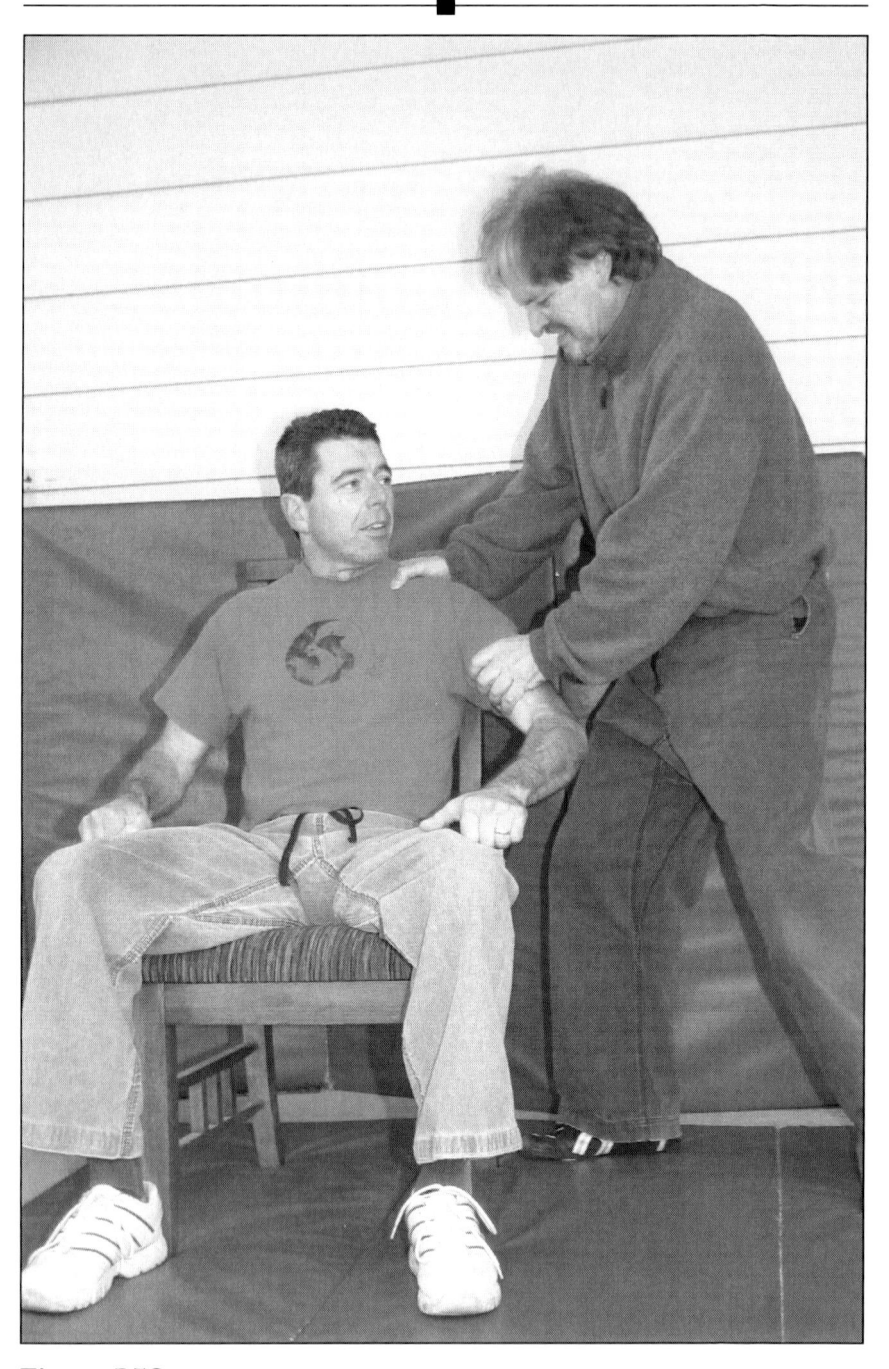

Figure 258

Arms and Shoulders

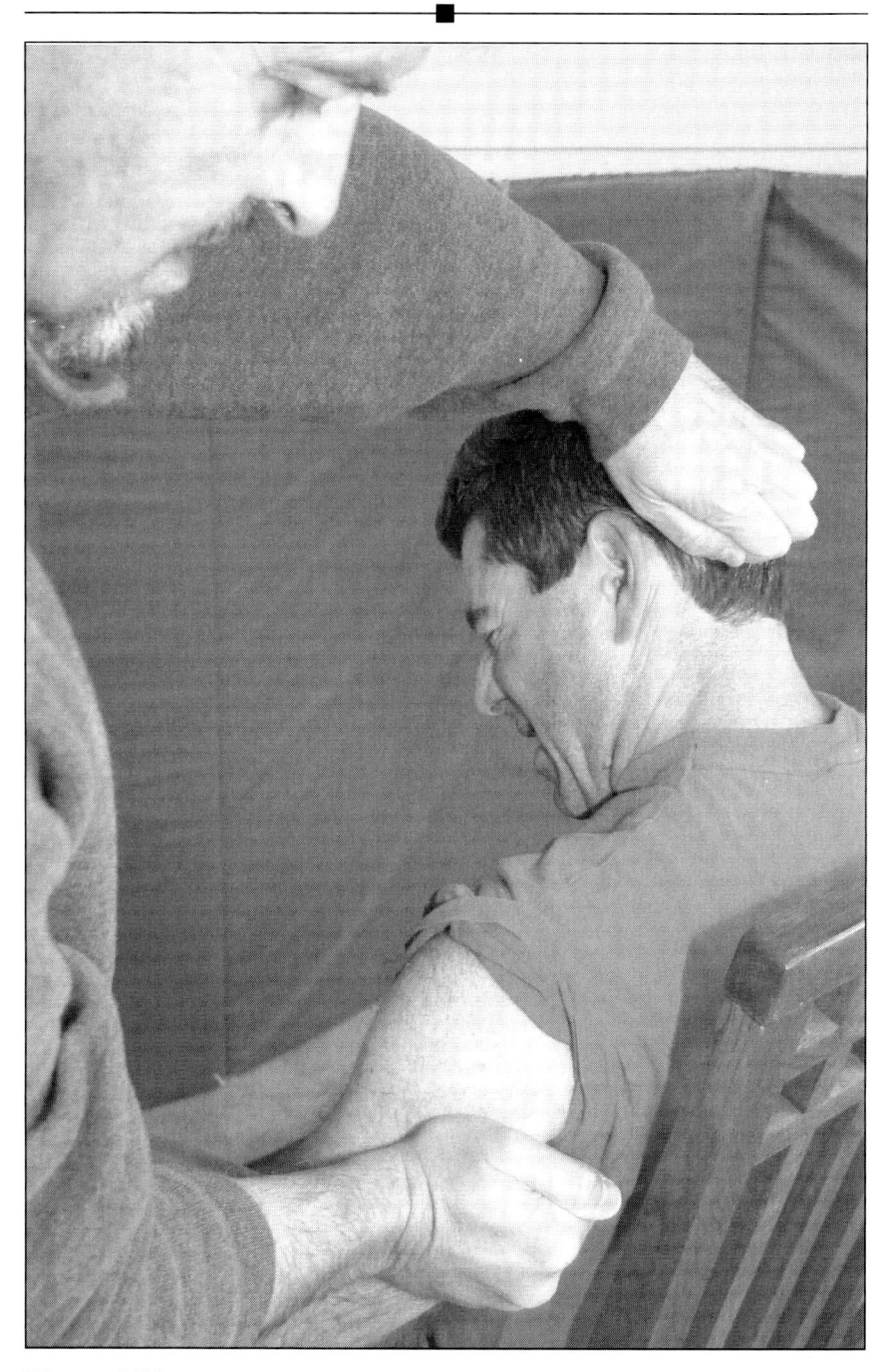

Figure 259

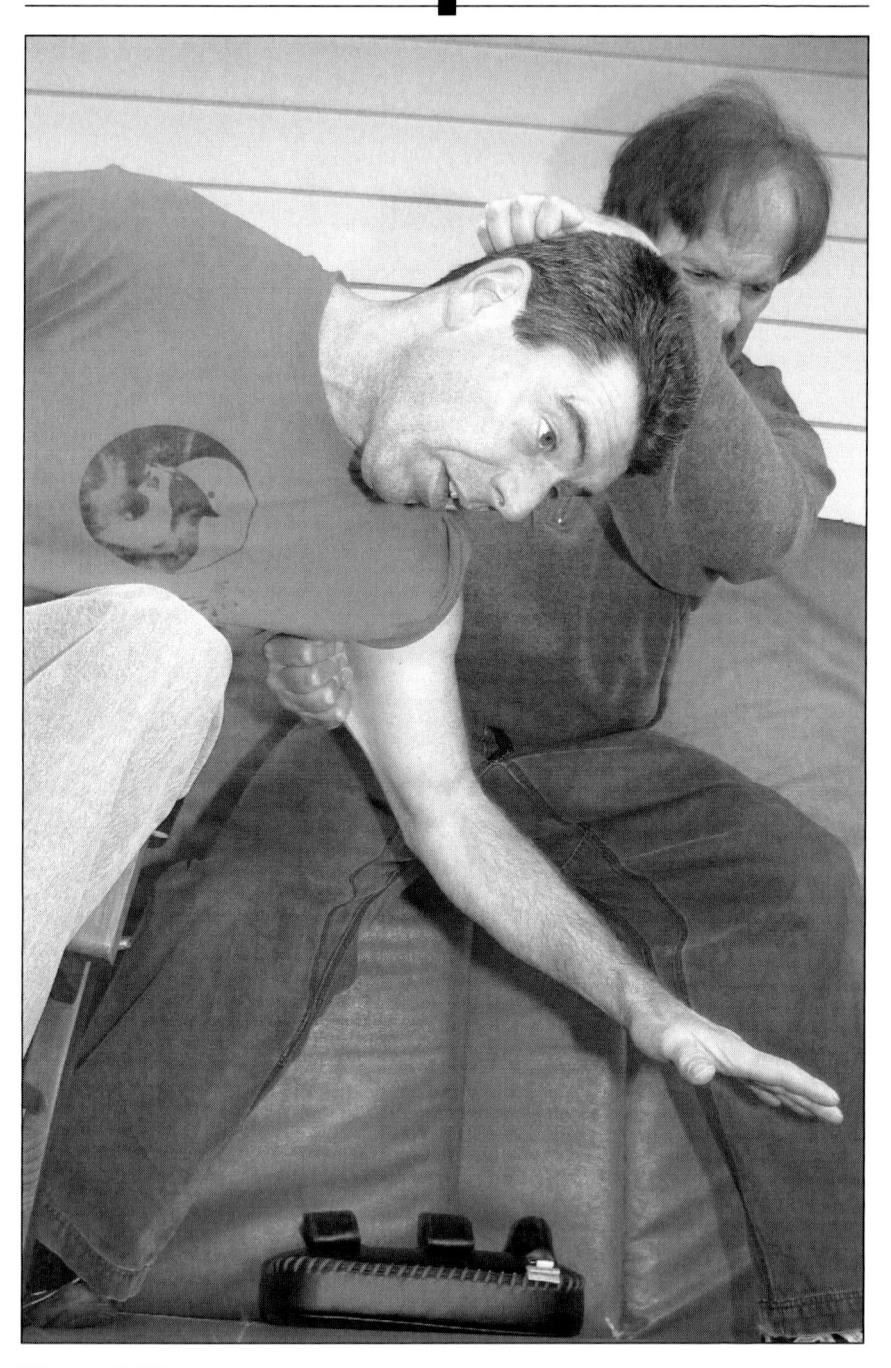

Figure 260

Arms and Shoulders

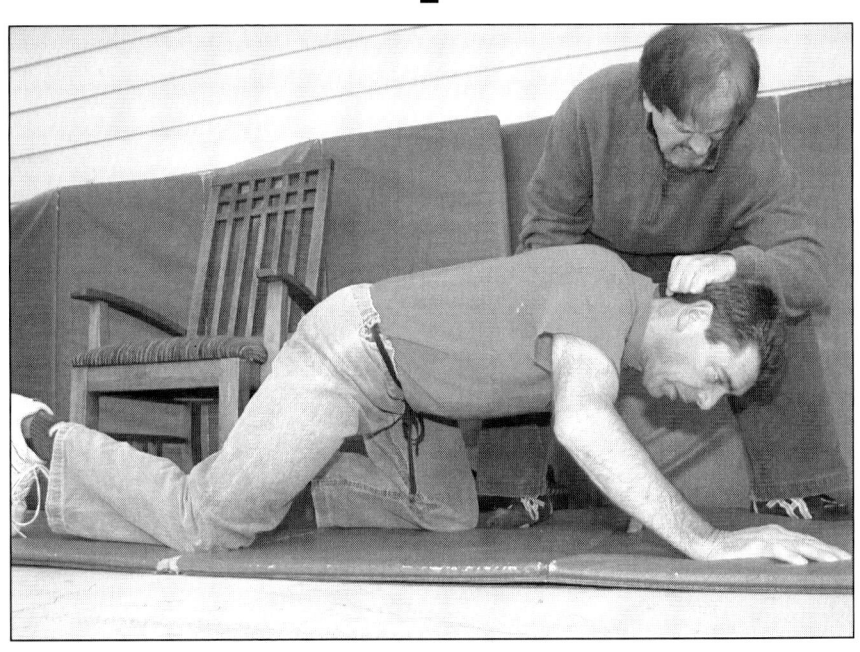

Figure 261

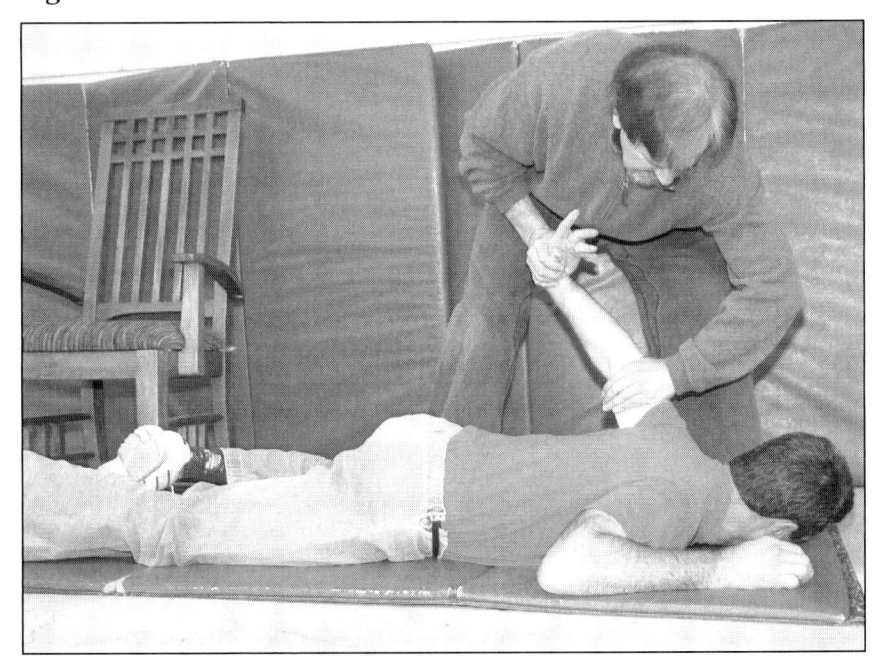

Figure 262

Prone Triceps Pinch with Knee

As a cop, I used this technique on people lying face down on the floor and refusing to bring one or both arms out from under them. It's dangerous when your attacker's arm is out of sight since he might be accessing a weapon from his waistband. You want his arm and empty hand in your control and you want it now.

Note: This is a dangerous situation to handle alone. Your best option is to flee the instant you see that he has landed with one or both arms under him. But if circumstances are such that you don't have that option and you have to deal with him, this is an effective technique.

You're alone and your attacker is down with *both* arms under his body.

- As one hand grips his forearm, press your knee into the triceps of his arm and press the thumb of your other hand into the corner of his eye. You don't have to press your thumb hard; he just needs to know it's there. Tell him, "Slowly pull out your *other* arm, the one I'm not holding. Do it slowly. If there is a weapon in your hand I will take out your eye. Understand?" (Fig. 263)

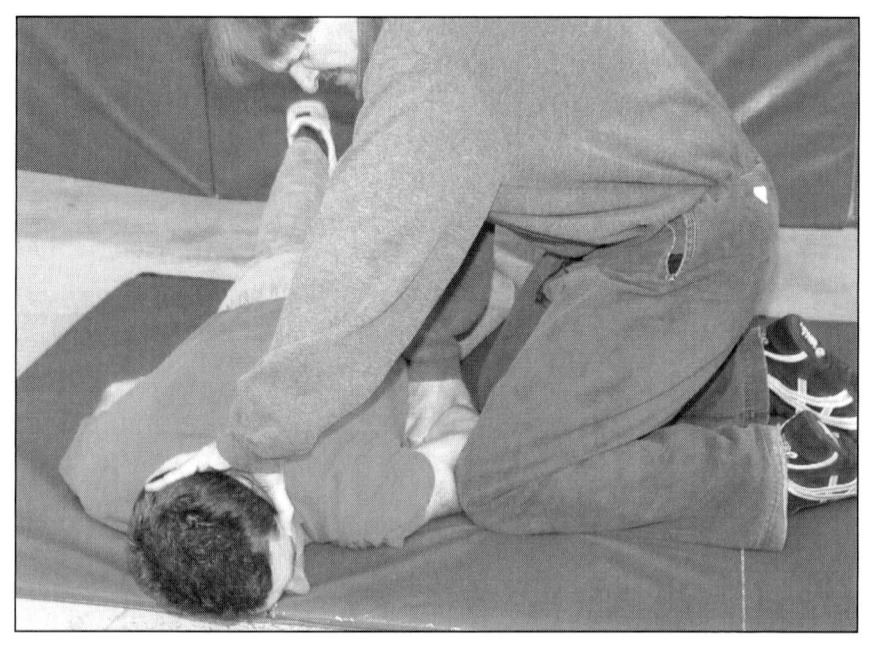

Figure 263

Arms and Shoulders

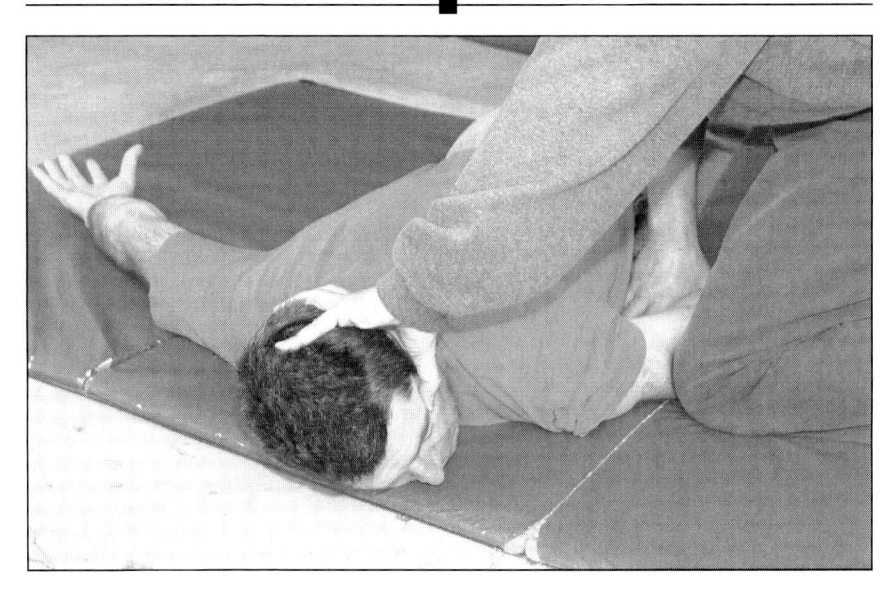

Figure 264

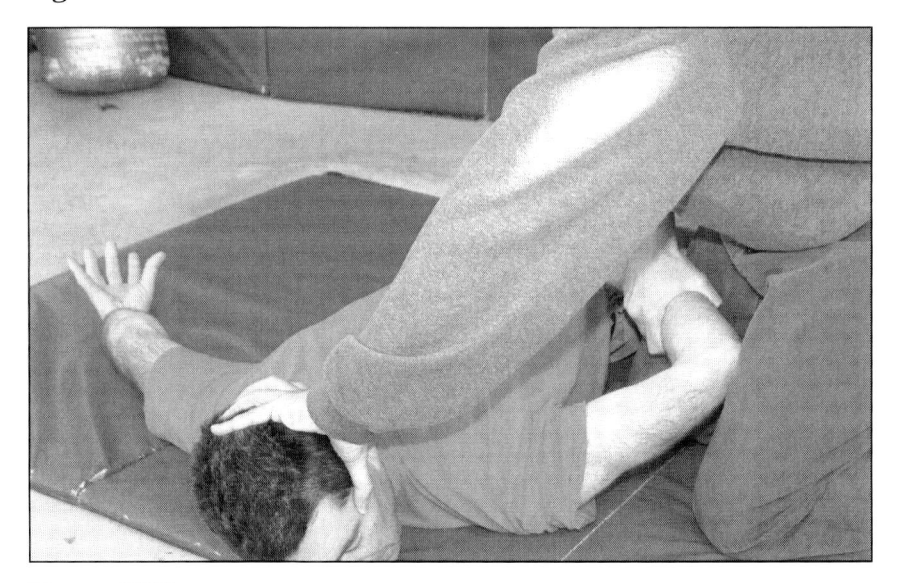

Figure 265

- When you see that it's empty, tell him to stretch it out at his side, palm facing up. (Fig. 264)
- Direct him to slowly pull out the arm you're holding. (Fig. 265)
- Apply an armlock as before. (Fig. 266)

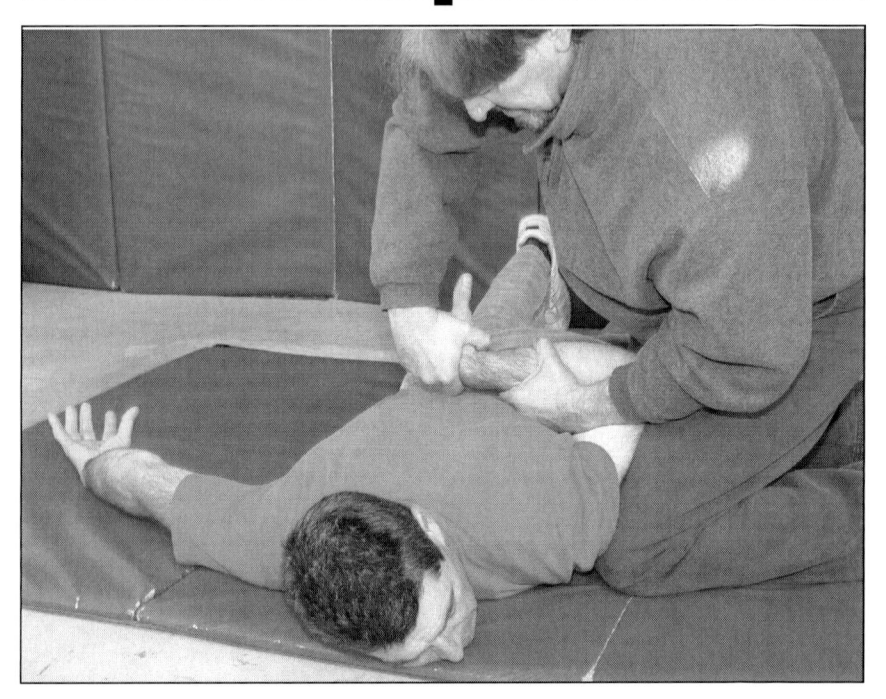

Figure 266

Variation:

Even when you have a partner you must proceed slowly and cautiously when the attacker has both arms under him.

- Each of you grips an arm and then you both apply the triceps pinch with one of your knees. Even with two people it's a good idea to use the thumb threat. The person he is facing should be the one to apply the thumb at the corner of his eye. (Fig. 267)
- The commands are given by one person. Tell him, "Slowly pull out your empty left hand. Do it slowly. If there is a weapon in your hand I will take out your eye. Any part of that you don't understand?" (Fig. 268)
- Stretch the extracted arm out to the side and hold it down with two hands and body weight. (Fig. 269)
- Give him commands to slowly extract his other arm as your partner holds onto it and then stretch it out to the side. Your partner then controls it. (Fig. 270)

Arms and Shoulders 177

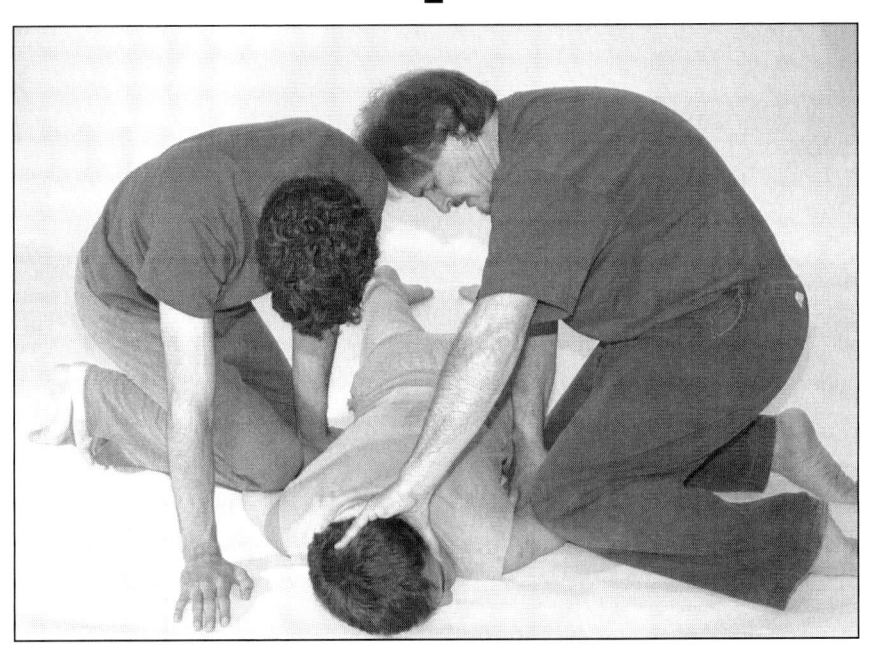

Figure 267

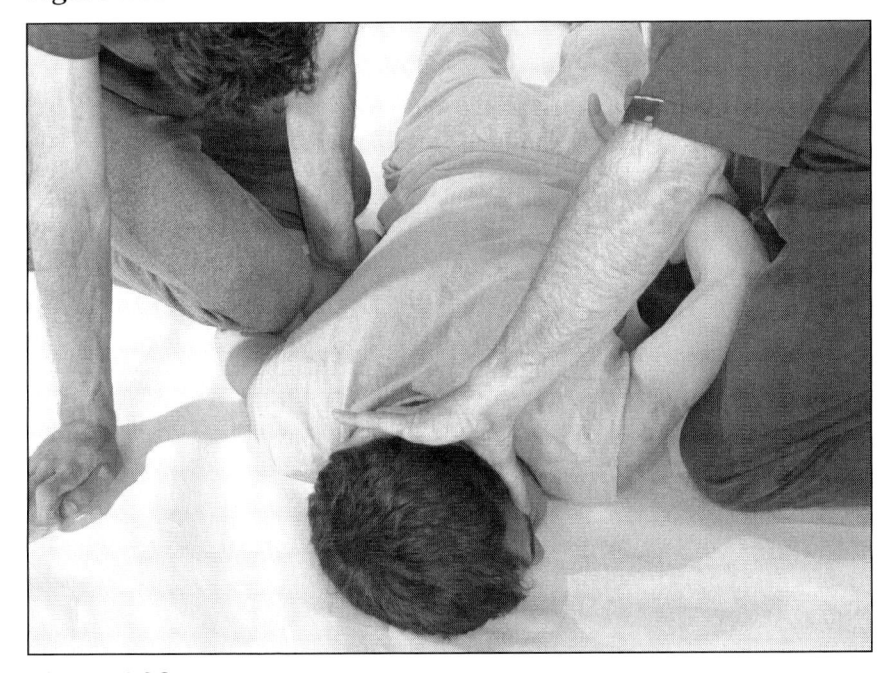

Figure 268

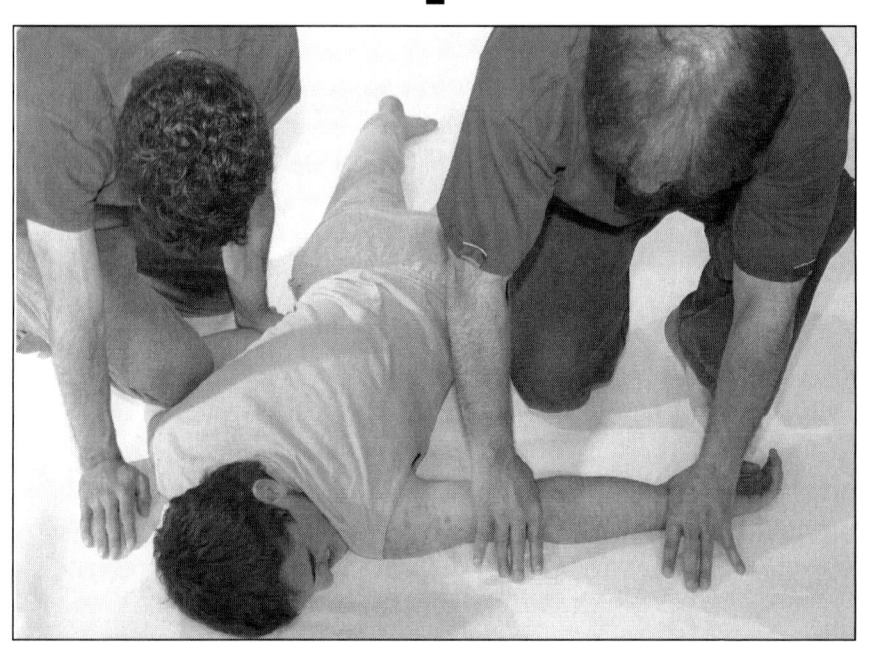

Figure 269

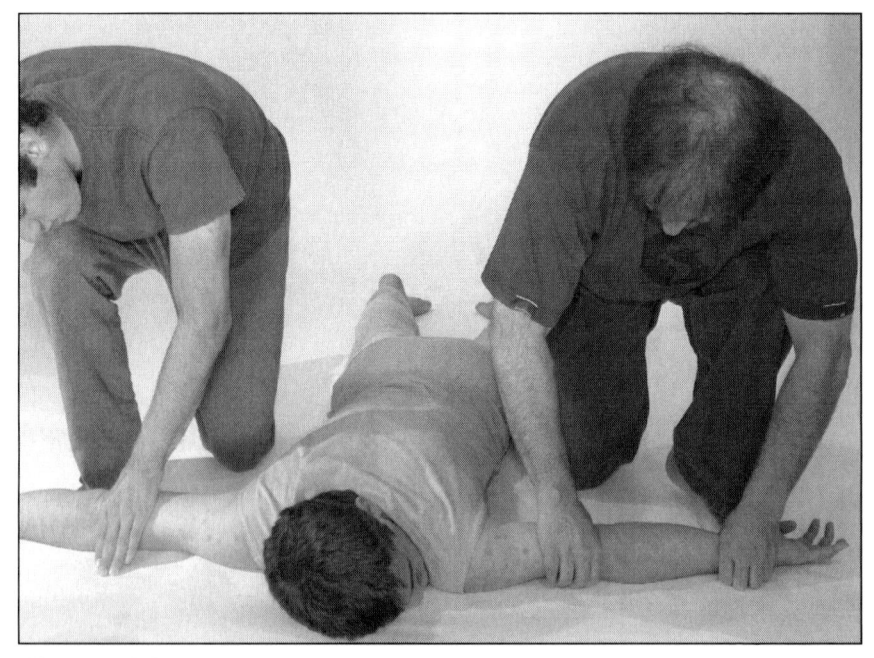

Figure 270

Elbow, Ulna, Triceps Press

I've used these successfully many times in the street. If you press too hard and too quickly with any of them, you're likely to cause structural damage. If that is your intention, you must be legally justified. Otherwise, press slowly and progressively harder until your attacker yields to the pain.

Elbow:
You have taken your attacker down onto his belly.

- Stretch his arm out to the side like the wing of an airplane, palm up. Place your foot under his wrist to create a bridge and then lean on his elbow with your hand or shin. To apply additional pain, use your shin or the heel of your hand to saw back and forth an inch or so in each direction. (Fig. 271)

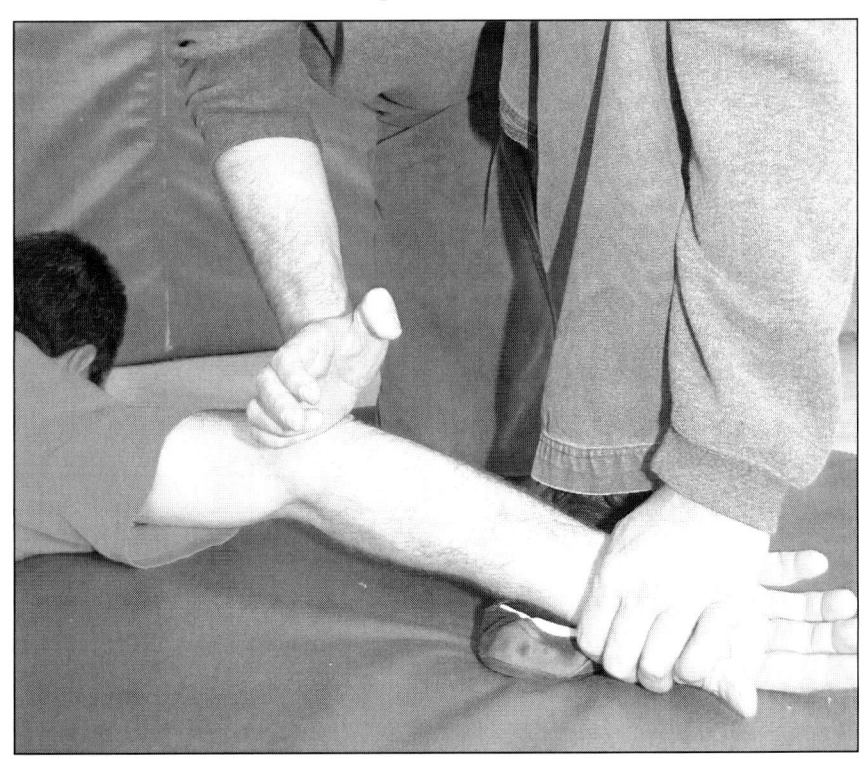

Figure 271

Ulnar:

The ulnar nerve is about an inch from the elbow on the shoulder side. Some people find that pressure on it hurts more than pressure on the elbow joint.

- Place your foot under your attacker's wrist and use your hand or shin to press and saw on the ulnar. (Fig. 272)

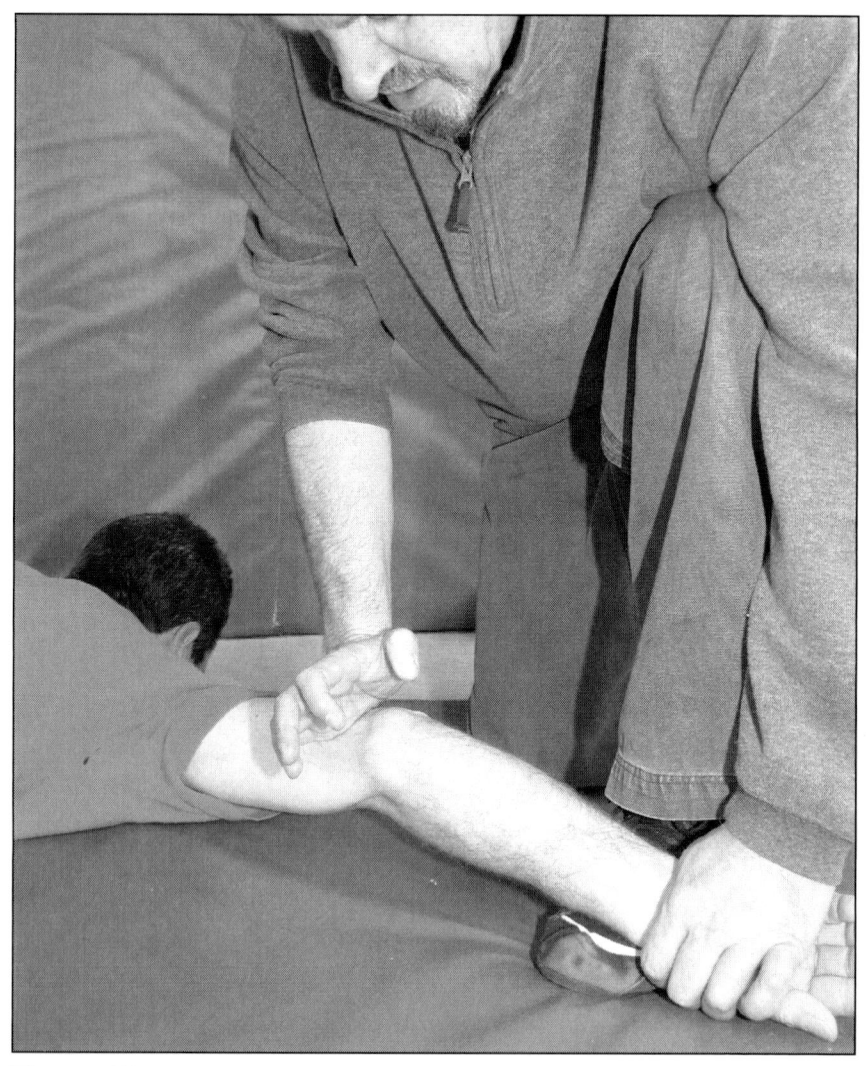

Figure 272

Arms and Shoulders 181

Triceps:
The large three-headed muscle on the back of the arm is quite tender when pressed, but not to everyone. Some people will shrug it off, while others will yelp like a startled puppy. Press and rub the muscle into the arm bone.

- Place your foot under your attacker's wrist and use your hand or shin to press and saw on the triceps muscle. (Fig. 273)

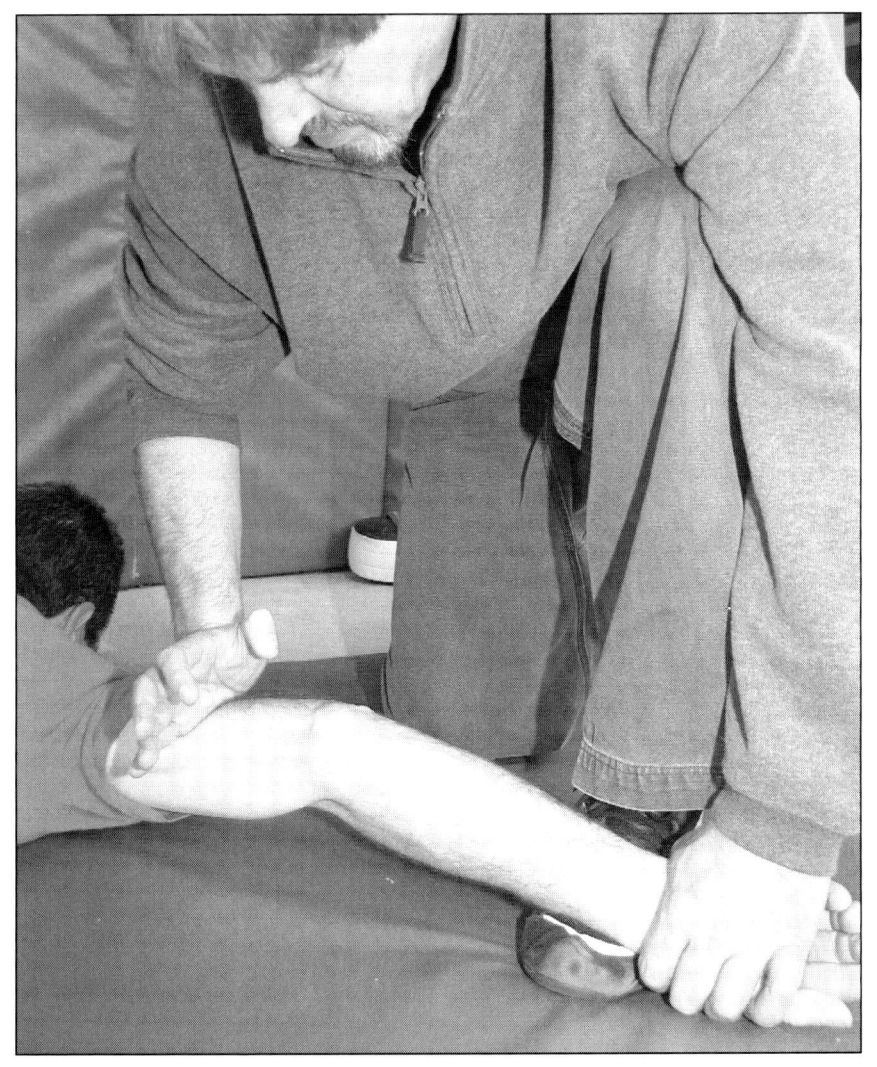

Figure 273

Biceps Press

This is a good technique when the attacker lands on his back ever so briefly with his arms extended out to his side. While it's best to get him onto his stomach where it's easier to control him, if his resistance is extreme, you might want to control him first on his back and then, when the timing is right, coordinate with your partner to roll him over. Your partner can use the same pressing technique as you. Should the attacker kick at you, press harder and order him to stop. Most will comply because of the intense pain in their biceps muscles.

- The instant his arm is flat on the floor, secure his wrist. There is no armlock in this position, so if he is strong he can curl his arm to defeat the hold. To prevent this, press the edge of your hand into his biceps muscle and apply your body weight to pinch/press his flesh against his upper arm bone. Saw your hand back and forth an inch in both directions. (Fig. 274)

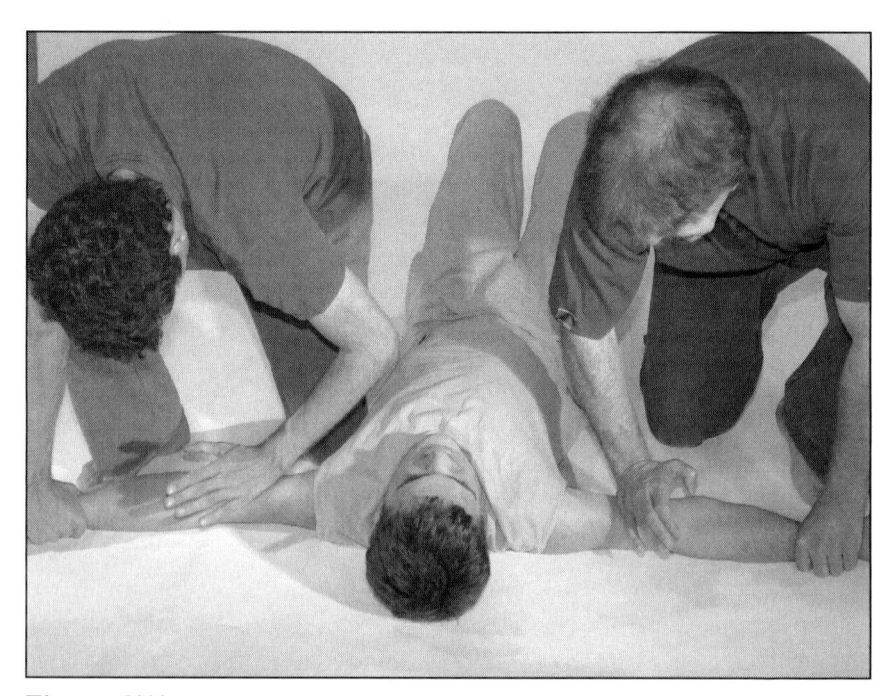

Figure 274

Biceps Pinch with Foot

You have taken your attacker to the floor but he is quick and grabs your ankle. You must react with speed before he can roll toward you.

- Reach down and wrap your hand around the hand that is gripping your ankle. (Figs. 275, 276)
- Step quickly over his upper arm and place your heel on the inside of his biceps. Press your heel down so that it pinches his soft flesh into the floor. (Fig. 277)
- When he raises his head in pain, backfist his face. (Fig. 278)

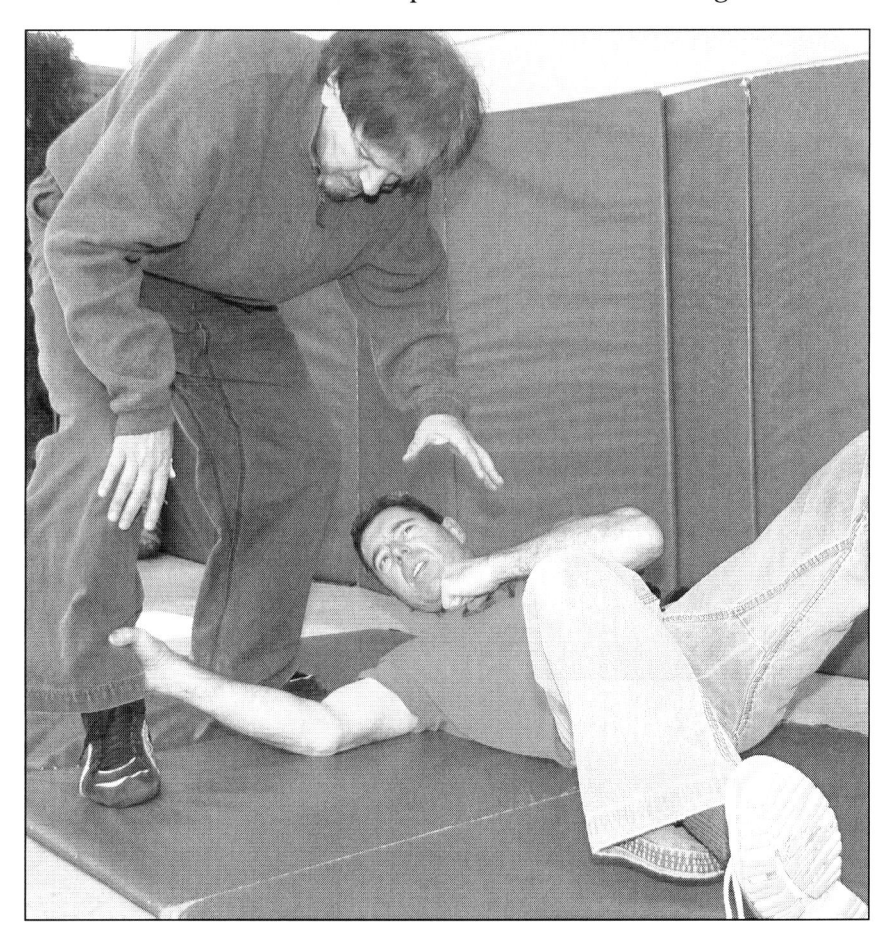

Figure 275

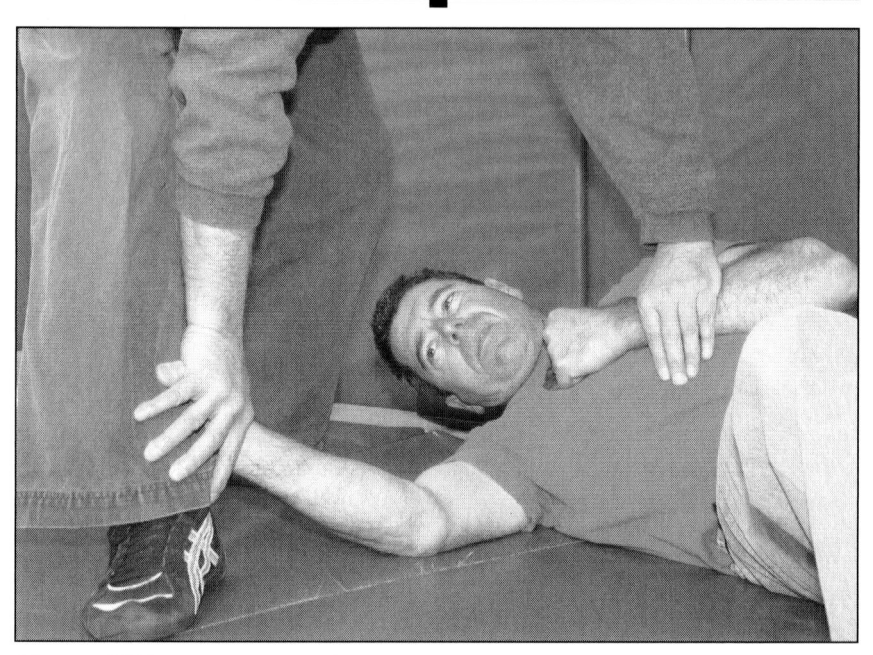

184　　　*The Brutal Art of Ripping, Poking, and Pressing Vital Targets*

Figure 276

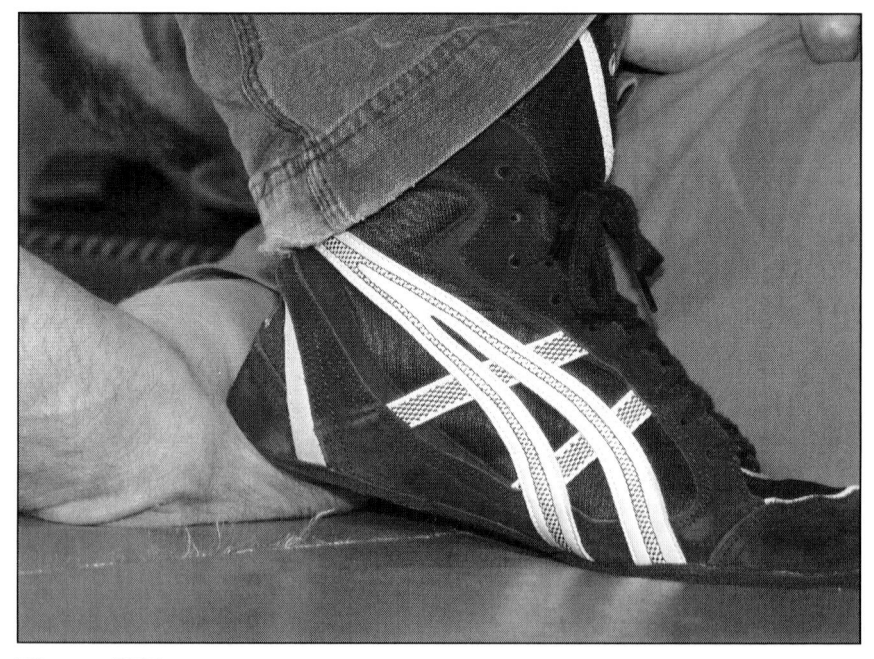

Figure 277

Arms and Shoulders 185

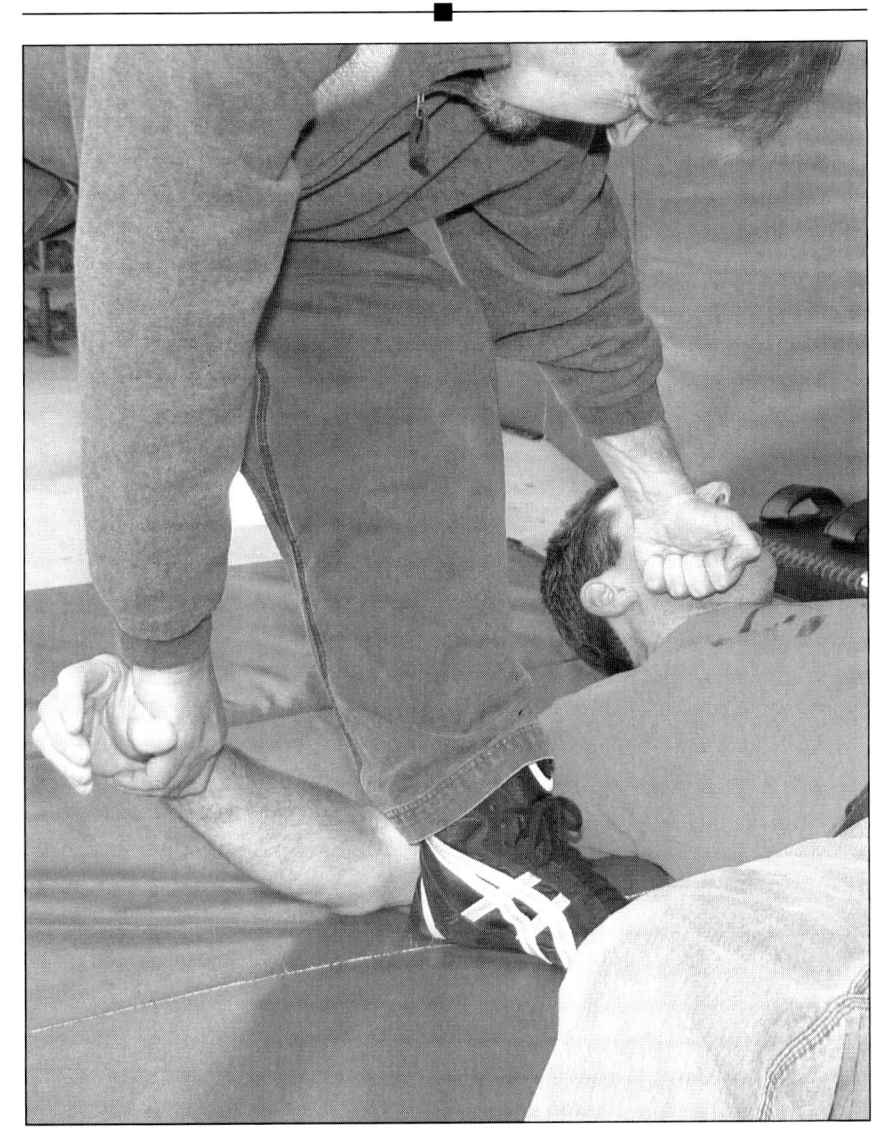

Figure 278

4
Torso

"Imagine yourself to be a jungle cat shredding its prey with multiple strikes."

The upper body has more padding—muscles and fat—than does the head, but it still contains many sensitive targets. If the attacker is wearing a heavy winter coat, you will have to move your defense to his head or lower body.

PEC SQUEEZE

It's been my experience that this technique delivers as much psychological shock as it does physical pain. The recipient's first thought is "What the heck are you doing to me?!" Then he transitions to "Agggh! That hurts!" It's not a technique that you use to restrain someone for a long minute but rather for a few short seconds to move him away from something or to get him to release his grip on you.

Standing Outer Pec Squeeze

You should always have a Plan B, another technique that you flow into when Plan A falls apart. But Plan B can also be a device that makes Plan A work better.

- You're attempting to lock in a bent-arm wristlock, but your attacker is beginning to defeat your hold. (Fig. 279)
- Keep hold of your attacker's hand with your closest hand and grab his outer pec with your other, with either a four-fingers-to-palm grip or a five-finger claw. Squeeze hard as you simul-

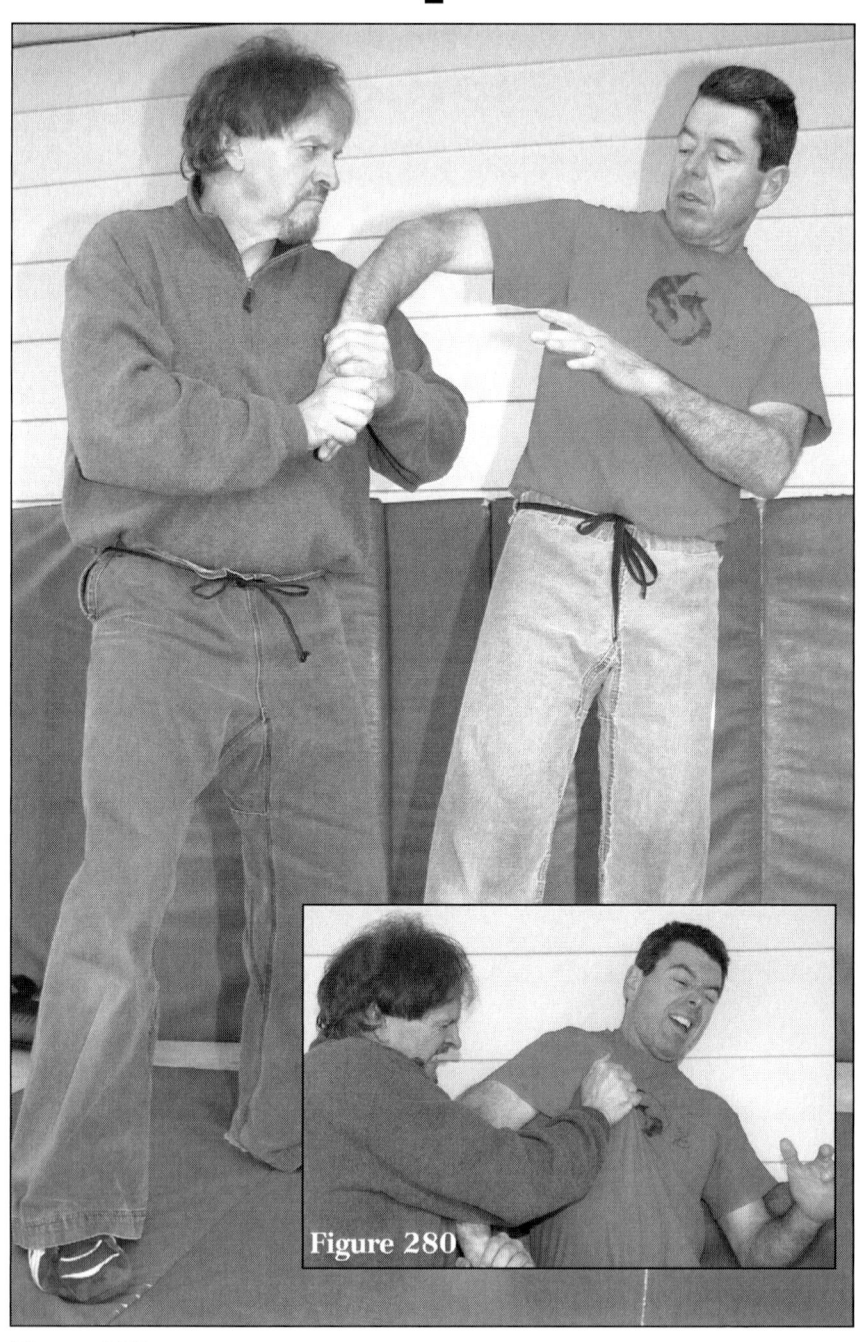

The Brutal Art of Ripping, Poking, and Pressing Vital Targets

Figure 280

Figure 279

Torso 189

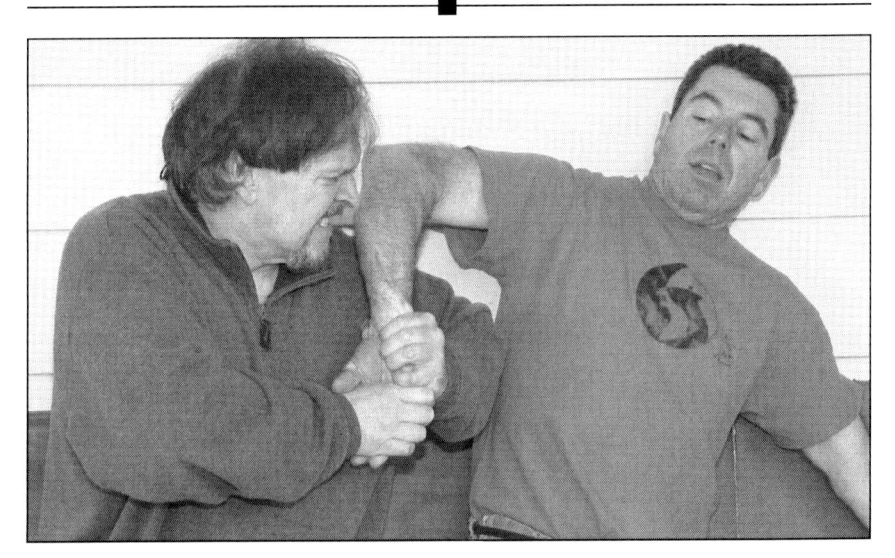

Figure 281

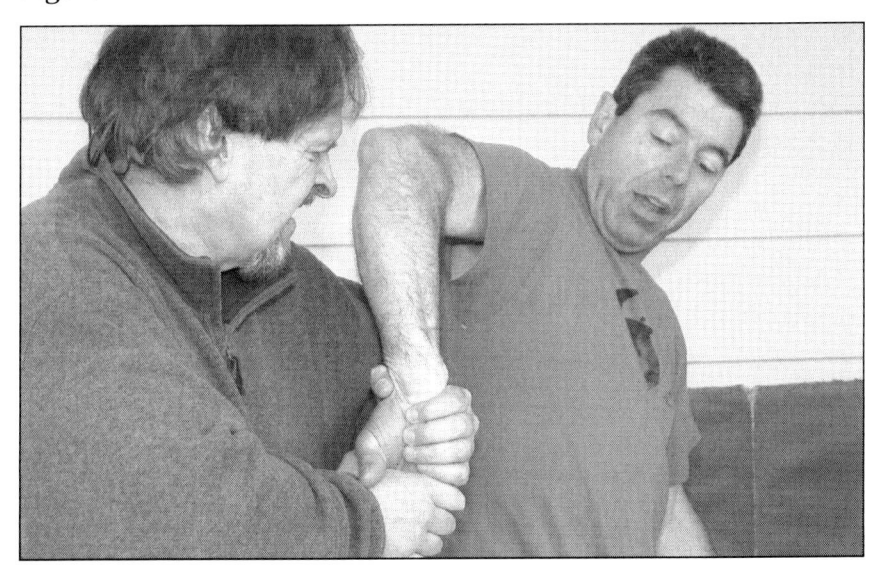

Figure 282

taneously slam him into a wall. You want to distract him from his resistance. (Fig. 280)
- Upon impact with the wall, reapply your hold (Fig. 281)
- Move him away from the wall so he can't push off of it and into you. (Fig. 282)

On the Floor Outer Pec Squeeze

This works well as a distraction device so you can re-establish another hold.

- You have taken your attacker to the floor and onto his side. Your intention is to lock his arm, but he grabs your clothing with his hand. (Fig. 283)

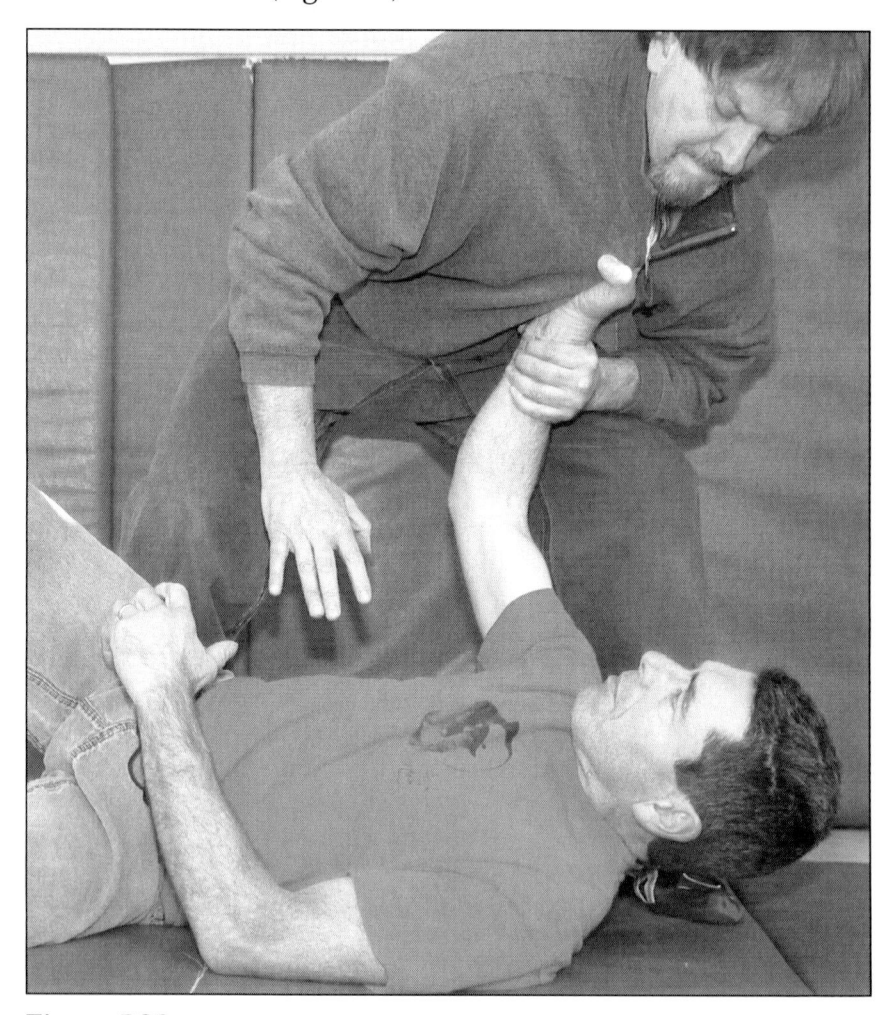

Figure 283

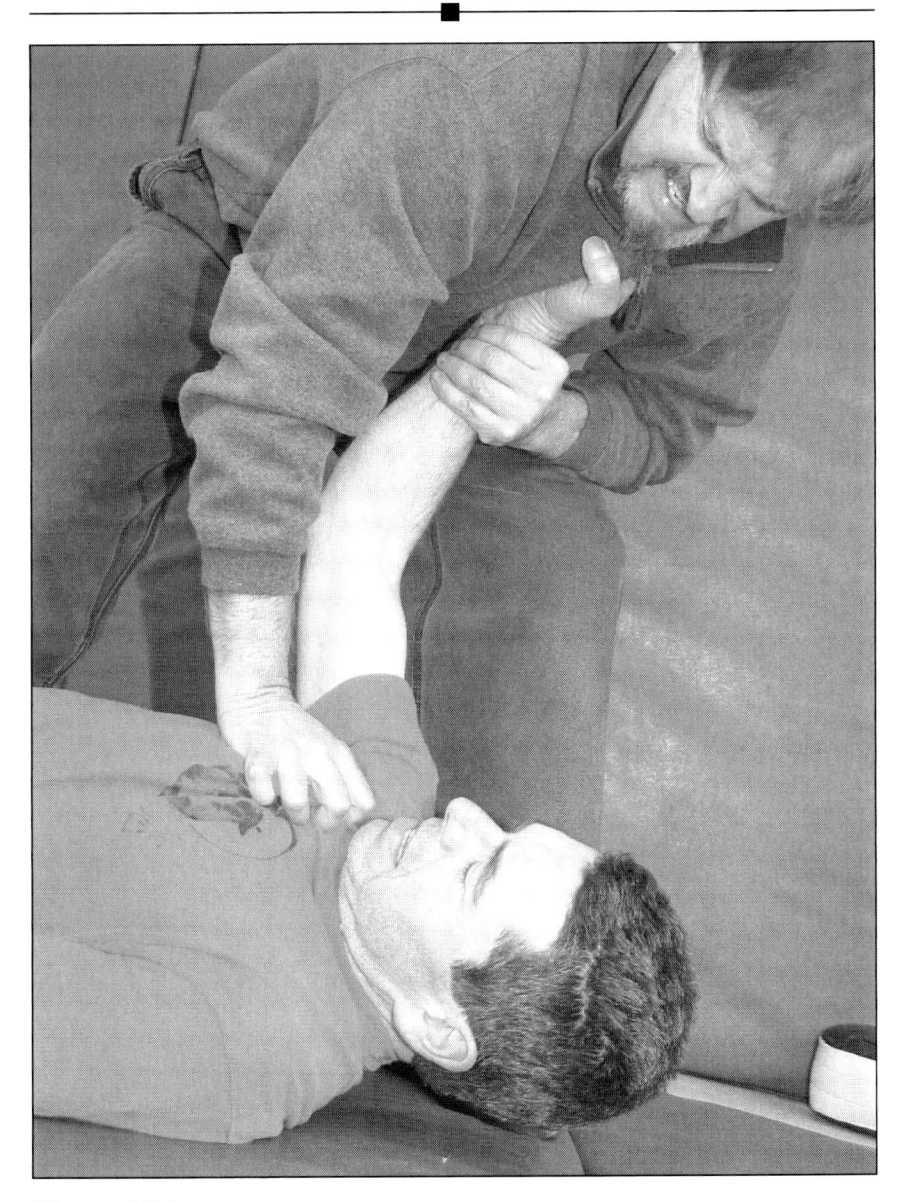

Figure 284

- Maintain the hold, grab his outer pec with your other hand, and squeeze. With his body braced against the floor, you can dig your fingers deeper into flesh. Use your five fingertips or dig in with your nails. (Fig. 284)

- Once you have a deep, firm grip, rotate your hand as if turning a doorknob. Your attacker will think his skin is ripping. (Fig. 285)
- This will distract your attacker long enough for you to secure a good lock on his other arm. (Fig. 286)

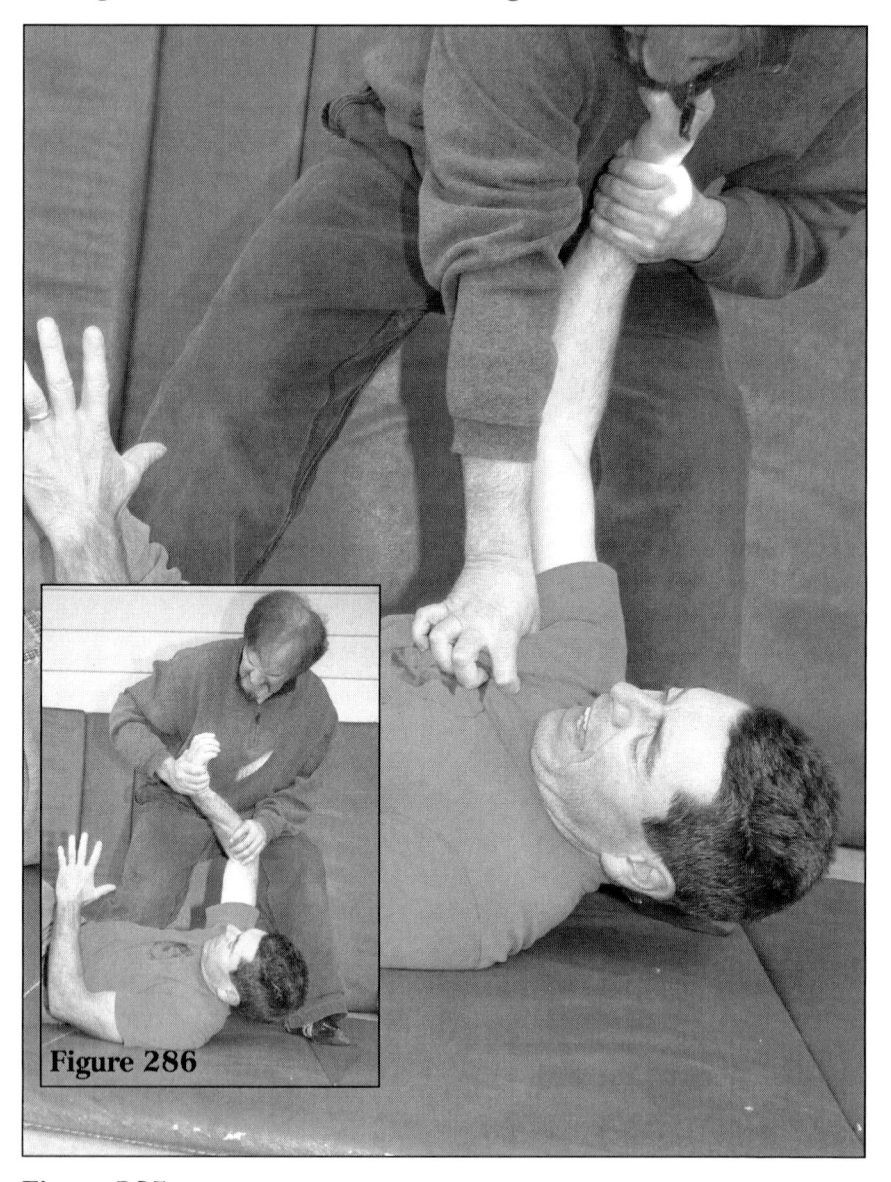

Figure 286

Figure 285

Torso

Chest Plate Press with Knuckles

There isn't a lot of padding on the center of the chest just above the pec muscles, even among the morbidly obese. The nerves directly underneath the skin there are painfully sensitive when pressed and rubbed.

- You're kneeling alongside your attacker applying a bent arm wrist flex. For whatever reason, you've lost the integrity of the hold and your attacker begins to bend his arm. (Fig. 287)

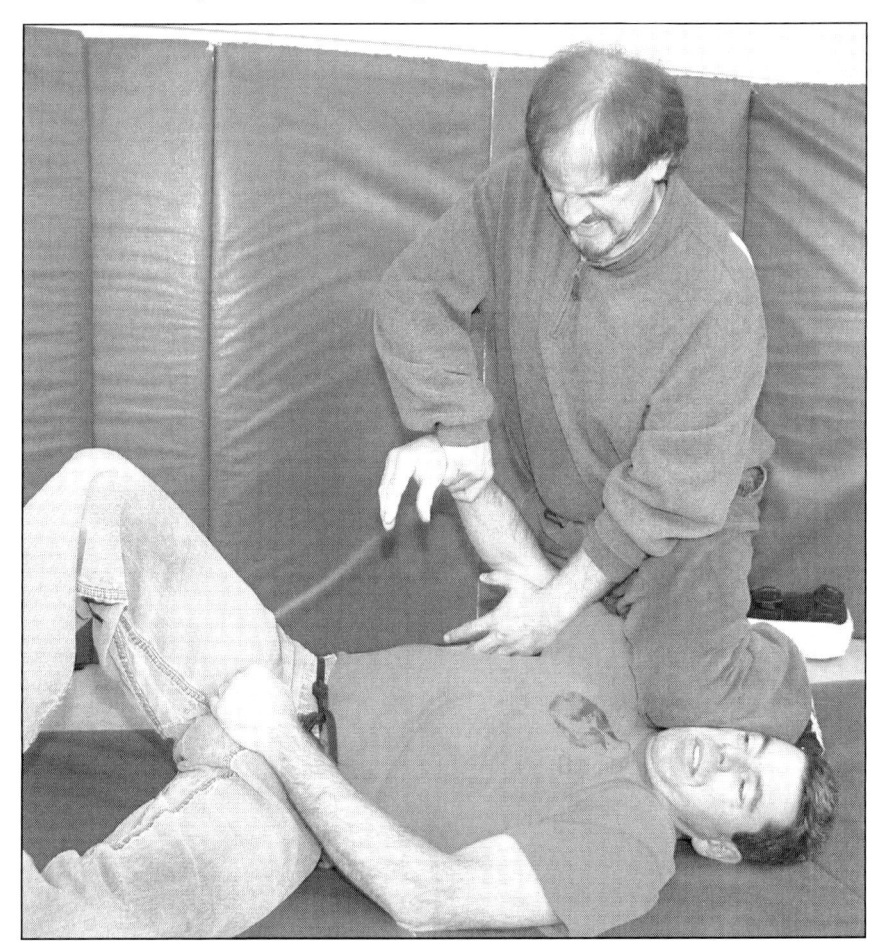

Figure 287

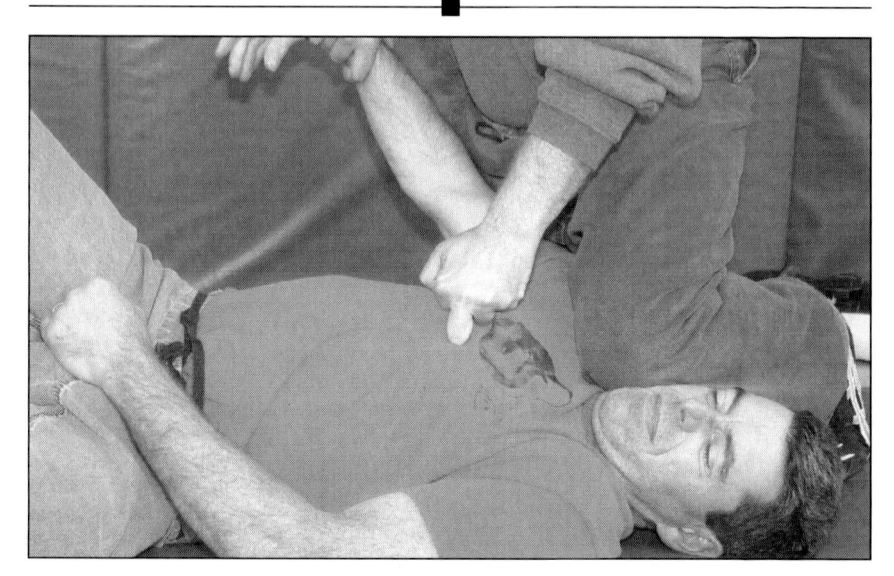

Figure 288

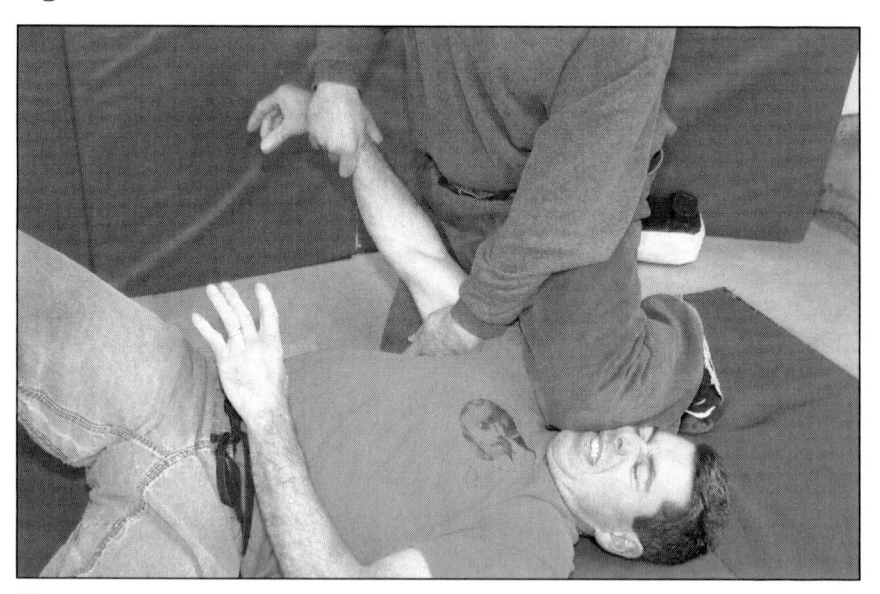

Figure 289

- Use the middle knuckles of your free hand to press into his chest plate. Lean your weight into it. (Fig. 288)
- This momentary distraction buys you a second or two to fix your wrist flex. (Fig. 289)

Torso 195

Chest Plate Press with Elbow

You've fallen on top of your attacker.

- Before you can apply a hold, he grabs you and pulls you into him. (Fig. 290)

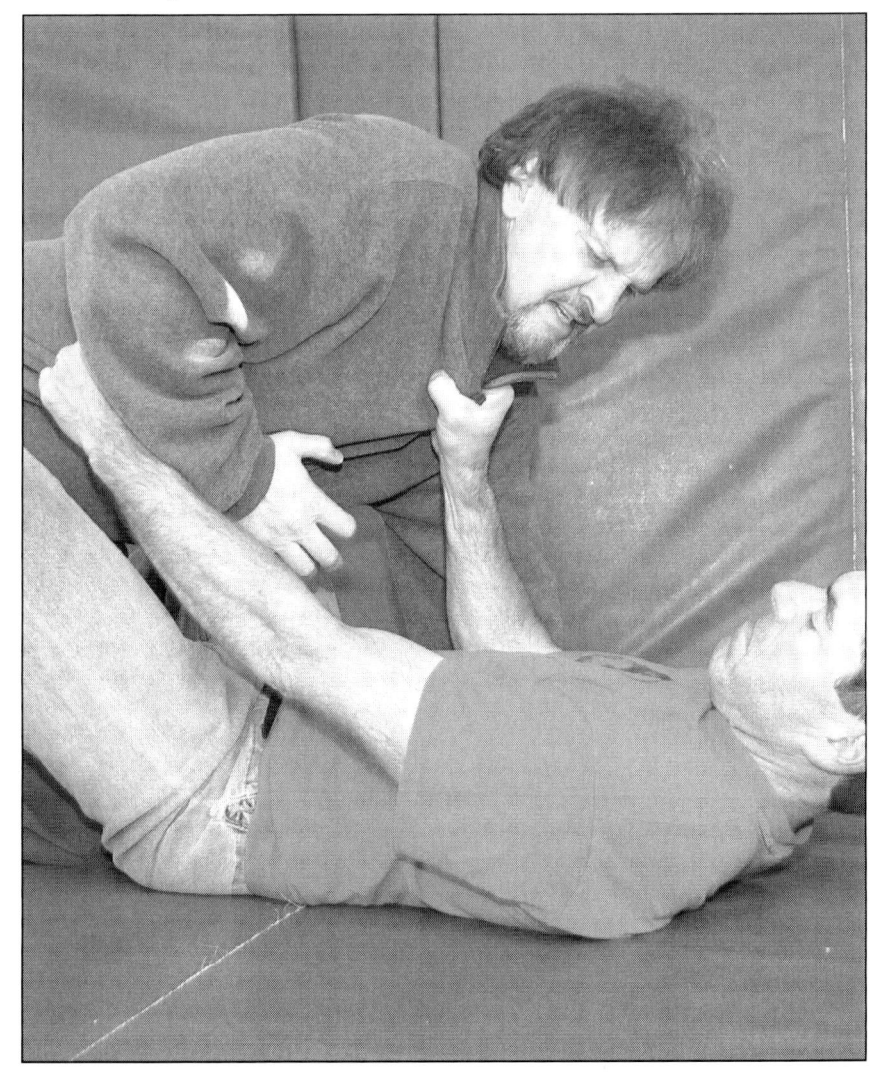

Figure 290

- Snap your forearm inward so that you land with the point of your elbow in his chest plate. (Fig. 291)
- Rub your elbow into his chest as you move your other hand up to his eyes. Poke his eyes until he turns his head to the side. (Fig. 292)
- Palm his face with your other hand. (Fig. 293)

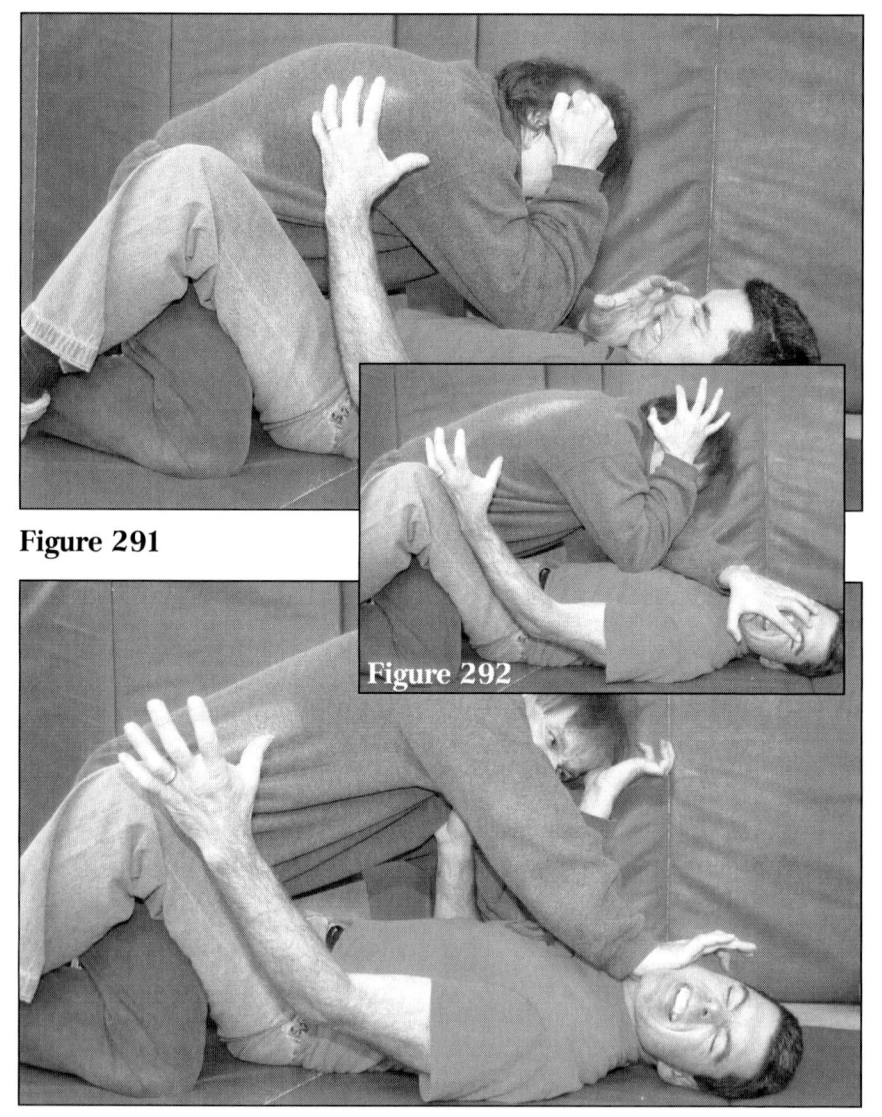

Figure 291

Figure 292

Figure 293

Center Pec Squeeze

This is similar to "On the floor outer pec squeeze," but in this situation it serves a different purpose. You have taken your attacker down, but he has landed on his back instead of on his side, a position from which he can hit you. He is too big or resisting too much for you to lift him, so make him do the work for you.

- Grab the center of his pec over the nipple with a five-fingered claw, dig in deeply, and squeeze with all of your fingers into the tender meat. With his back braced by the floor, the squeeze is more effective than if he were standing. (Fig. 294)

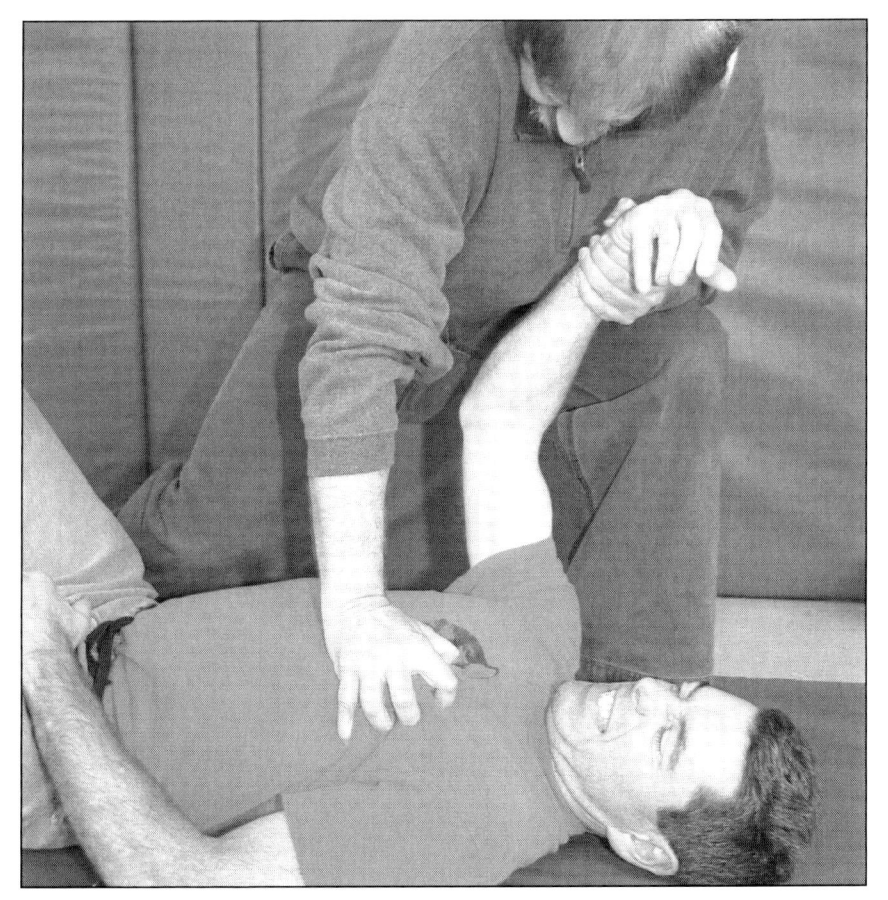

Figure 294

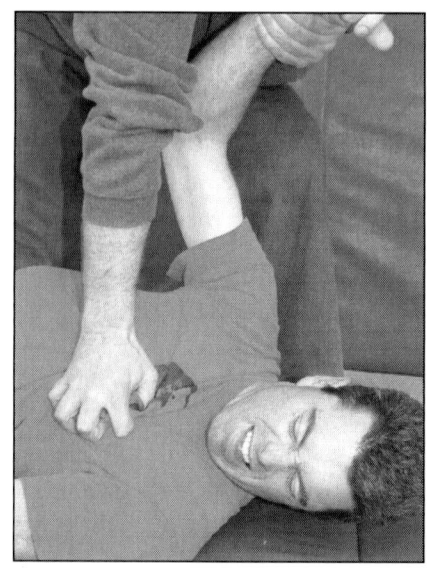

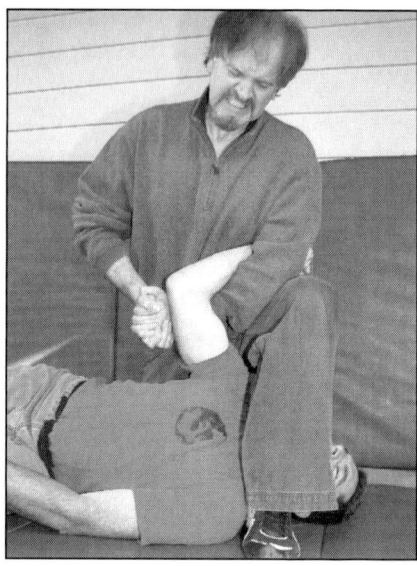

Figure 295

Figure 296

- After a second of pushing him into the floor, continue to squeeze and add a vigorous twist as you pull up on his flesh as if trying to lift him. He will follow your pull by rolling up onto his side. (Fig. 295)
- Now you're in a better position to secure a solid hold on his arm. (Fig. 296)

Downward Pec and Nipple Rip

Skip this one if the attacker is wearing a coat or a thick sweatshirt. Practice on a live opponent or a mannequin-style bag.

He launches a right cross.

- Block with your left backhand. (Fig. 297)
- Use the same hand in a five-fingered claw to rip downward over a nipple. (Fig. 298)
- Rip his other nipple with your other hand. (Fig. 299)
- Rip the first nipple again with your first hand. Strike as many times as you can. Imagine yourself to be a jungle cat shredding its prey with multiple strikes. (Fig. 300)

Torso 199

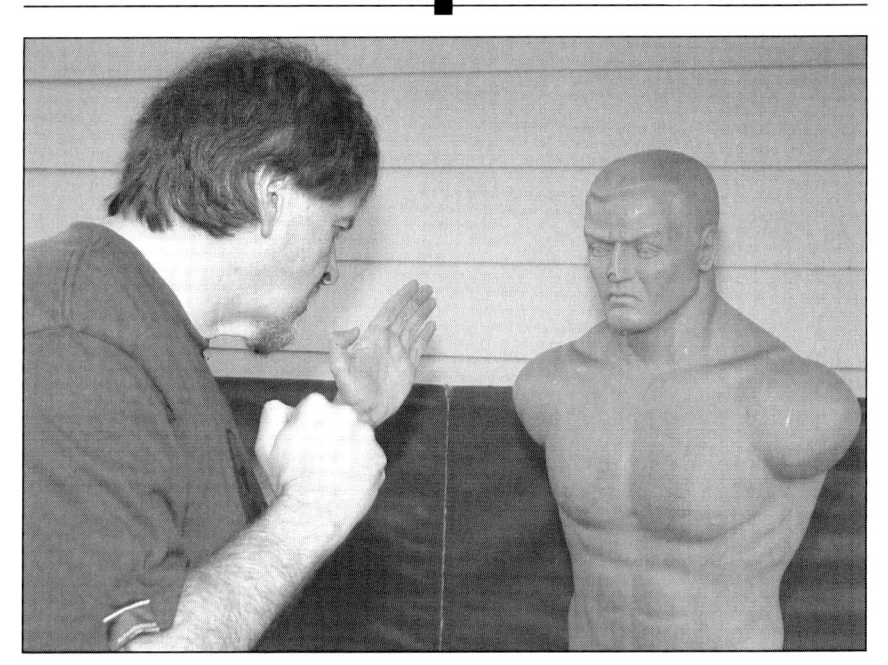

Figure 297

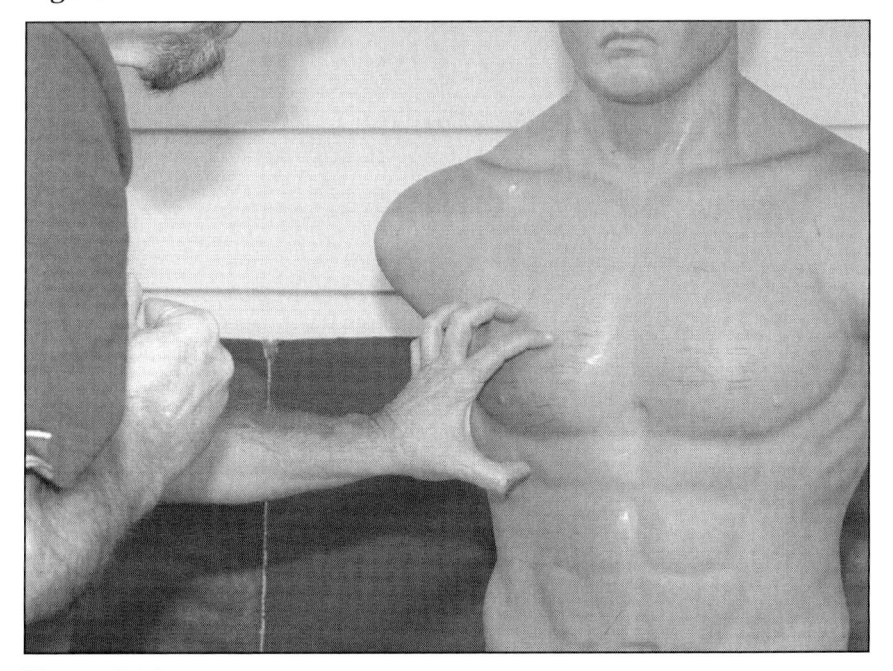

Figure 298

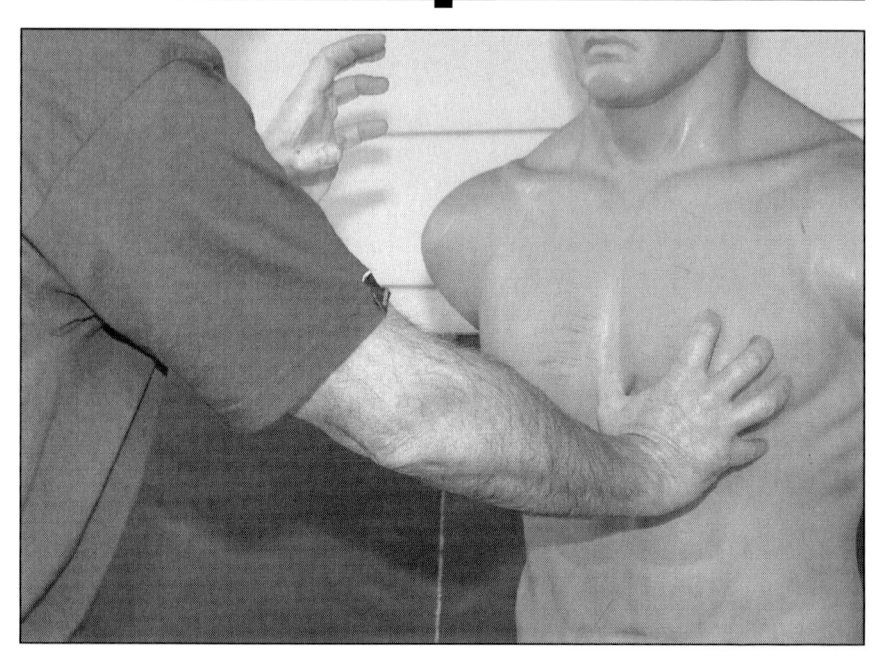

Figure 299

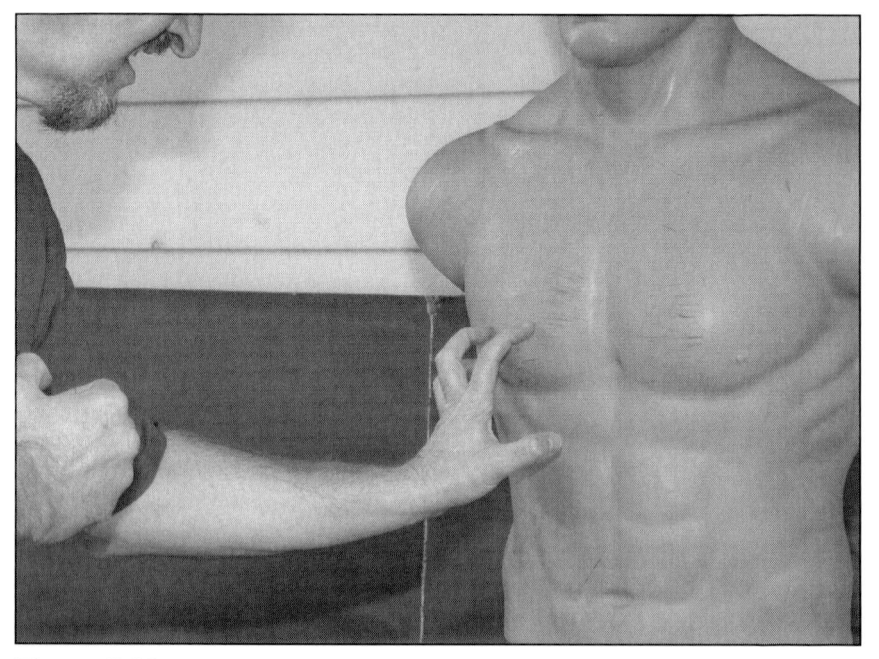

Figure 300

Torso 201

Horizontal Nipple Rip

This works well when your arm is stretched out across your attacker's chest. As long as you have to retract it anyway, you might as well rip it across his nipples. Practice on a live opponent or a mannequin-style bag.

- During the course of the fight, one of your arms is stretched across your attacker's chest for a fraction of a second. (Fig. 301)

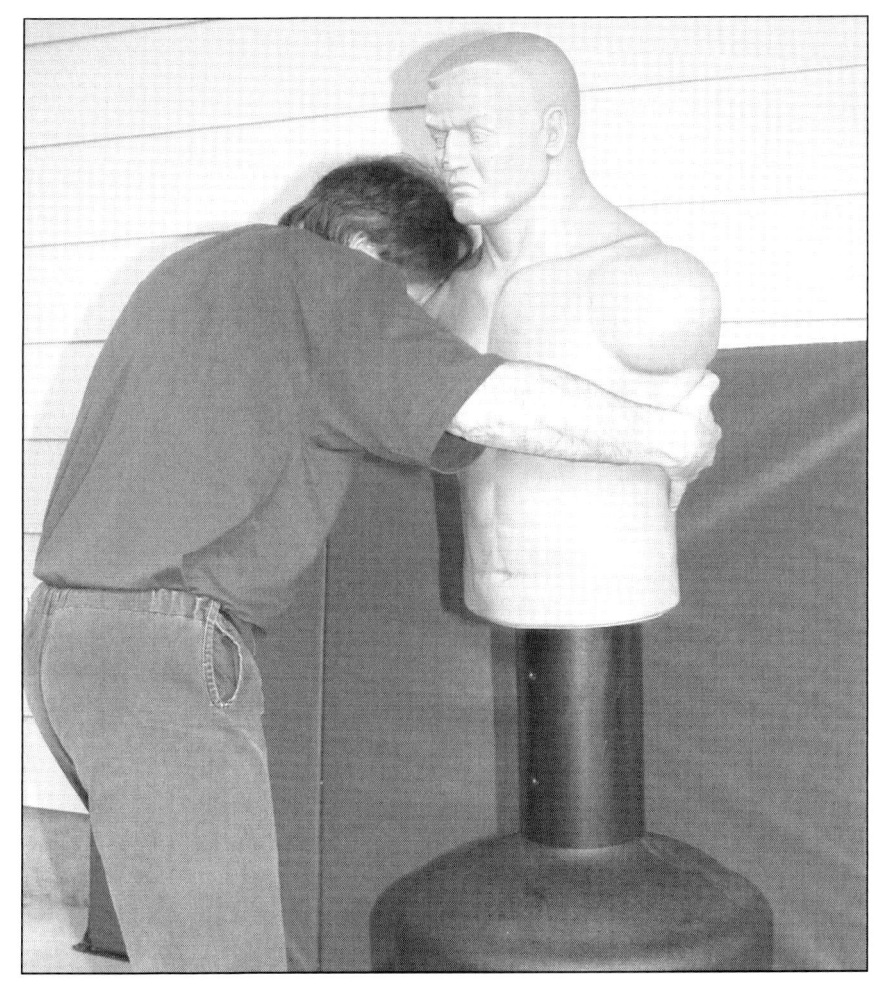

Figure 301

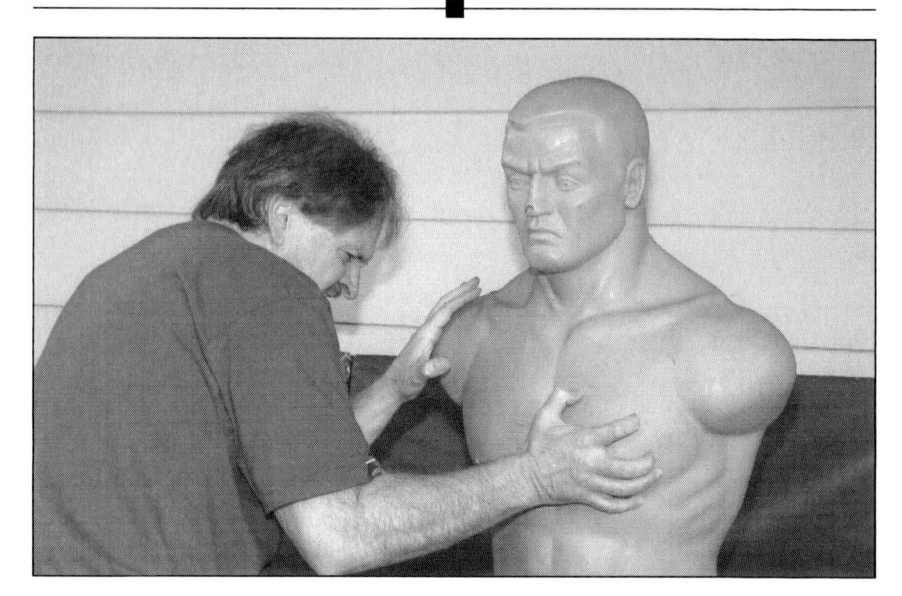

Figure 302

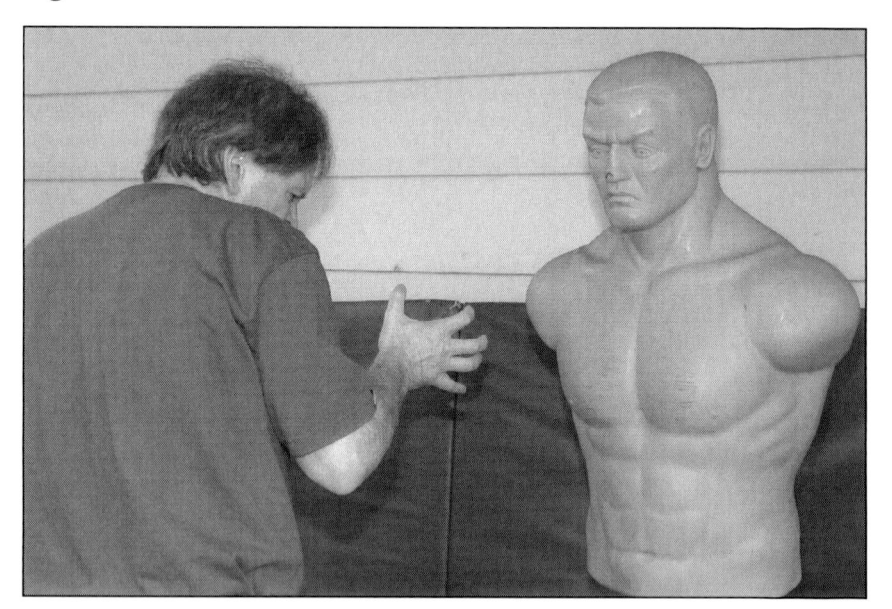

Figure 303

- Retract it by raking your five-fingered claw across his chest. (Fig. 302)
- Chamber your hand. (Fig. 303)
- Backfist an opening. (Fig. 304)

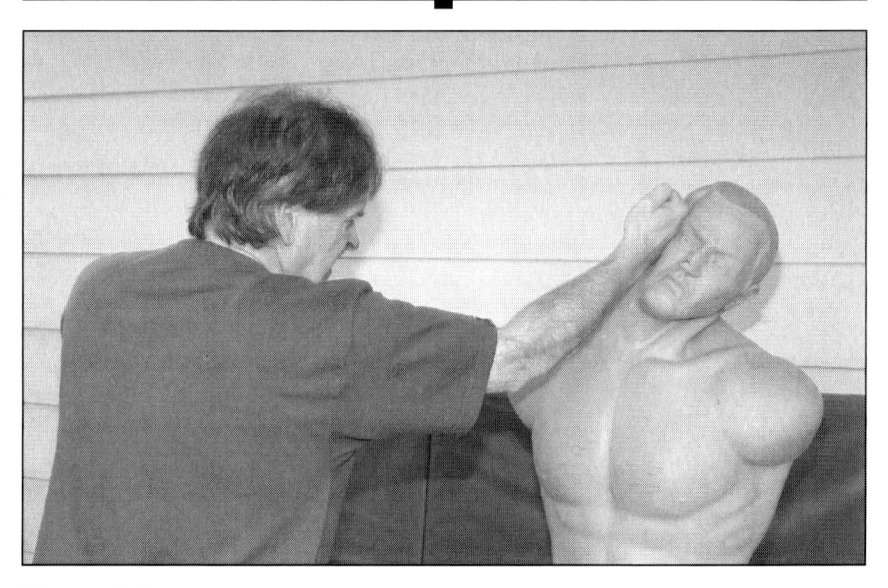

Figure 304

Lat Squeeze and Push

This is a surprise technique that gives your attacker direction for a few steps. It can't be applied for long because the recipient can easily wiggle free once the shock wears off.

A drunk throws a sloppy jab at your midsection.

- Sweep his arm to the inside. (Fig. 305)
- Grasp his closest lat (upper back muscle) with the four-fingers-to-palm grip or five-fingered claw as you step behind him. (Fig. 306)
- Grab his other lat muscle with your other hand and squeeze both. (Fig. 307)
- Lower yourself a little to gather power and drive him into a wall, through a door, or over furniture. (Fig. 308)

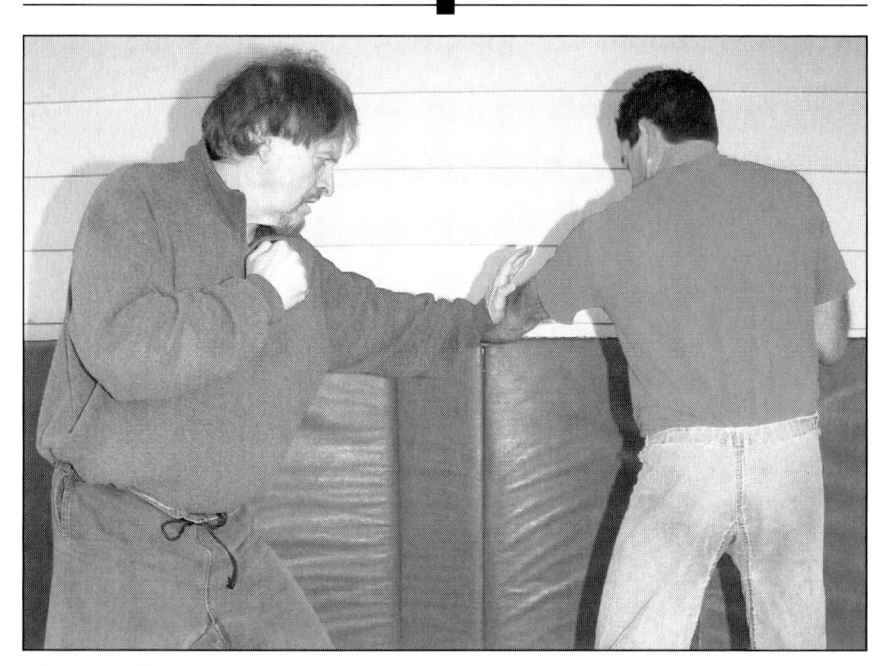

Figure 305

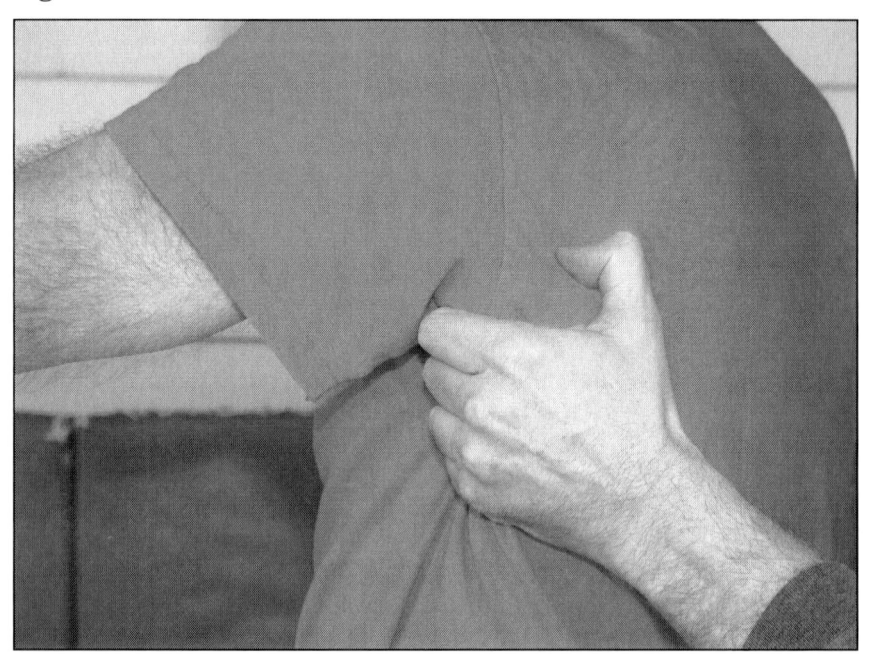

Figure 306

Torso 205

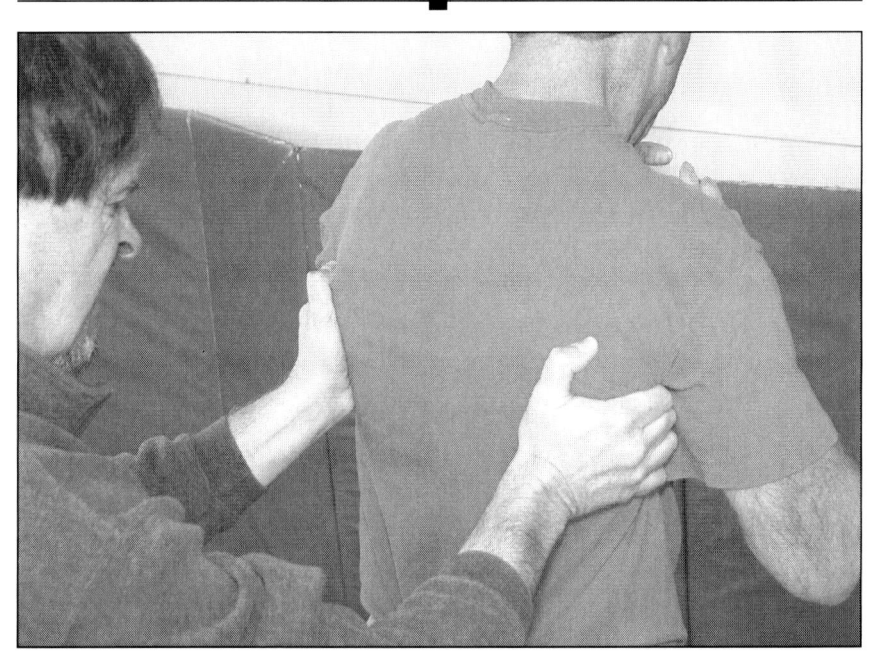

Figure 307

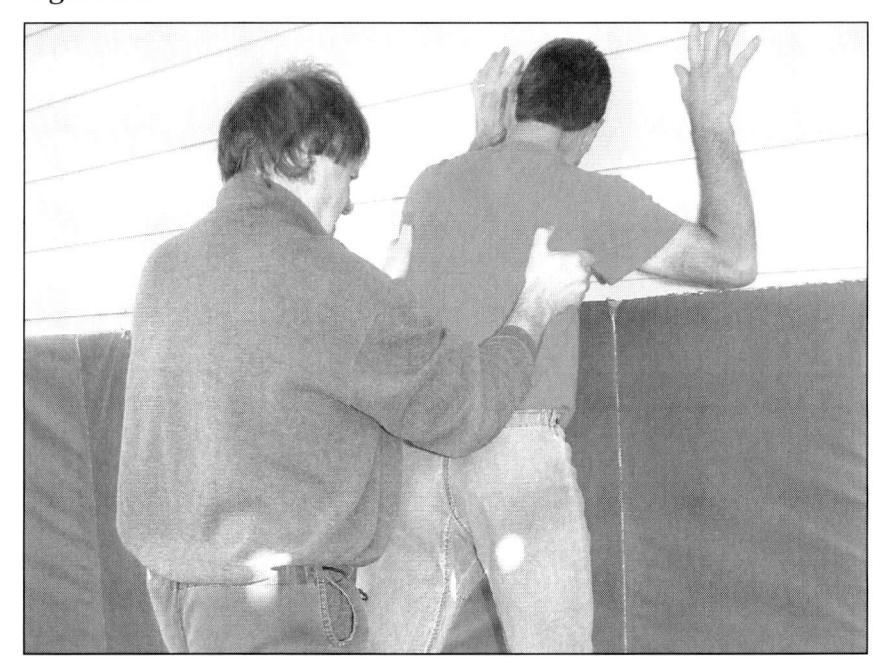

Figure 308

Side Crab Bite

As has been noted earlier, a crab bite is a great technique to use anytime you need a quick distraction to improve a technique you're applying. In this case, it's a standing wristlock.

- You're just about to lock in a wrist hold when your attacker begins to muscle out of it. (Fig. 309)
- Brace his arm against your upper body to hold it briefly with one hand, and then reach toward his side with your other hand. (Fig. 310)
- Using the nails of your index finger and thumb, crab bite the tender flesh over his ribs. For added pain, twist your fingers as if turning a key (skin exposed to better show technique). (Fig. 311)
- When he winces, slam his hand into the wrist flex. (Fig. 312)
- Support it with your other hand. (Fig. 313)

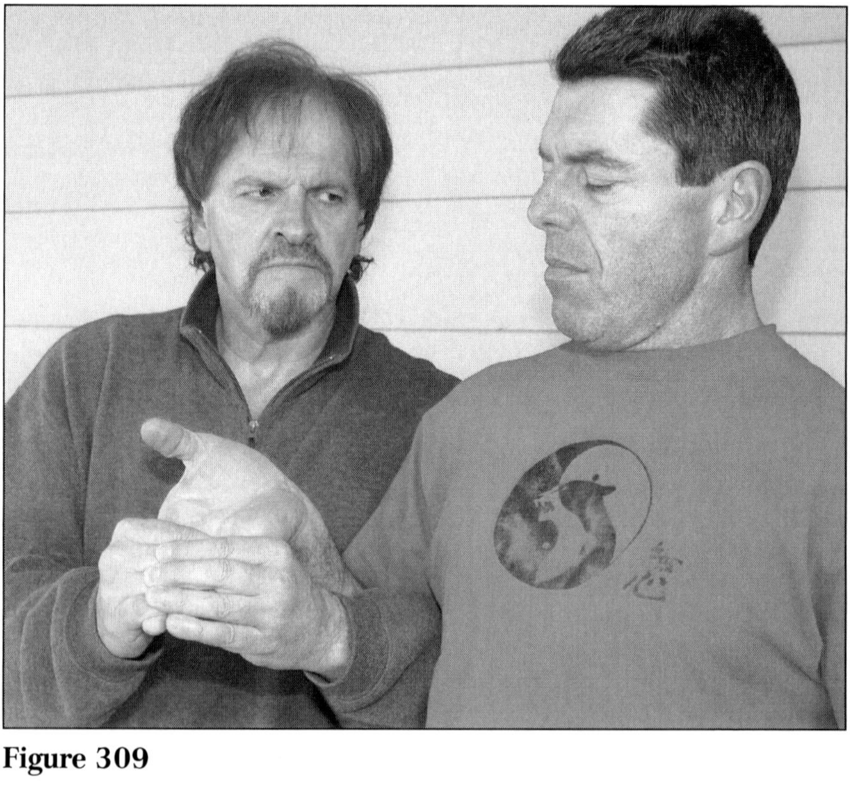

Figure 309

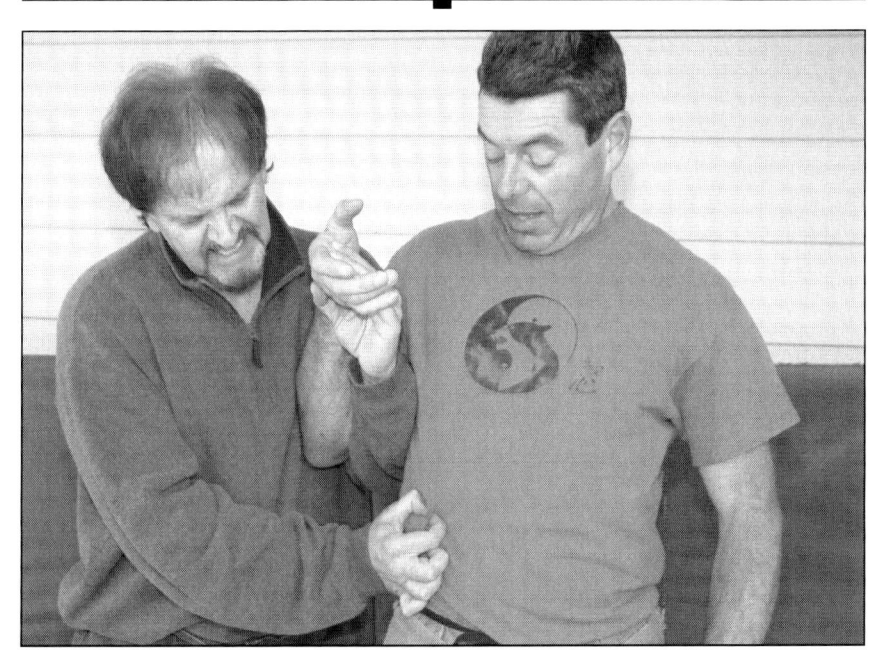

Figure 310

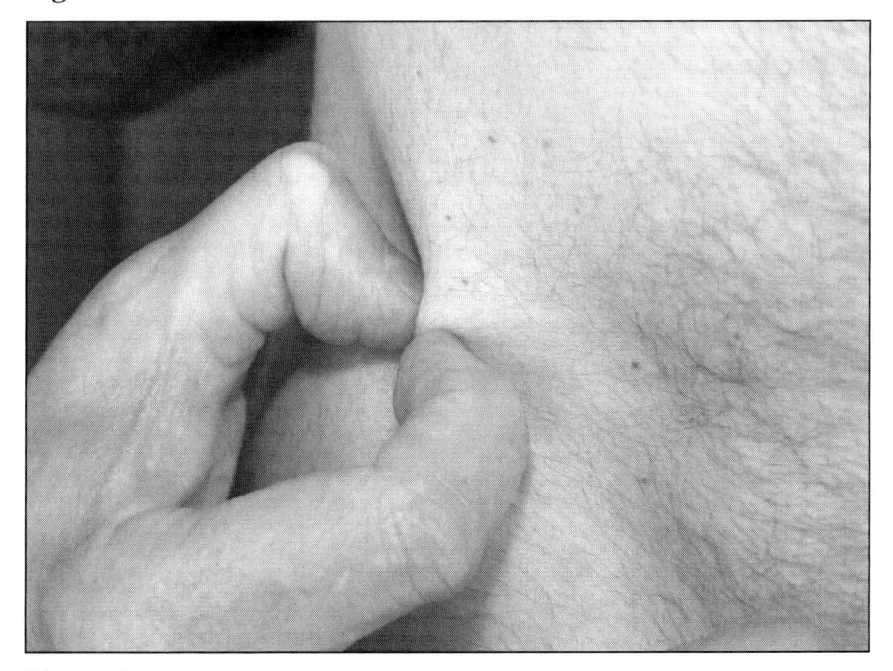

Figure 311

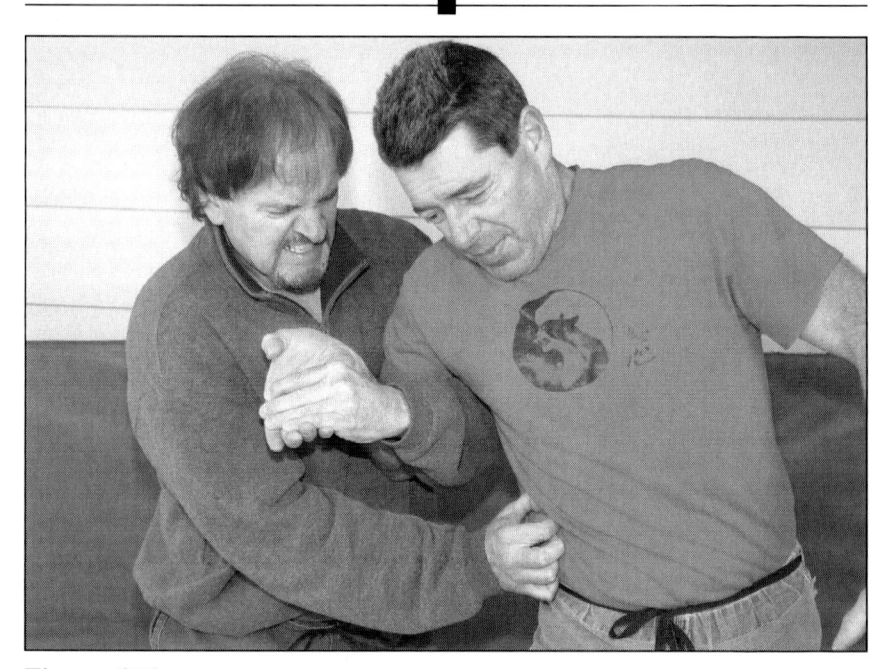

Figure 312

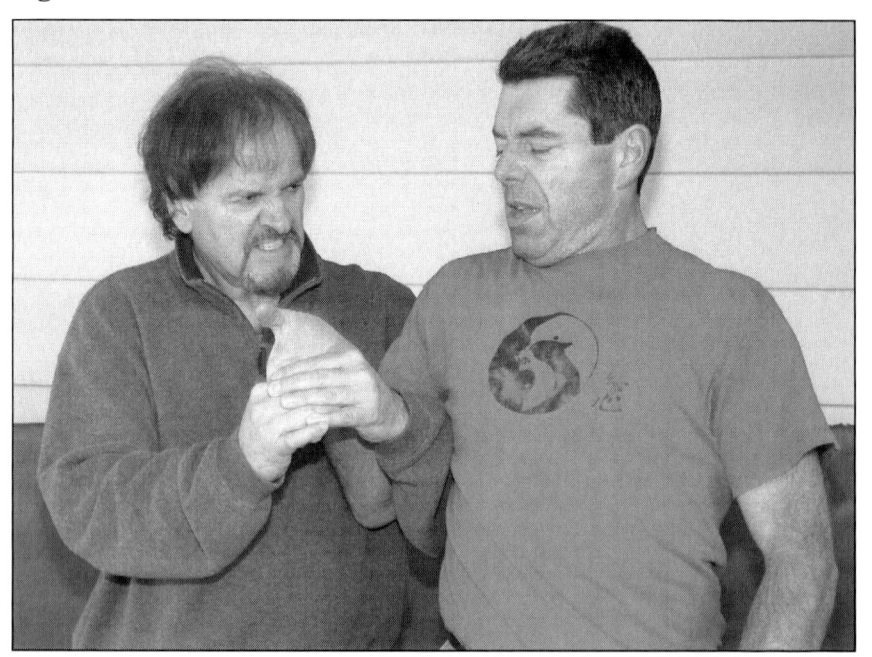

Figure 313

Standing Love Handle Pinch

This will make your attacker grit his teeth and curse like a sailor. It's especially effective because, along with the pain and indignation, it provides clear direction. Most people go up on their tiptoes in a feeble attempt to escape the sharp, excruciating pinch, while others twist, writhe, and stumble forward to get away from you. That is what makes it a good technique to move your attacker across a room and through a doorway. Should he grab hold of the door facing, an extra hard pinch will make him release his hold in a hurry.

Unless your attacker is a real dope, he isn't going to let you do this to him for more than a few seconds before he squirms out of your grip or smacks your hands away. So your goal destination—into a wall, through a door, away from someone he was bullying—should be under 10 feet away.

A bully threatens your friend.

- Approach him from behind and grab his love handles with both hands. Use the four-fingers-to-palm pinch or the five-fingered claw. (Fig. 314)
- If you have especially strong fingers (the love handles tend to be thick), use your thumb and index finger. (Fig. 315)
- Squeeze hard and push him in the direction you want him to go, in this case a wall. (Fig. 316)
- When he hits it, grab his trapezius muscles (muscles on top of the shoulders) and jerk your elbows downward to dump him on the floor. (Fig. 317)

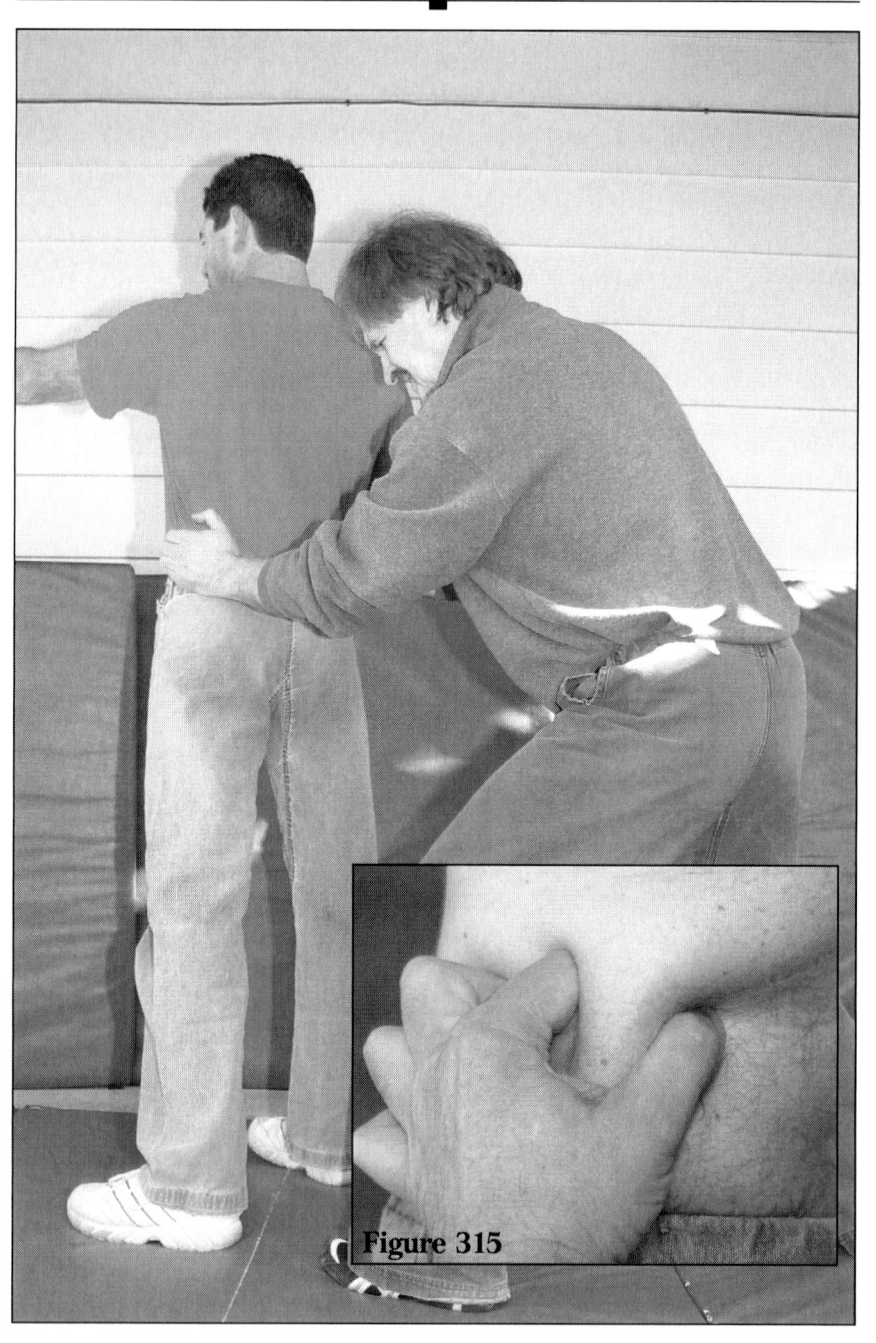

210 *The Brutal Art of Ripping, Poking, and Pressing Vital Targets*

Figure 315

Figure 314

Torso 211

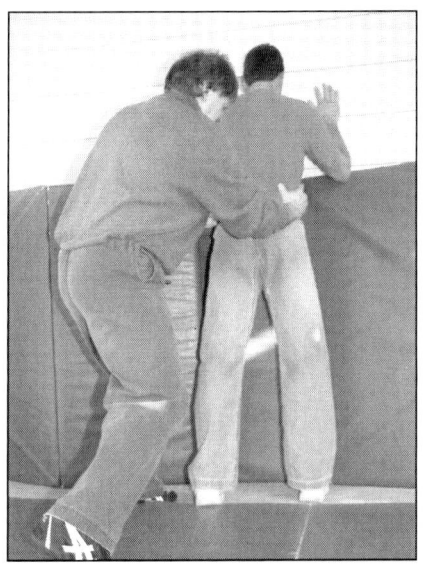

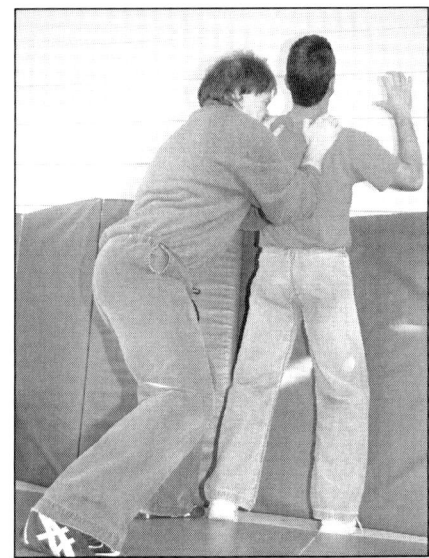

Figure 316

Figure 317

Lying Love Handle Pinch

The argument against using a relatively weak technique in a serious situation where, say, a brawler or rapist is on top of you, is that such moments call for greater force than what a pinch can deliver. This is true. But if your arms are pinned at your sides or in some other way restrained, a seemingly mild technique such as this is a way to open a window of opportunity for you to attack a better target.

The attacker is on top of you.

- Work your hands down to his sides. (Fig. 318)
- Squeeze his love handles. (Fig. 319)
- Buck your hips in whatever direction he leans. (Fig. 320)
- Follow with powerful counters, such as eye claws. (Fig. 321)

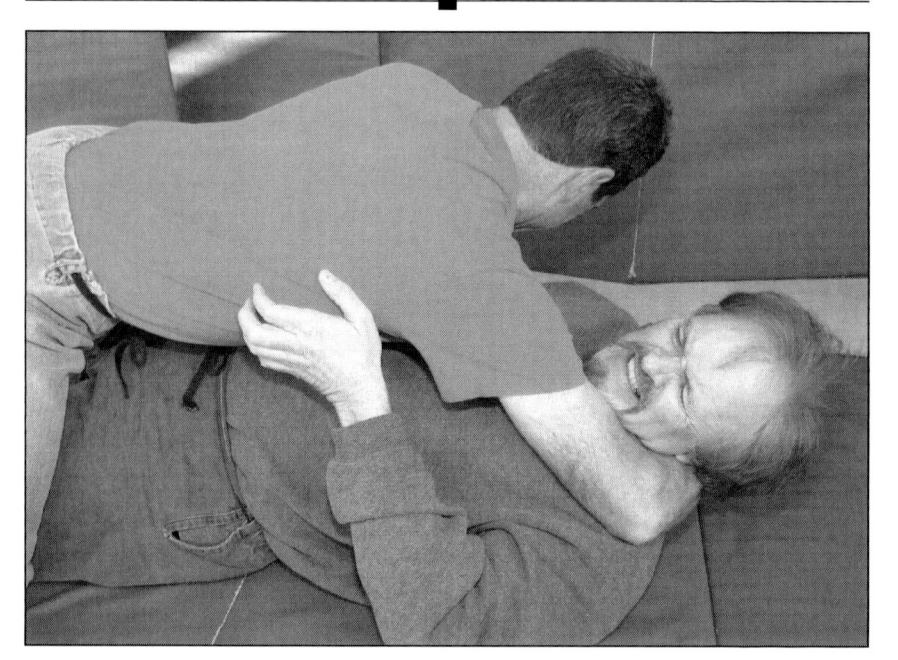

Figure 318

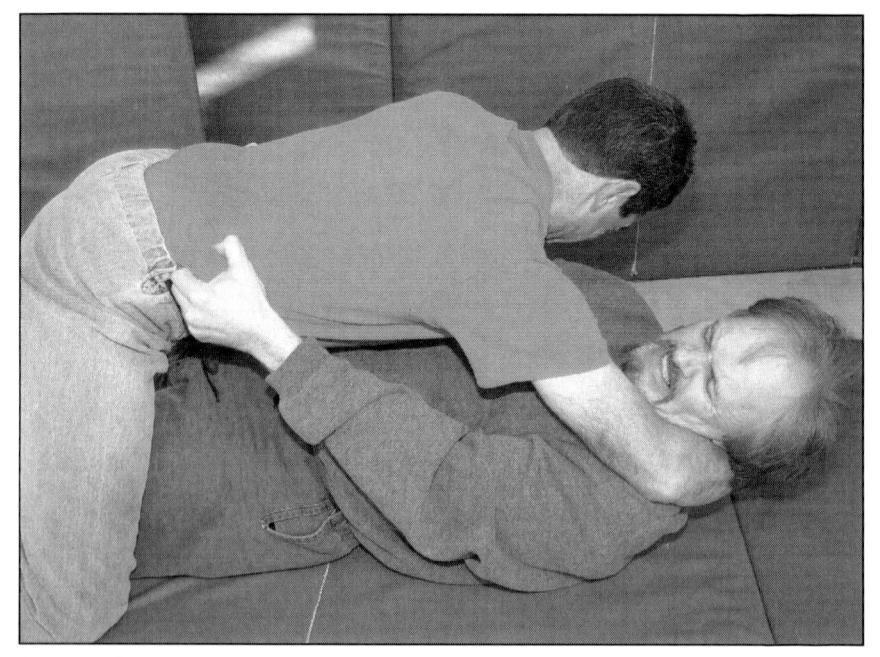

Figure 319

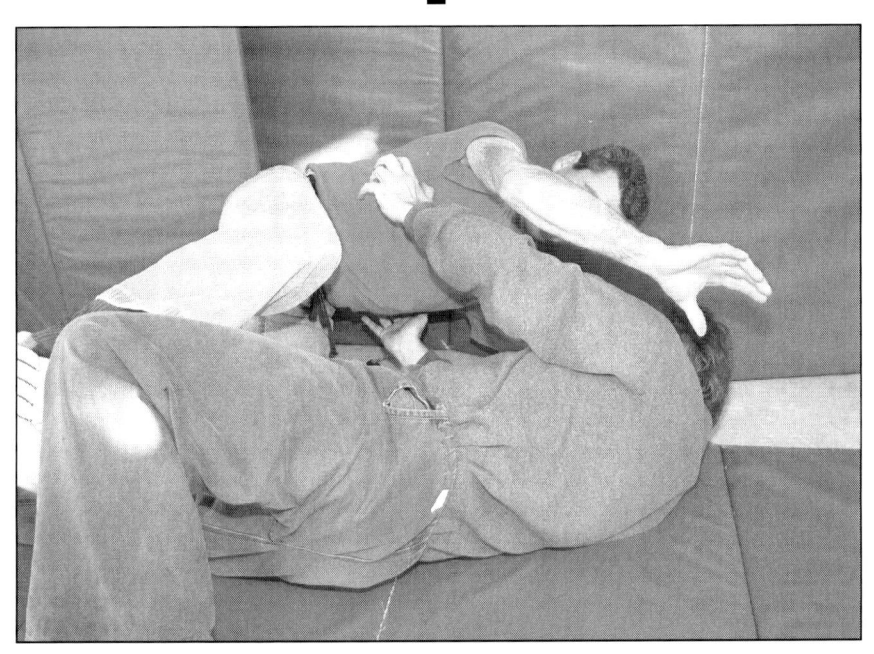

Figure 320

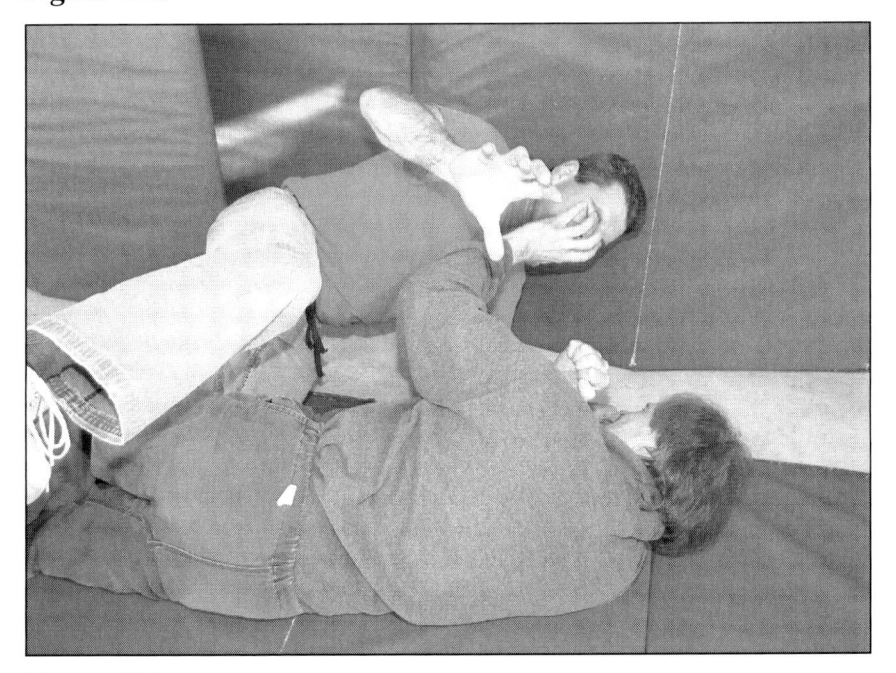

Figure 321

Use Objects in the Environment

Unlike your neat training space, the environment out in the cruel world isn't as tidy. Sometimes this can be used to your advantage.

You take your attacker to the ground.

- You see too late that he has landed on a fist-sized rock. (Fig. 322)
- Since you have control of one arm and his other one is out to his side, you decide to use the rock. Drop your knee and your weight onto his back to press his tender chest more intensely into the hard lump. (Fig. 323)
- If he tries to reach for the rock or you need to apply more pain, increase your weight on his back with your knee and crank hard on your pain compliance hold. (Fig. 324)

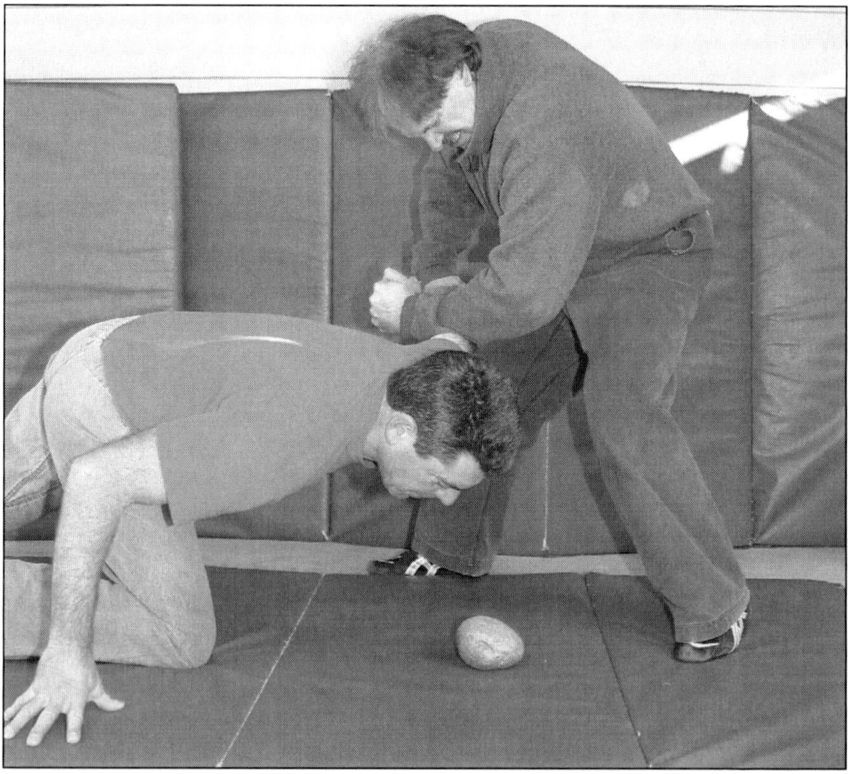

Figure 322

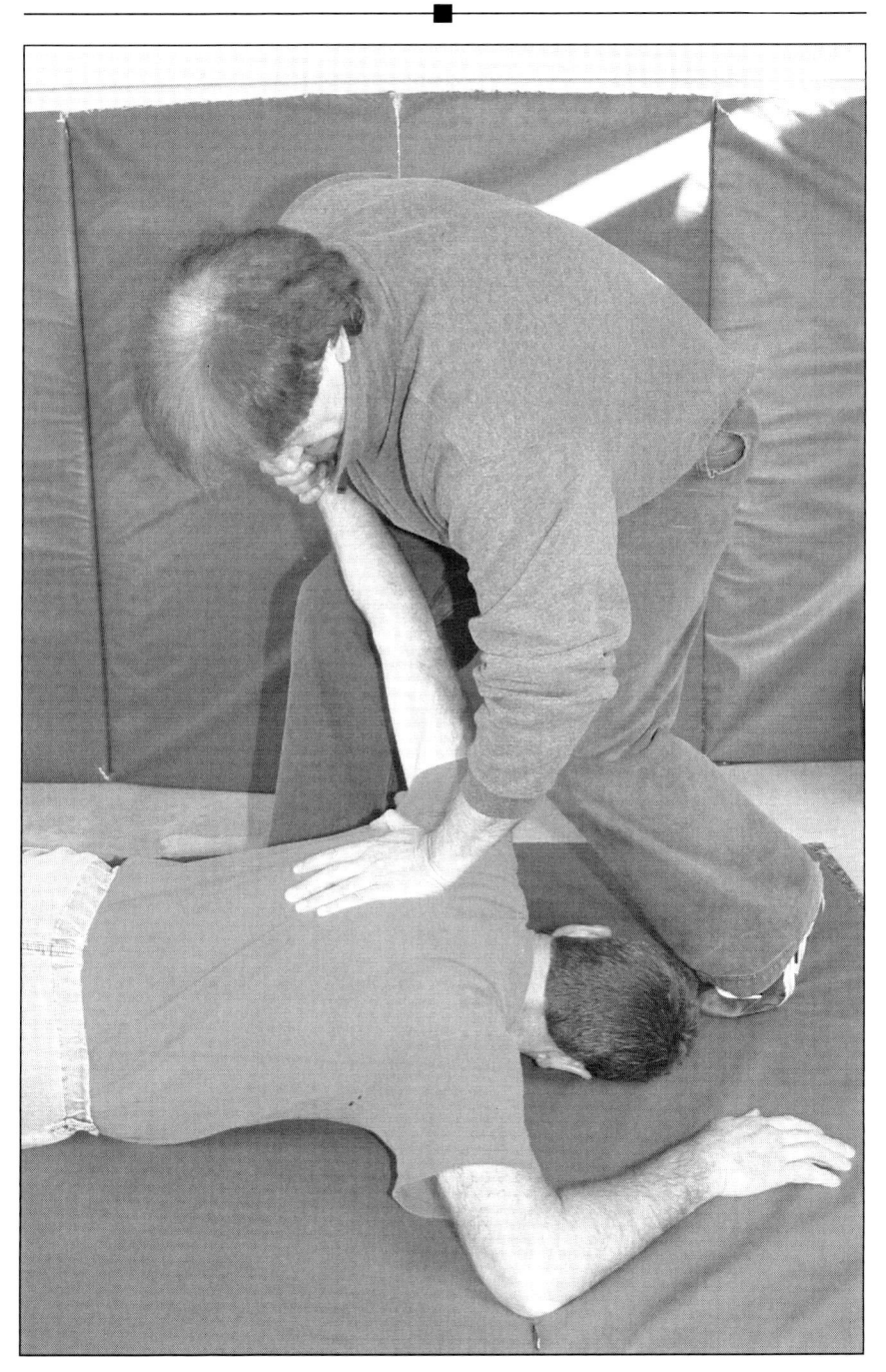

Figure 323

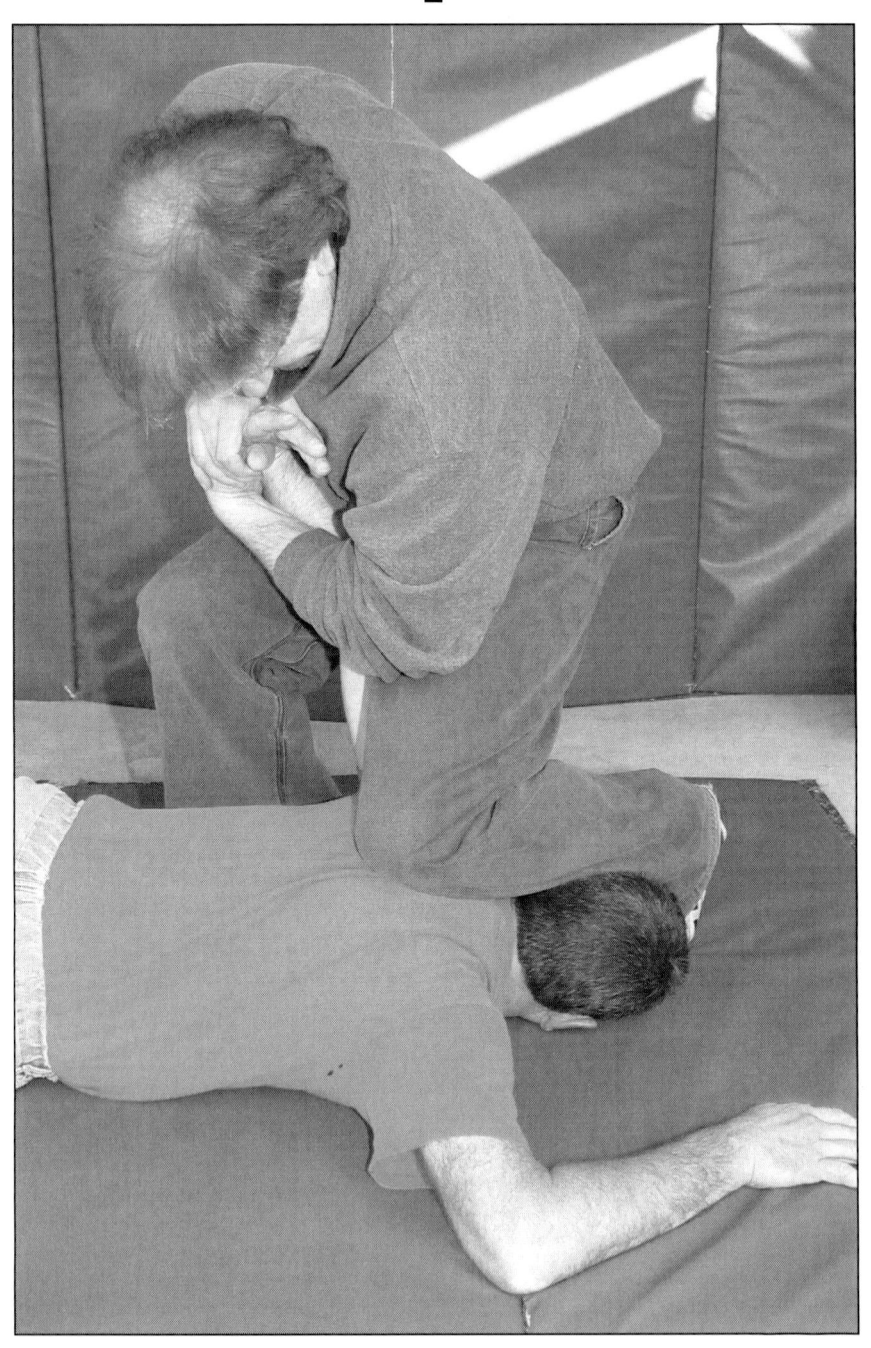

Figure 324

5
Groin

". . . rip his groin toward you as you push his upper body away."

I've always felt that many women's self-defense classes do a disservice to students by telling them that if they kick a man in the groin he will be down for the count. This is not always true. Yes, it hurts to get hit there in class, and it's common to see a kicked student drop into a fetal position and moan in agony.

However, my experience in the street has been just the opposite. A person pumped on adrenaline can often take a groin kick and keep on going. I got kicked hard there once as I was brawling with a big ape in the lobby of a police precinct. It wasn't an intentional kick but rather an inadvertent one that happened during the beef. As hard as it was, I didn't feel it until about 10 minutes later after I'd drug the violent man down a hall and lodged him into a holding cell. Then the nausea flooded in like a tsunami.

While we are going to hit the groin in this chapter, mostly we are going to crush it, rip it, and pinch it. Hey, if you're justified, do all three.

Belgian martial arts experts and my good friends Wim Demeere and Rock Dehon demonstrate in the photos. Demeere acts as the defender.

Foot Rip Back

This has the best effect when your attacker is wearing loose fitting pants because the, uh, target will be ripped more. The technique will still work, but to a lesser degree, when the attacker is wearing tight pants.

Your attacker launches a big, arcing haymaker.

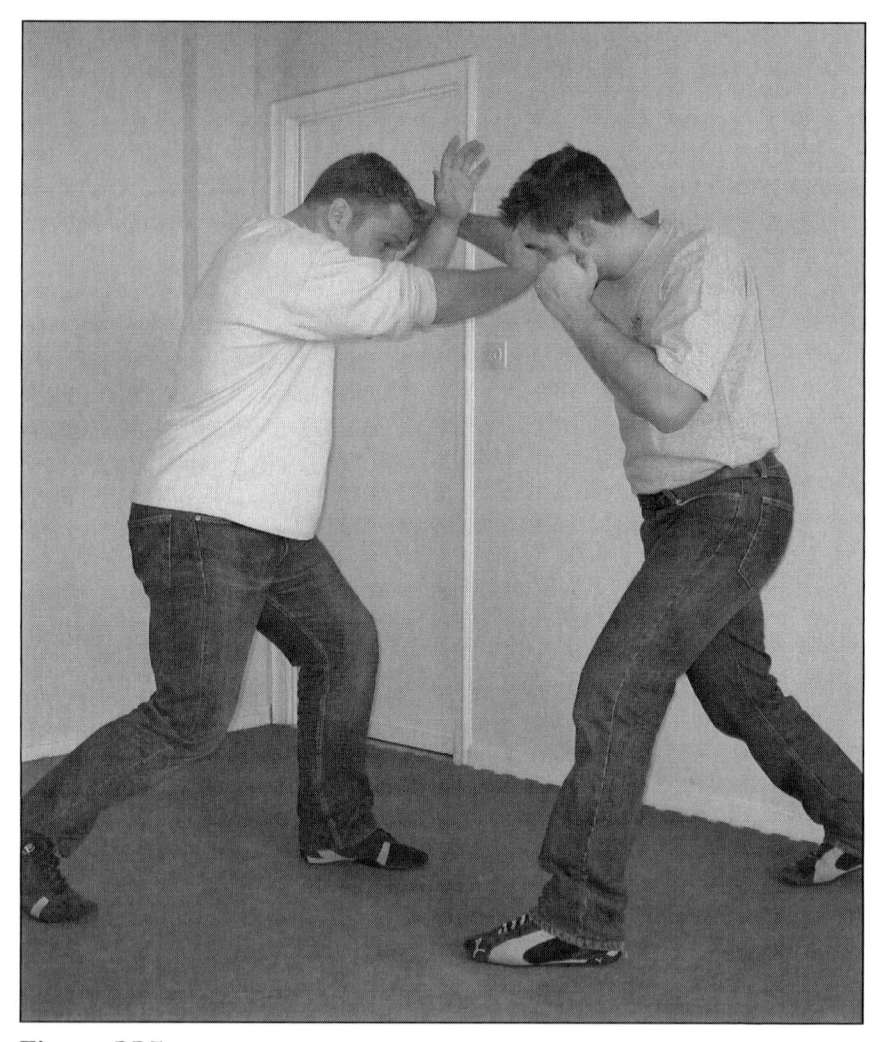

Figure 325

- Lower yourself for stability and block it with one or both arms. (Fig. 325)

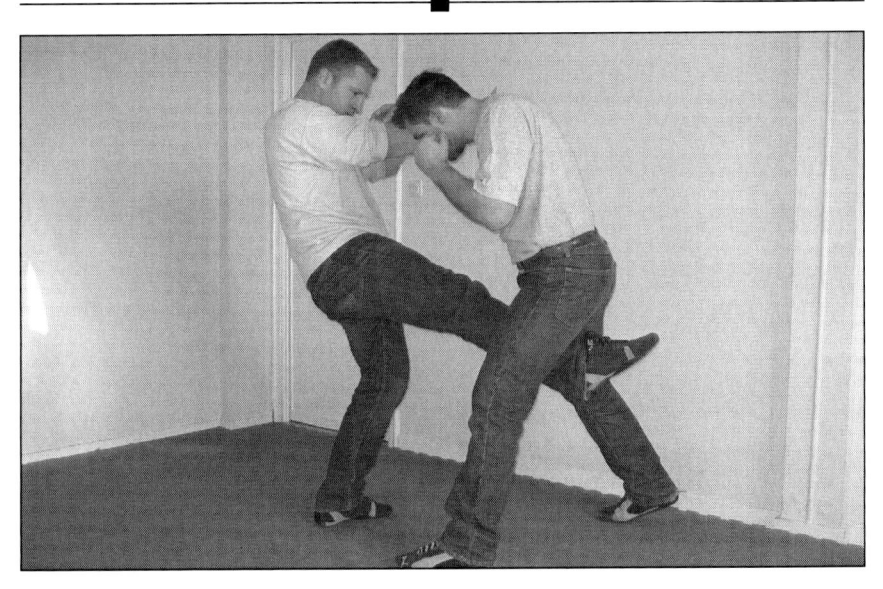

Figure 326

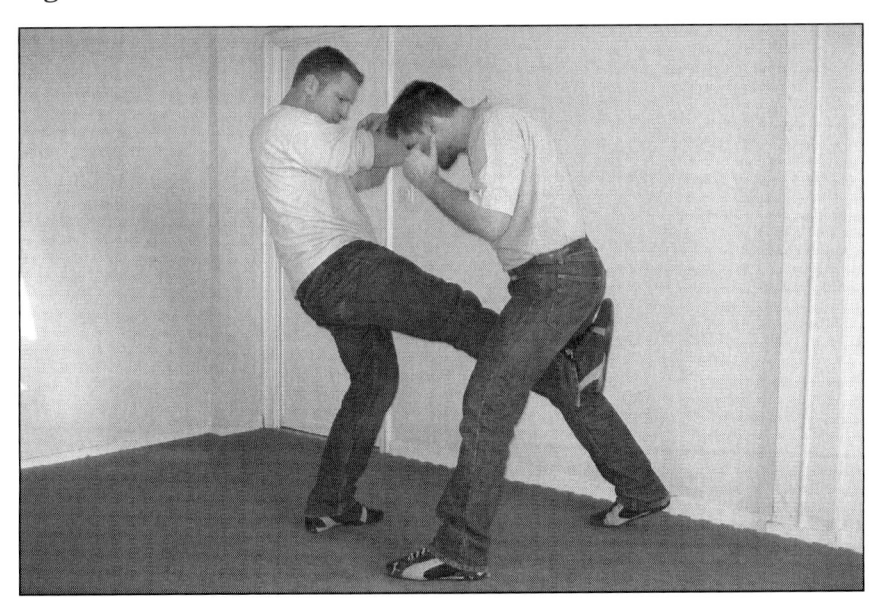

Figure 327

- Snap either foot between his legs—the front is fastest and the rear is strongest—impacting with your lower shin. (Fig. 326)
- Turn your toes upward to form a hook of sorts. (Fig. 327)

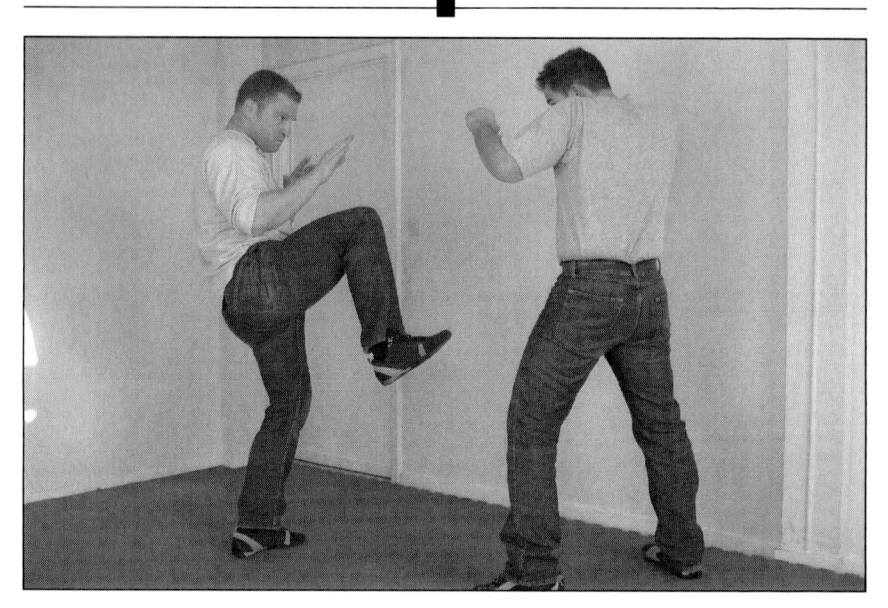

Figure 328

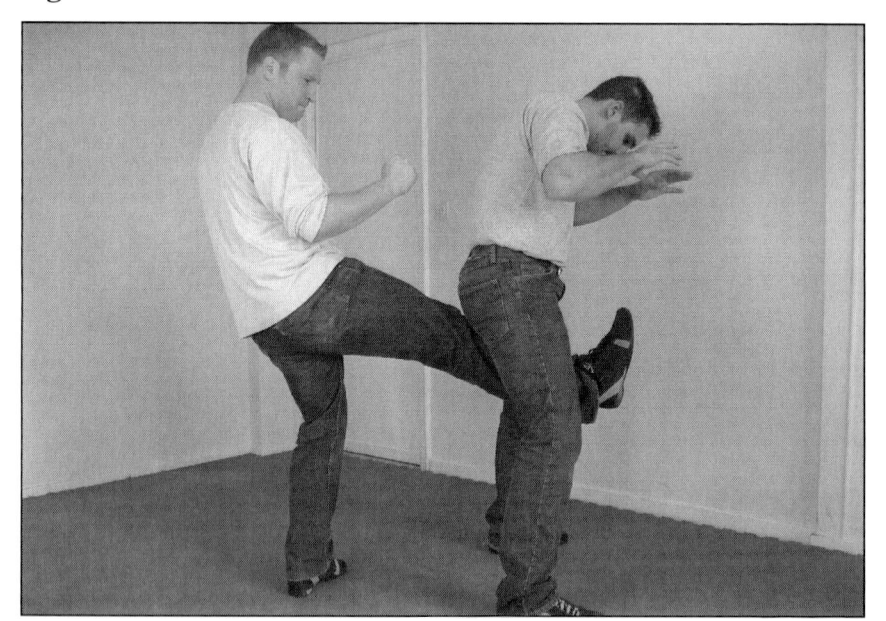

Figure 329

- Forcefully jerk your foot toward you to rip his groin. (Fig. 328)
- You can also kick and rip it from behind. (Figs. 329, 330)

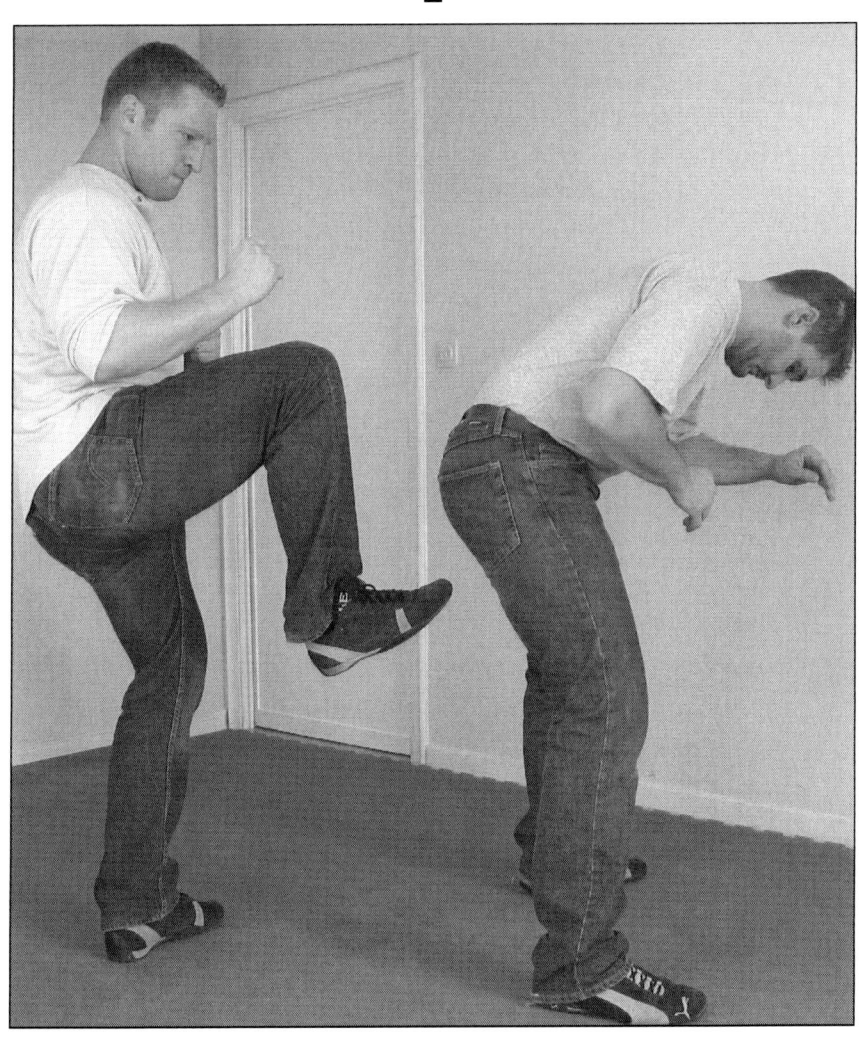

Figure 330

Foot Rip Forward

This technique, which works even at close range, will give your attacker some absolute misery.

Your attacker moves toward you with clenched fists.

- Imagine that you're standing before a set of stairs and lift your leg

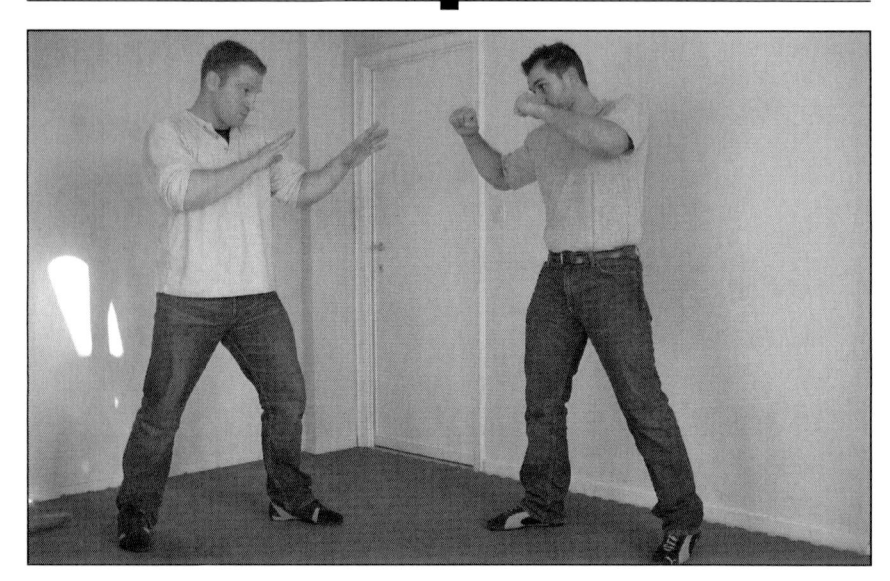

Figure 331

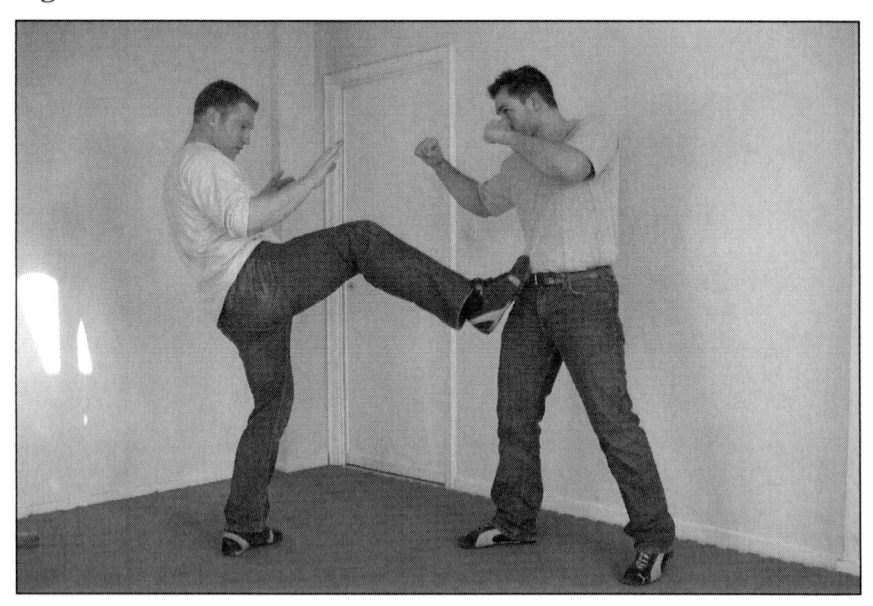

Figure 332

high enough to clear three steps. But instead of landing on a step, use this stepping motion to land with the ball of your foot just above your attacker's privates. (Figs. 331, 332)

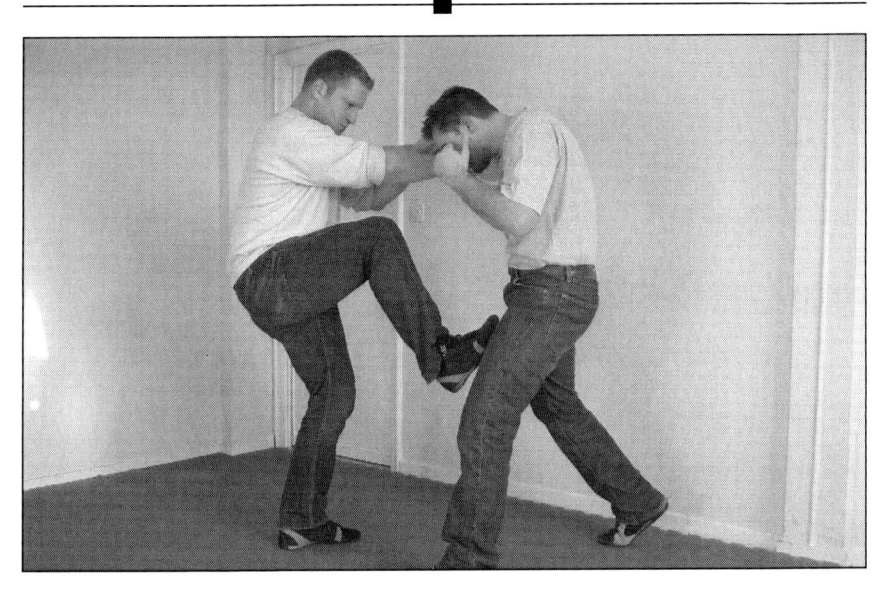

Figure 333

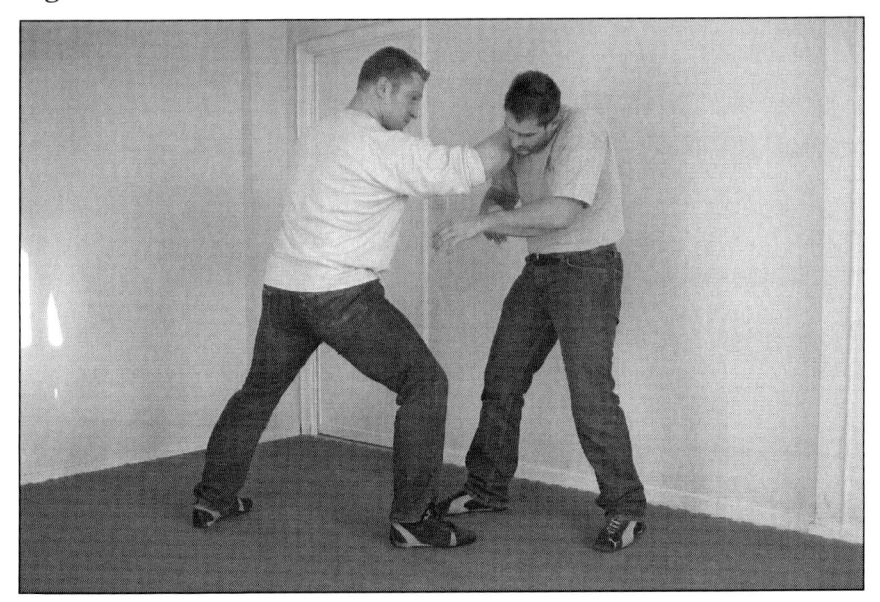

Figure 334

- Press down hard with the ball of your foot to rip through his groin. (Fig. 333)
- Follow with a forearm smash as your foot lands on the floor. (Fig. 334)

Calf Press and Groin Rip

You are trying to apply a figure-four lock on your attacker's calf muscle, but he resists by turning his leg.

- Shoot the heel of your foot into his groin. (Figs. 335, 336)

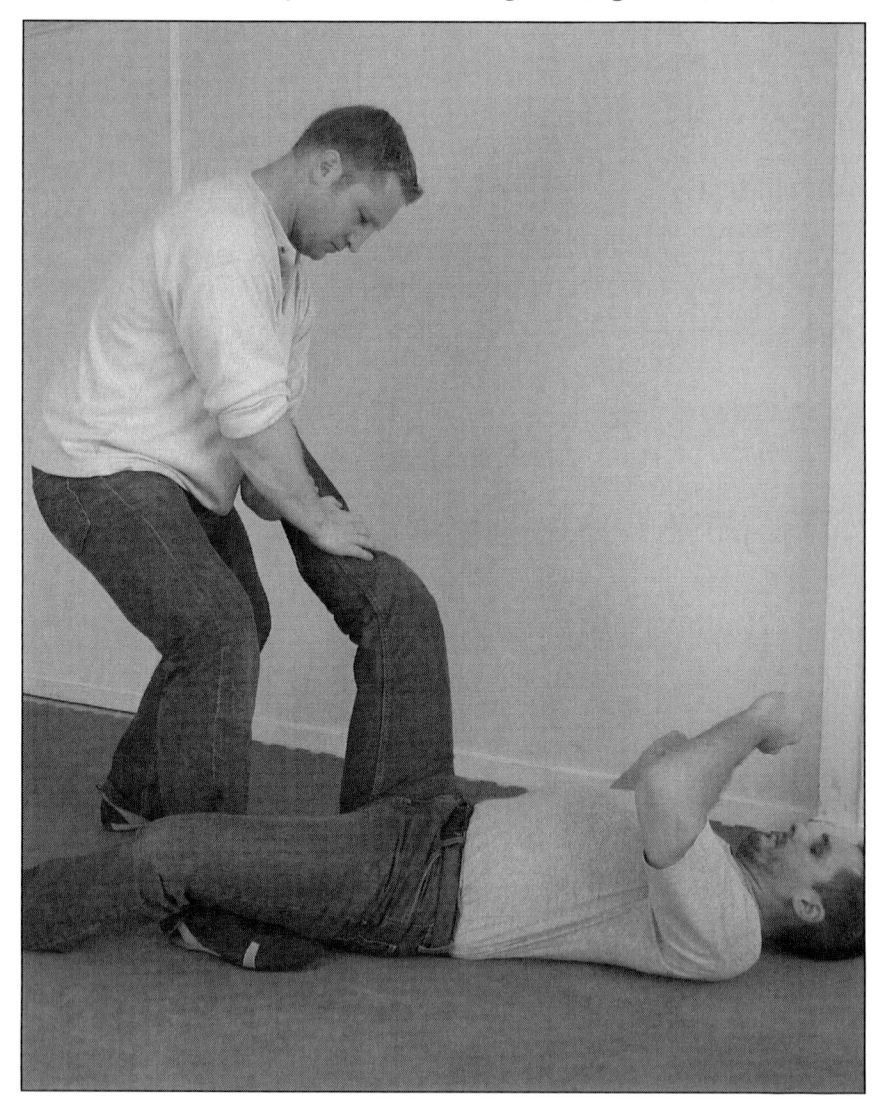

Figure 335

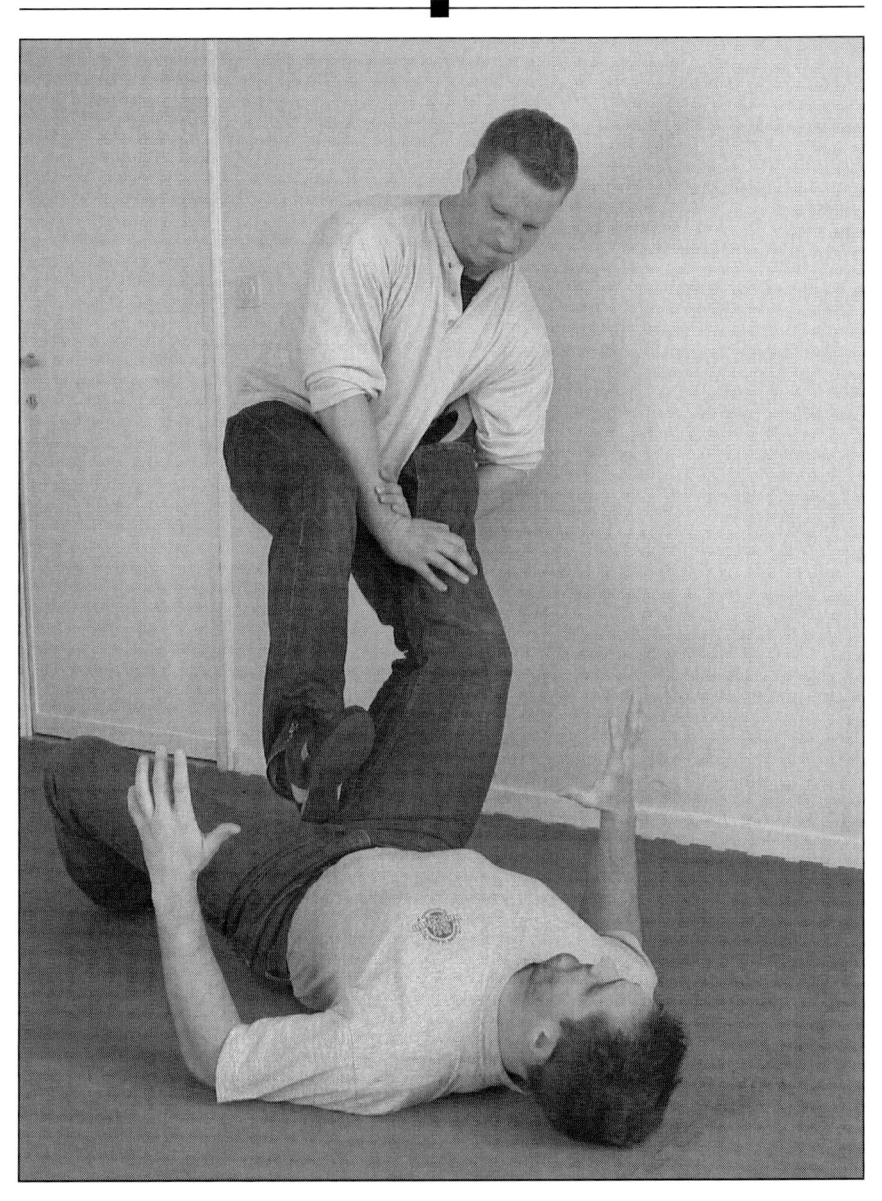

Figure 336

- Press into it as you pull his leg toward you to underscore the pressure on his groin. Then forcefully rip your heel off of it to give him a major shock of pain. (Fig. 337)
- Quickly apply a better figure-four lock. (Fig. 338)

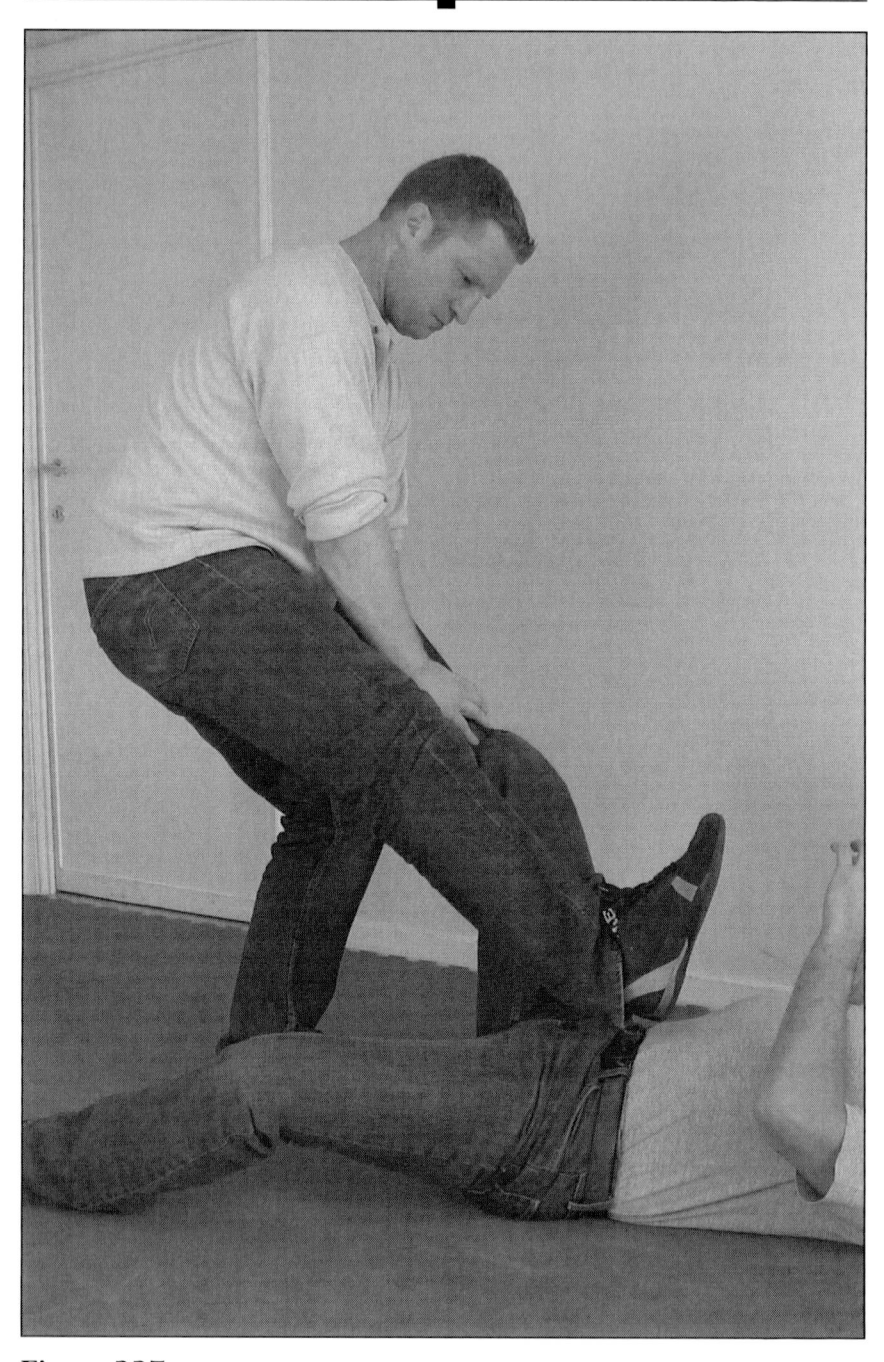

Figure 337

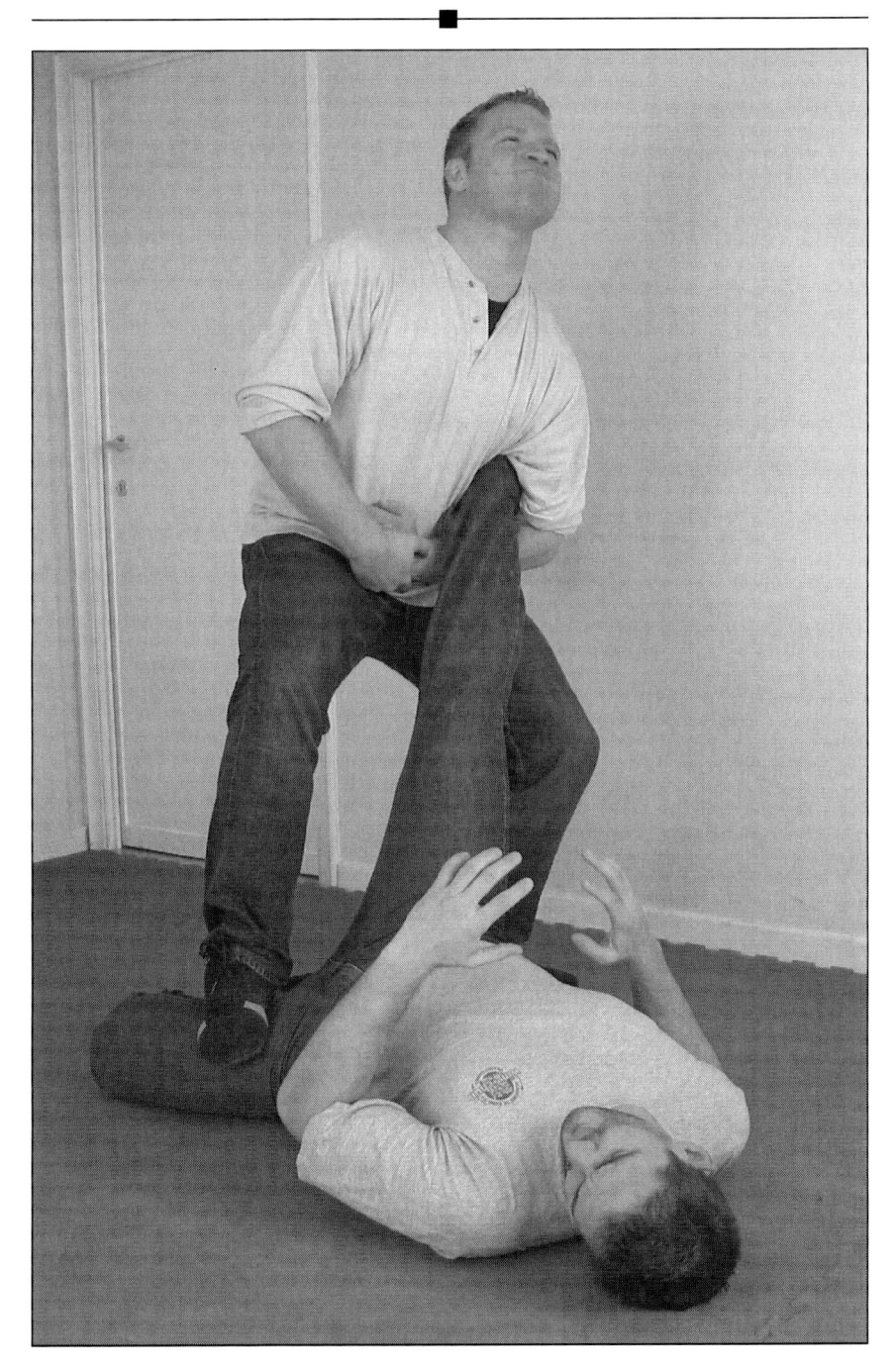

Figure 338

Five-Fingered Claw Rip

Your attacker throws a right cross at you.

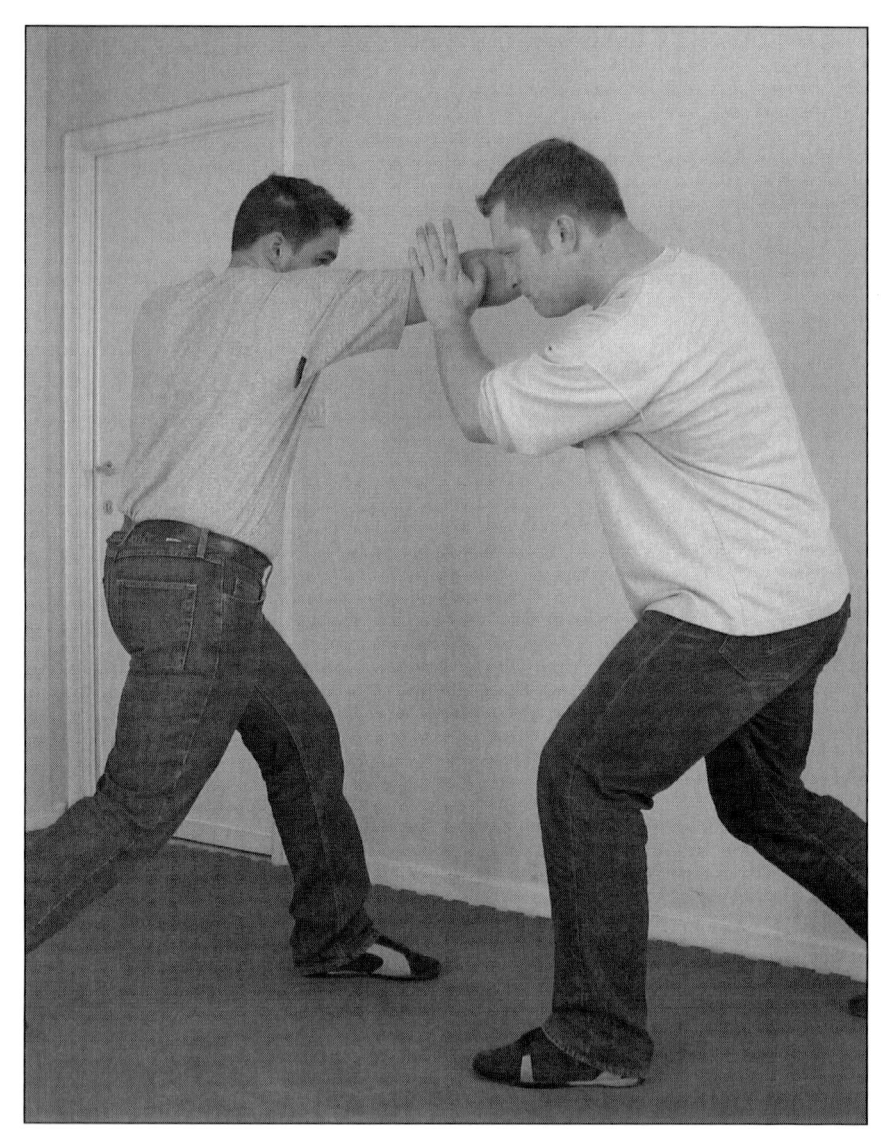

Figure 339

- Block his punch with a left sweep (Fig. 339)

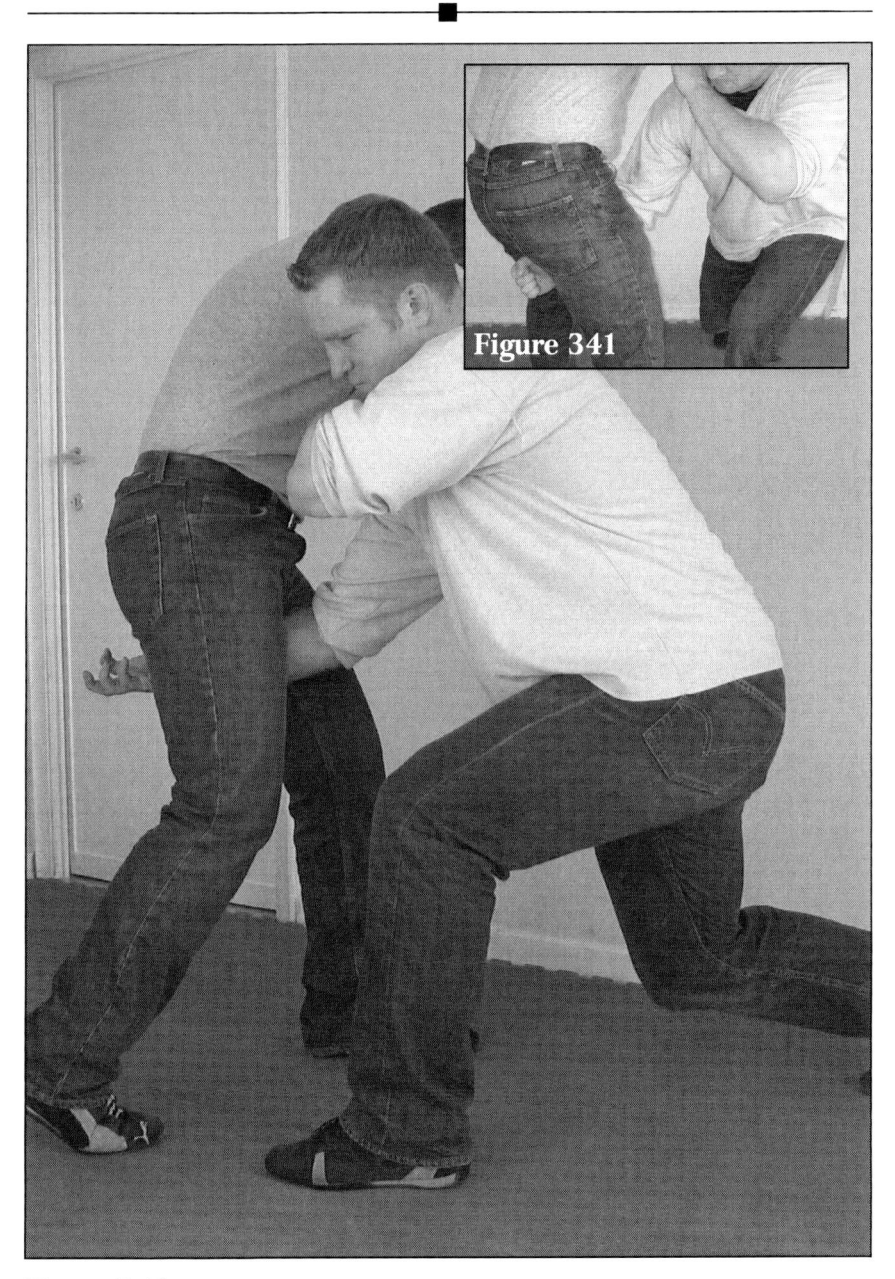

Figure 340

- Slam your right wrist up into his groin. Your hand should be extended slightly past his crotch. (Figs. 340, 341)

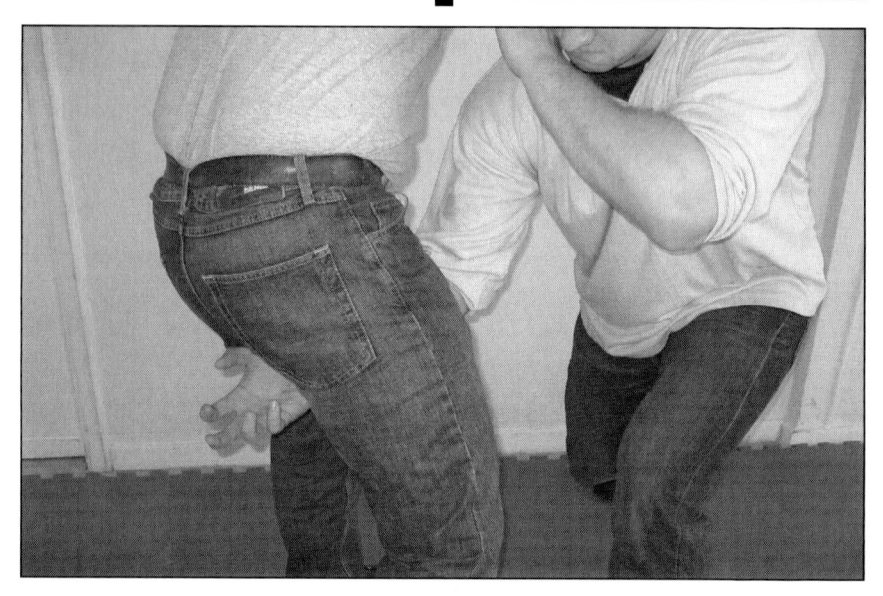

Figure 342

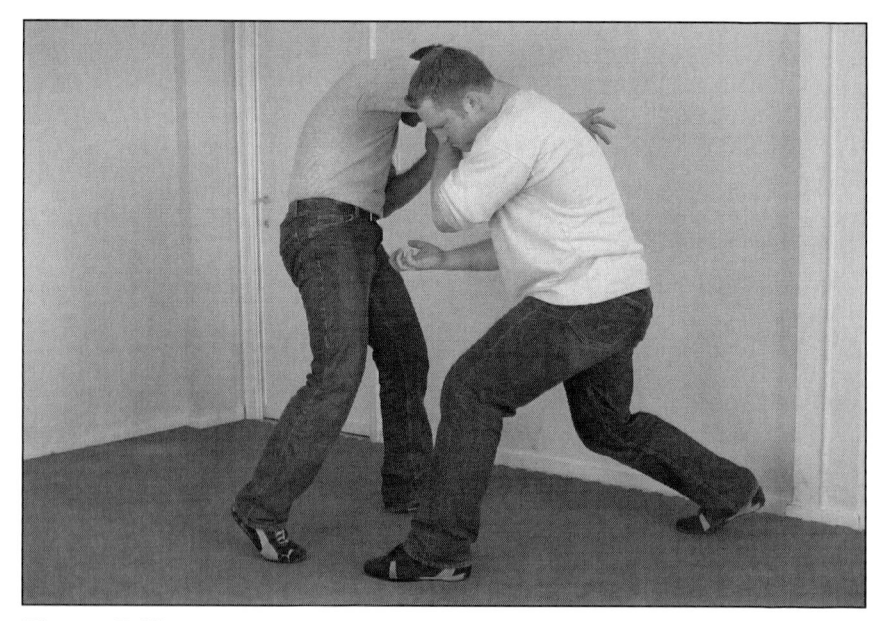

Figure 343

- Curl your fingers upward into a stiff claw. (Fig. 342)
- With upward pressure, yank your hand back toward you. (Fig. 343)

Grab, Squeeze, and Rip

A bully approaches your table as you sit.

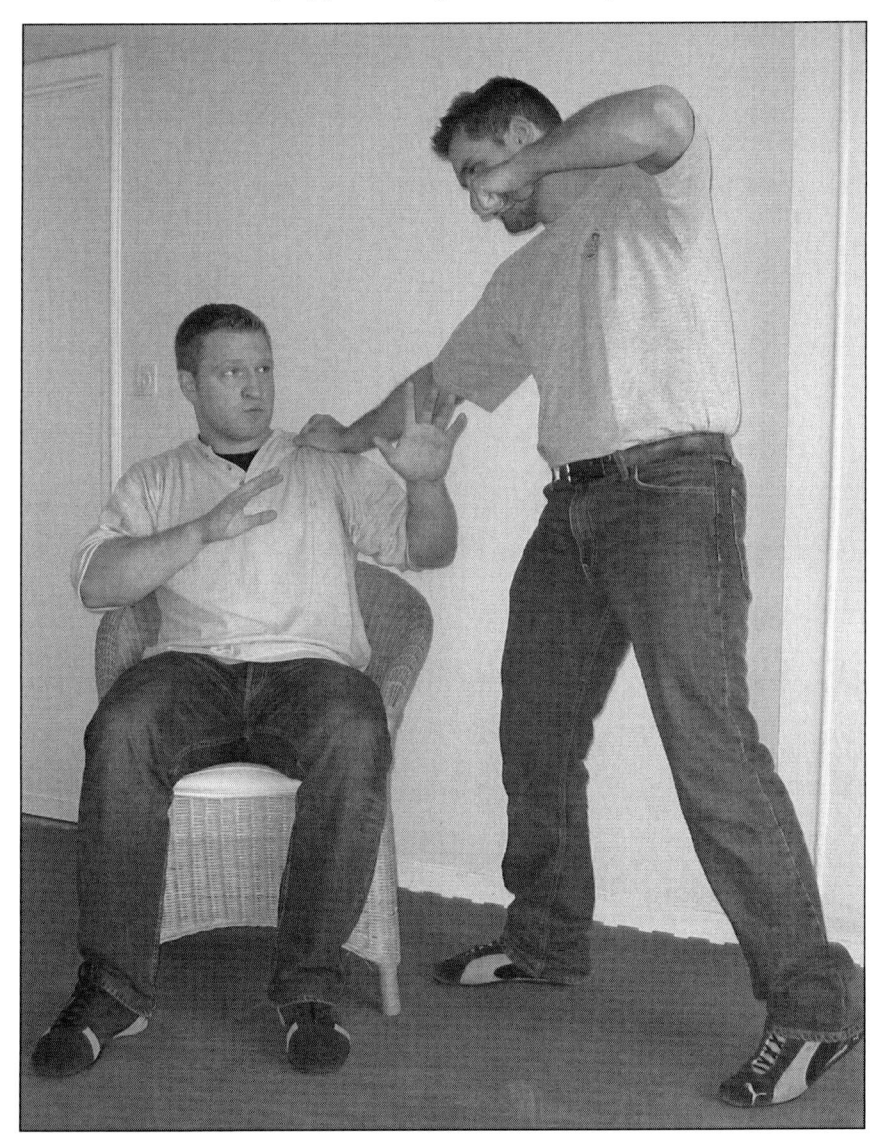

Figure 344

- He puts his hand threateningly on your shoulder. (Fig. 344)

- With your farthest hand, grab his groin and squeeze as you brace your other hand or forearm on his chest or abdomen for support. (Fig. 345)
- Rip his groin toward you as you push his upper body away. Even if he is too heavy to move or you're in a poor position to move him, the ripping effect still works to some degree. (Fig. 346)

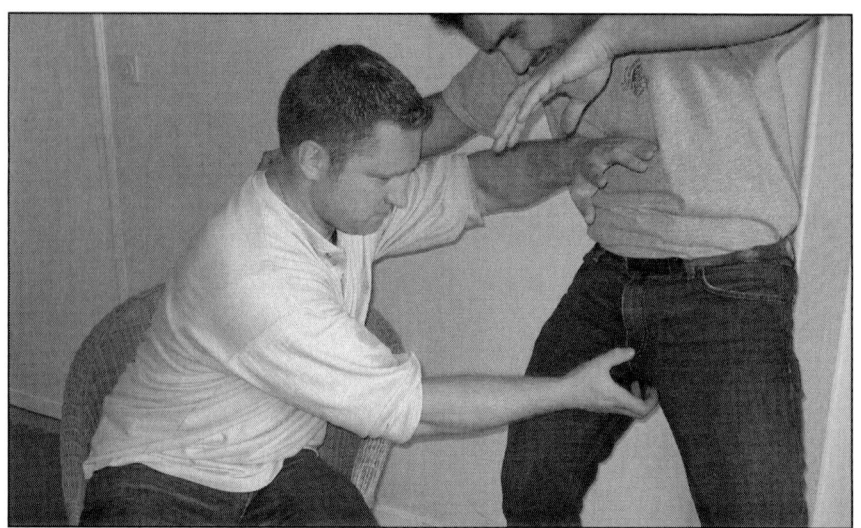

Figure 345

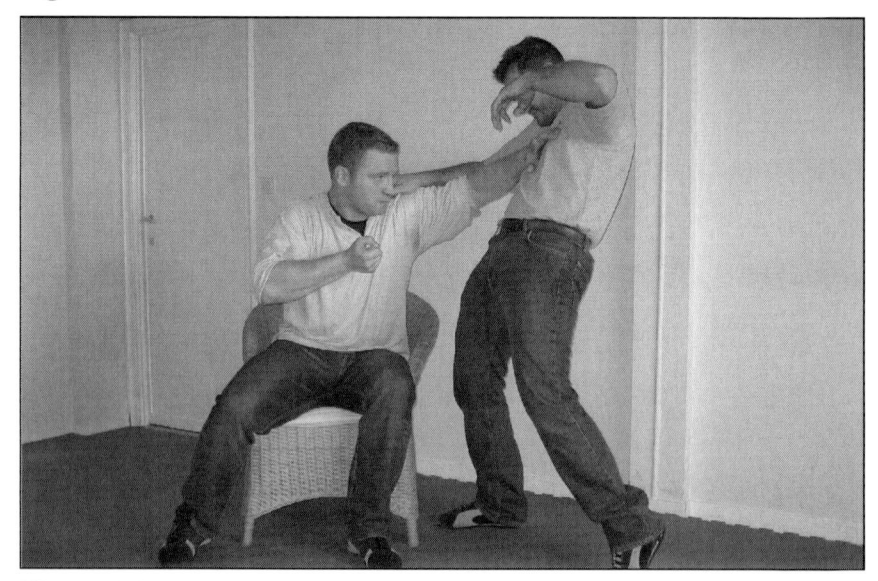

Figure 346

Variation:

- Just before you rip your hand away . . . (Fig. 347)
- . . . rotate it and then rip. (Fig. 348)

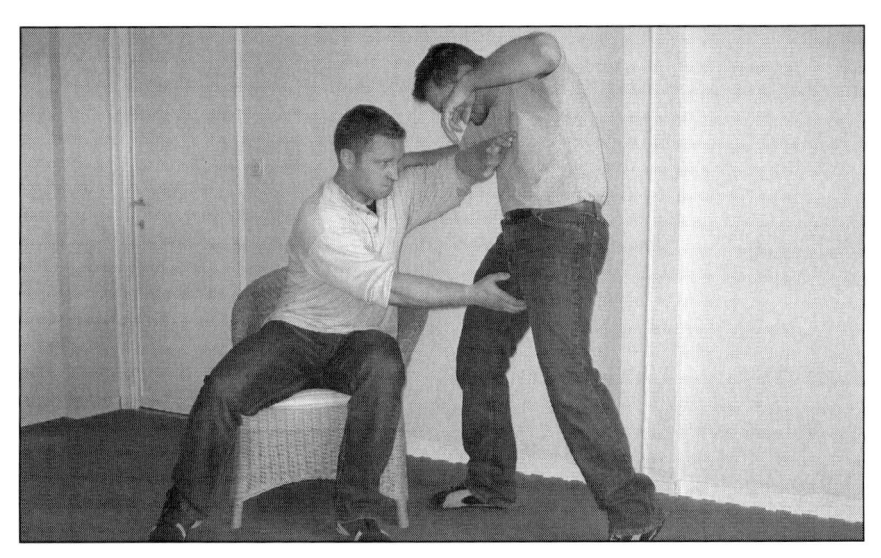

Figure 347

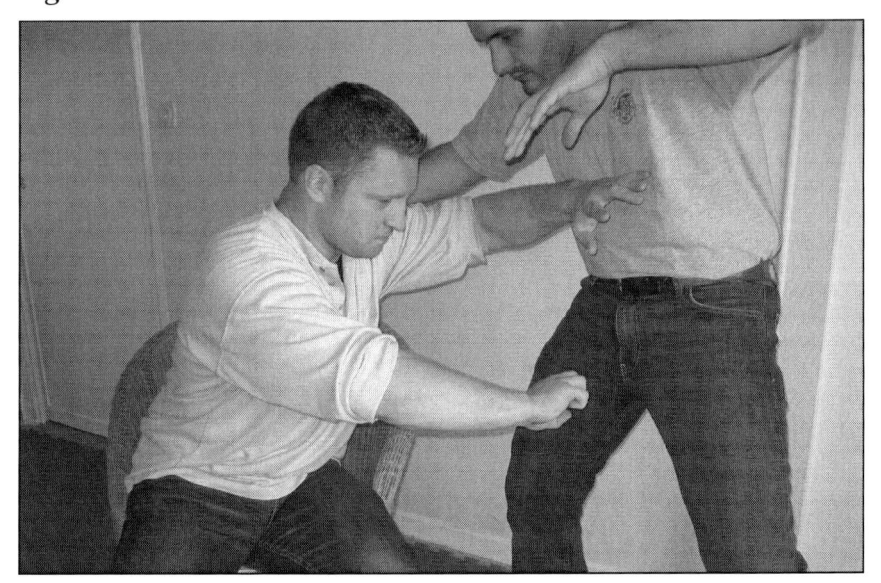

Figure 348

Groin Press with Knee and Shin

Your attacker is on his back trying to scissor you with his legs.

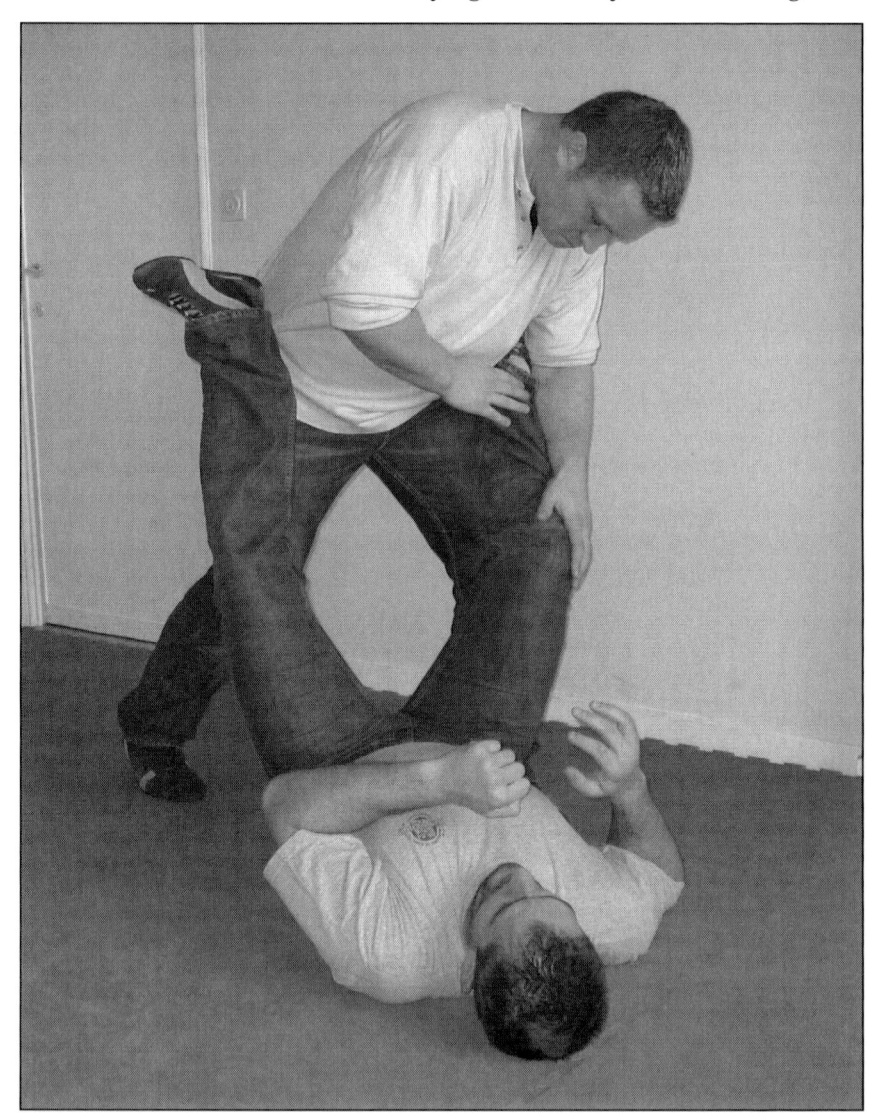

Figure 349

- Drop your knee or shin between his legs. (Fig. 349)

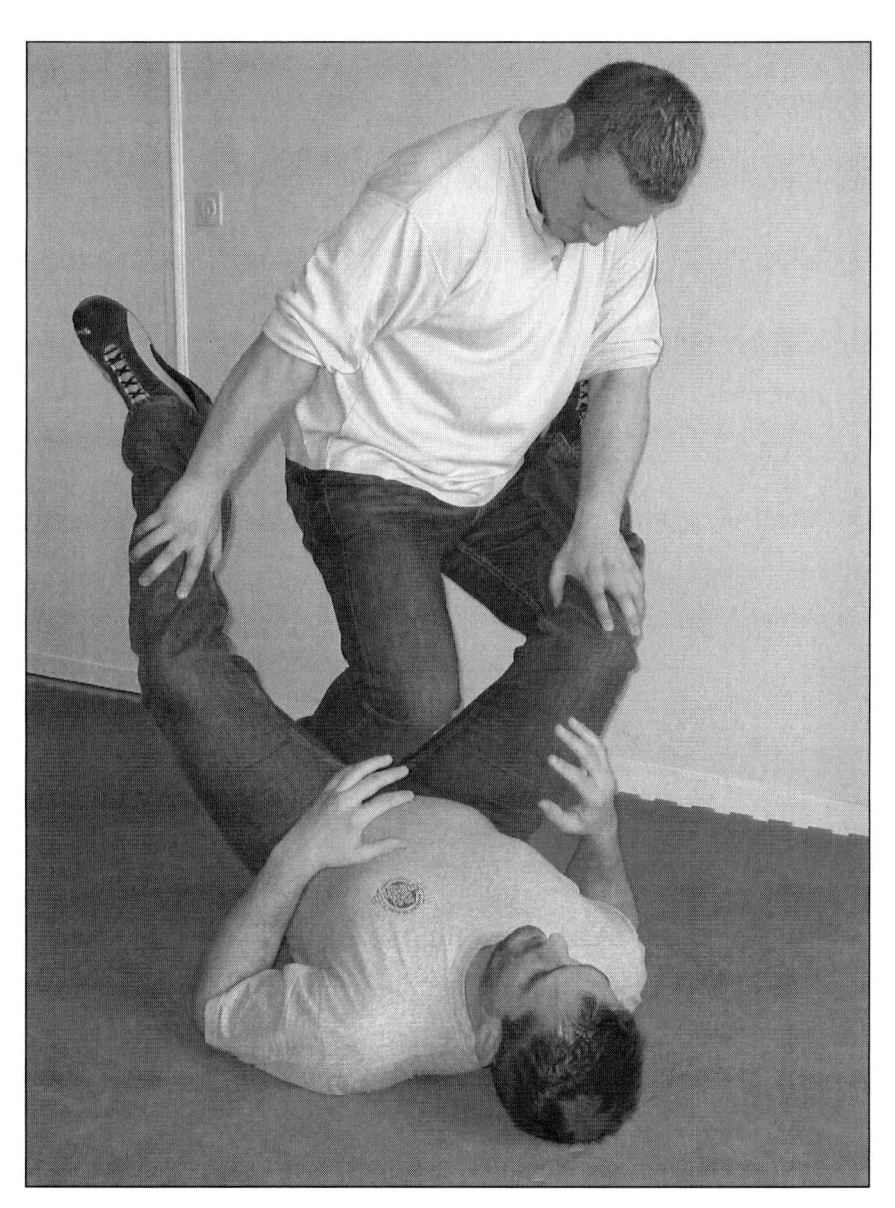

Figure 350

- Hold his legs for support and press your leg into him. If you have an extra two seconds, saw your knee or shin back and forth an inch or two in each direction. (Fig. 350)

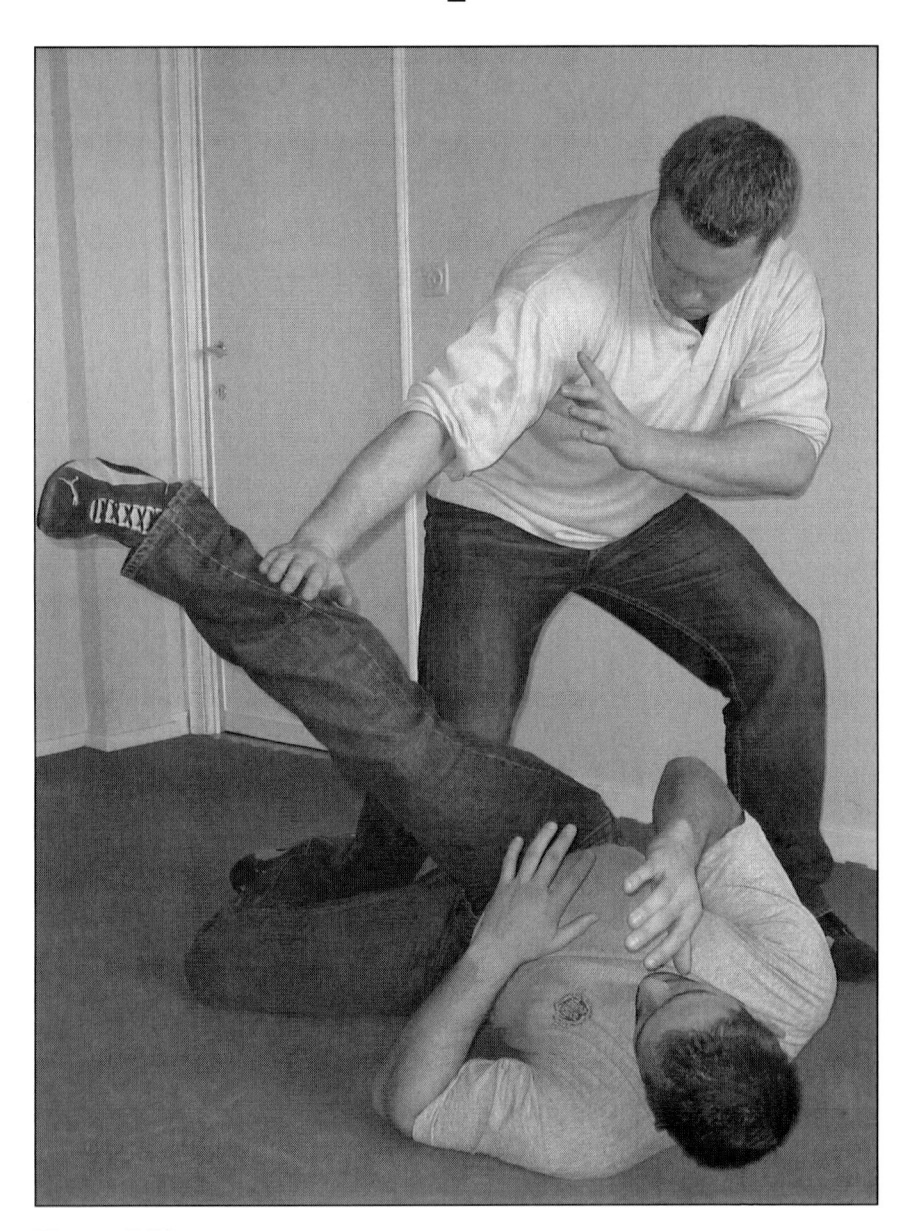

Figure 351

- Besides inflicting pain, your purpose here is to distract him from his scissors so that you can apply a hold or knock his legs aside. (Fig. 351)

6

Legs

". . . control his lower half by pressing one or both of his shins into the edge of the cement step."

The muscles of the legs, though large and powerful, nonetheless contain "hot" spots that are vulnerable to pressing, ripping, and twisting. Most of these techniques won't debilitate your attacker, but they will distract him long enough for you to counter with a stronger technique or escape. As always, intoxication, mental illness, and extreme rage can make these techniques ineffective.

Inner Thigh Pinch

This one often makes even the most macho man scream like a little girl. As a cop I used it to distract people who stiffened their arms to resist being handcuffed. It worked like a charm on sober people, inconsistently on those high on intoxicants.

You're escorting your drunken brother-in-law out of the family gathering.

- You have him in a wristlock but, when he gets to the doorway, he braces himself against the doorjamb with his free arm. (Fig. 352)
- When he pushes against the jamb you start to lose the wristlock. (Fig. 353)
- Quickly reach down and pinch his closest inner thigh with your thumb and index finger, or with the four-fingers-to-palm grip. (Fig. 354)
- As soon as he jerks in pain, slam your wrist hold on tighter and push him the rest of the way through the door. (Fig. 355)

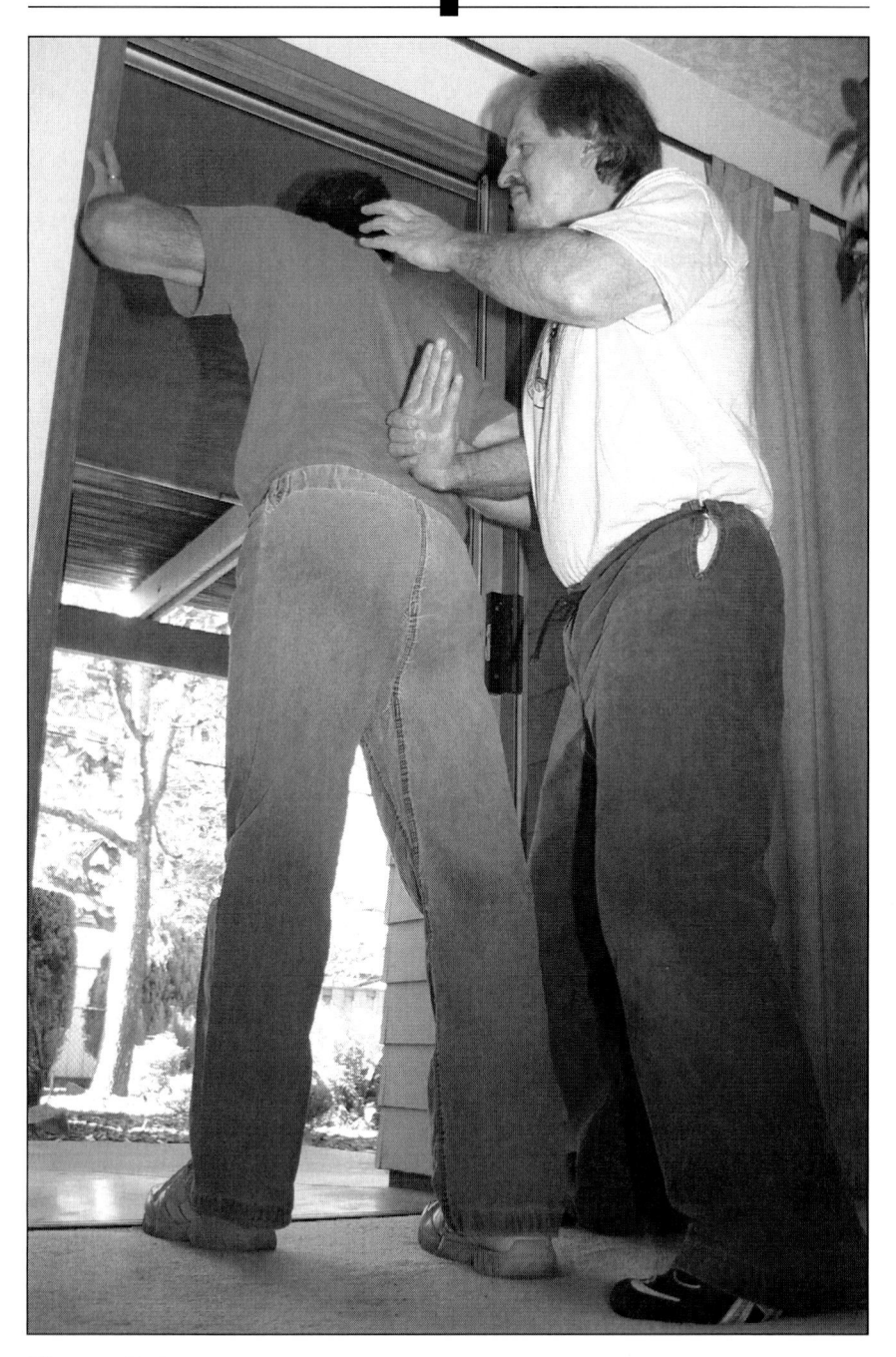

Figure 352

Legs 239

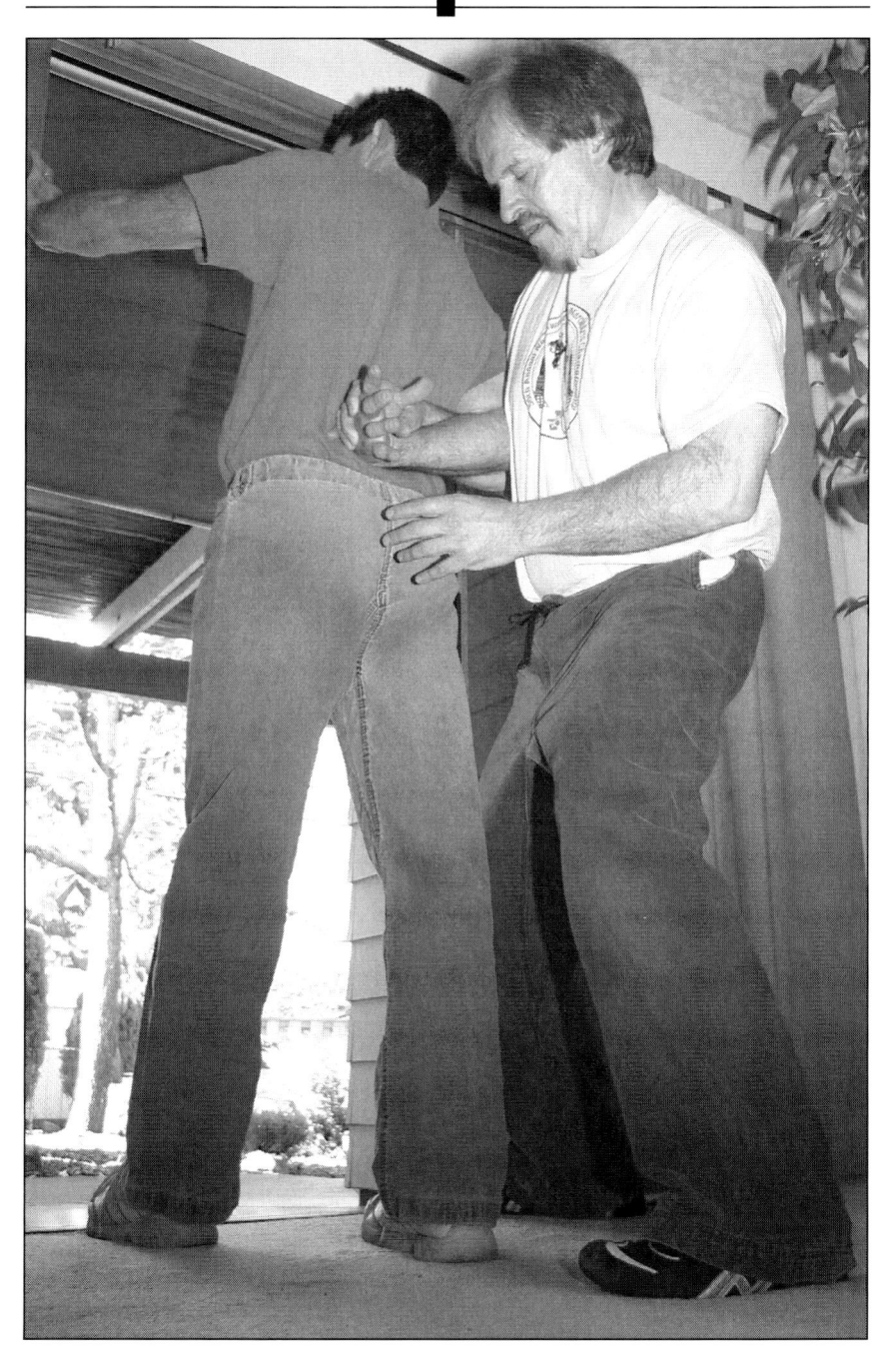

Figure 353

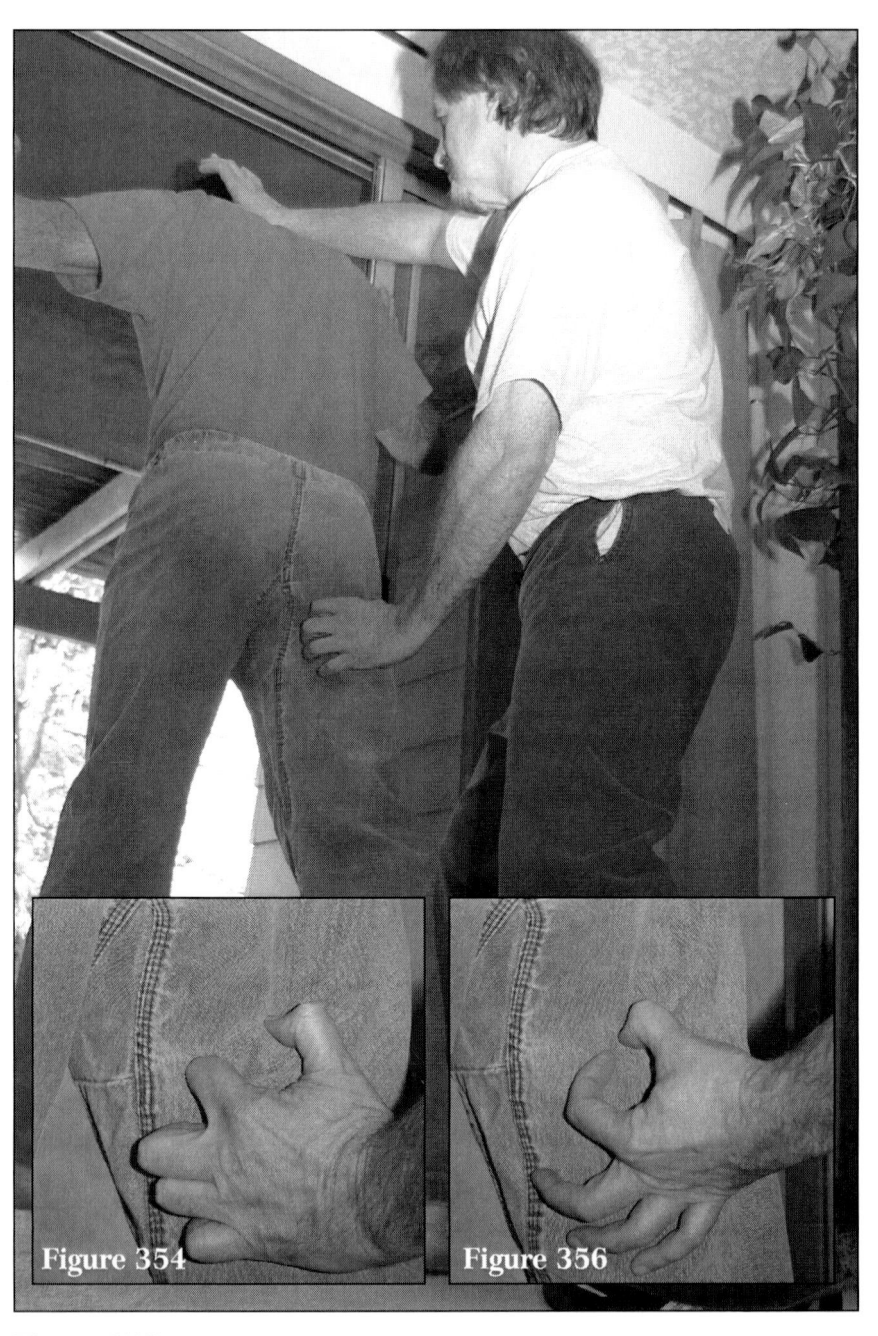

240 *The Brutal Art of Ripping, Poking, and Pressing Vital Targets*

Figure 354

Figure 356

Figure 355

Legs 241

Variation:

- Crab bite with the fingernails of your index finger and thumb. As intensely painful as this is to you and me, keep in mind that it might be ineffective on some people numbed by intoxicants. (Fig. 356)

Back of Thigh Pinch

Let's say you're again trying to get an unwanted person through a doorway, but this time you don't have a control hold on him. Of course this is never a good idea, but for any number of reasons, including that you simply messed up, that is the situation and now he has braced both hands against the door frame.

- Before he has time to do anything else, press your palm on the back of his head and grab a wad of flesh on his upper thigh just under his butt cheek. Pinch with your thumb and index finger or the tips of all five fingers. (Fig. 357)
- Pinch hard and push his head hard until you get him through the doorway. (Fig. 358)

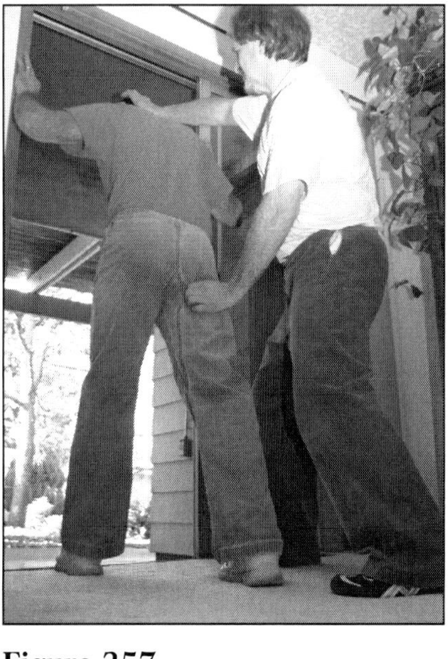

Figure 357 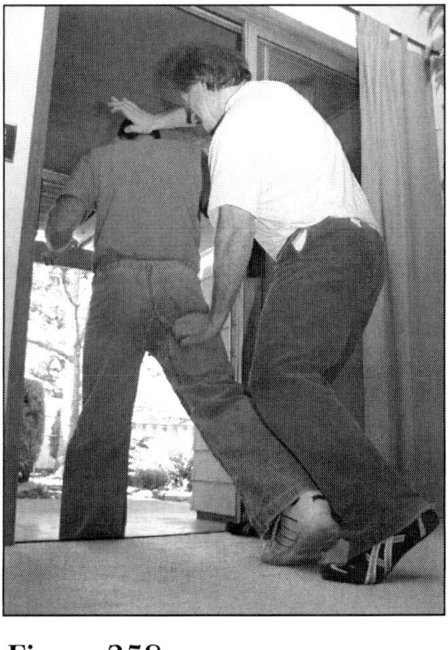   Figure 358

Variation:

- Grab his forearm as you pinch his upper leg with a five-fingered claw. (Figs. 359, 360)

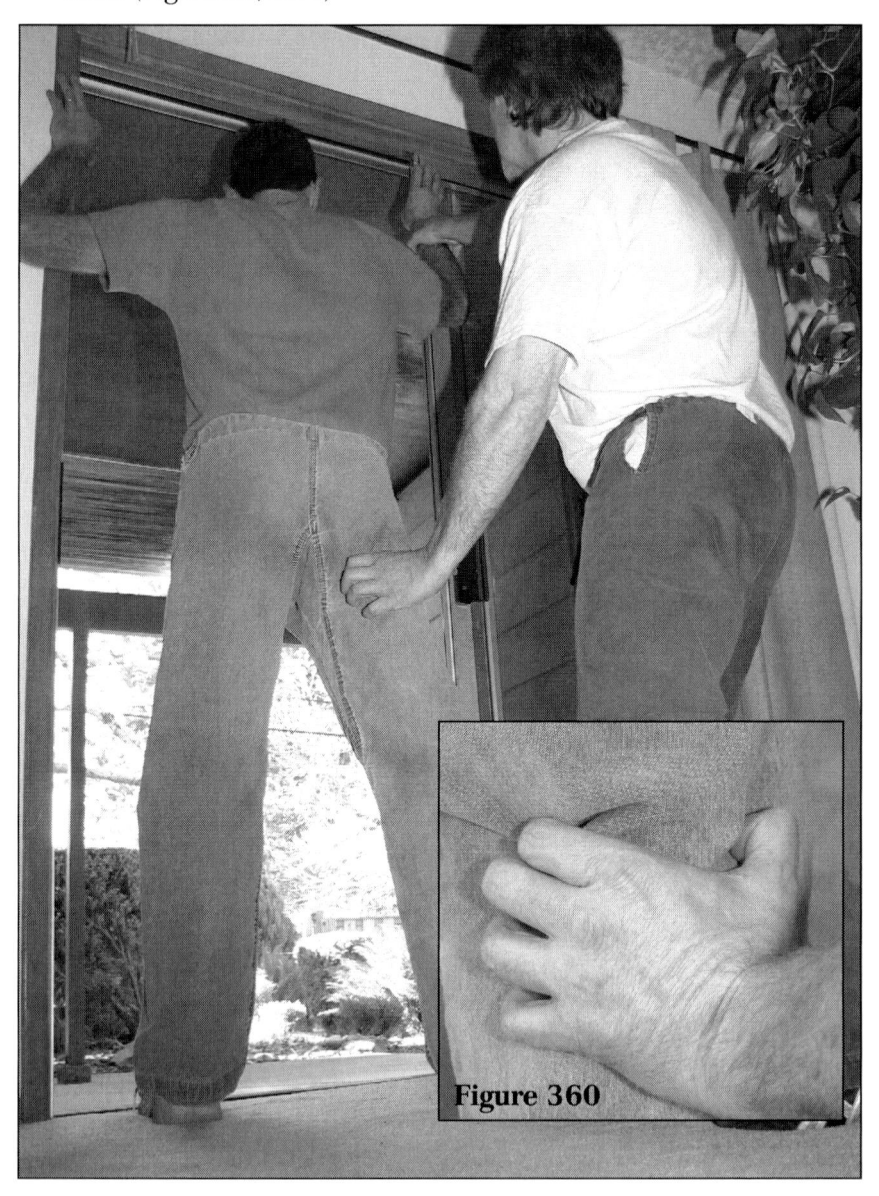

Figure 359

Figure 360

Legs 243

- When he yelps and releases his hold on the jamb, jerk his arm behind his back as you push him through the door. Immediately apply a wristlock of your choice. (Fig. 361)

Note: This is by no means a de-escalation technique. He will likely be quite angry after getting pinched, but at least you got him through the door.

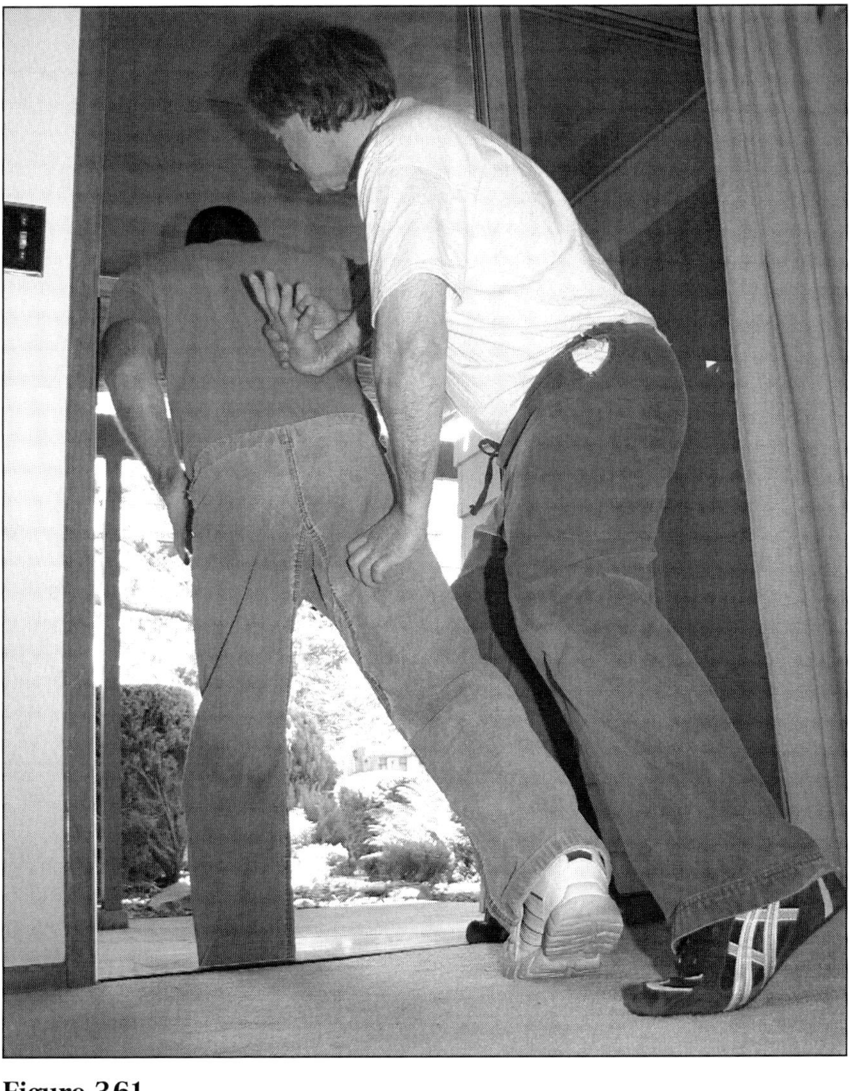

Figure 361

Back of Thigh Press

Most people squeal like a stuck pig when this press is done on them. I'm sure there are some who can tolerate it, but I'm guessing they are few in number.

You and your attacker have crashed to the floor, with you on top of the back of his legs.

- You try for a leglock but he jerks away, knocking you off balance. (Fig. 362)
- Land with the point of your elbow in the hamstring muscles of one of his legs. If you can't land elbow first, press your elbow into the muscles as quickly as you can. (Fig. 363)

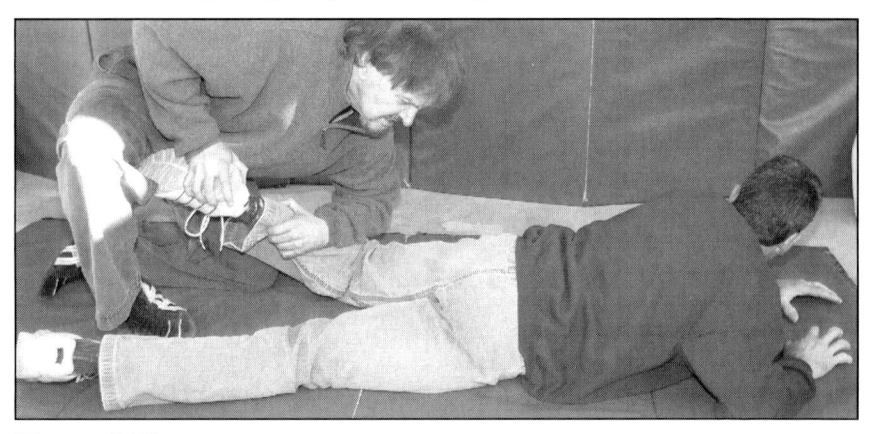

Figure 362

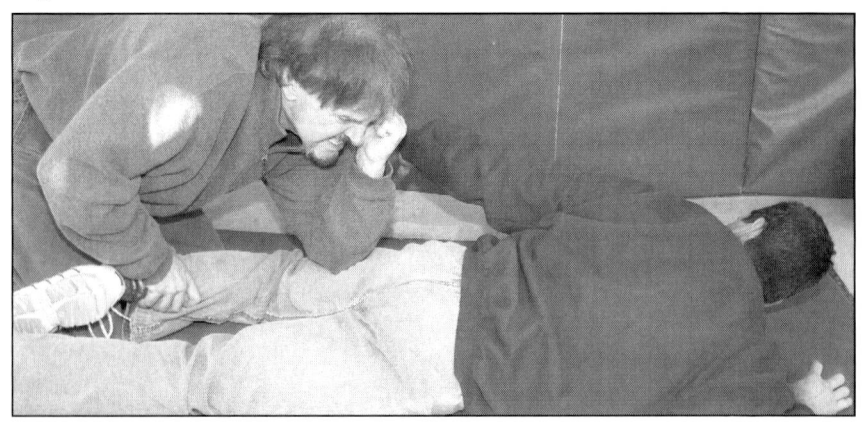

Figure 363

Legs 245

- Use this as a transition and distraction as you move up his back to secure an arm. He might even unintentionally help you out by reaching back to push you off his leg, inadvertently presenting his arm for an easy grab. (Fig. 364)
- Apply an arm hold. (Fig. 365)

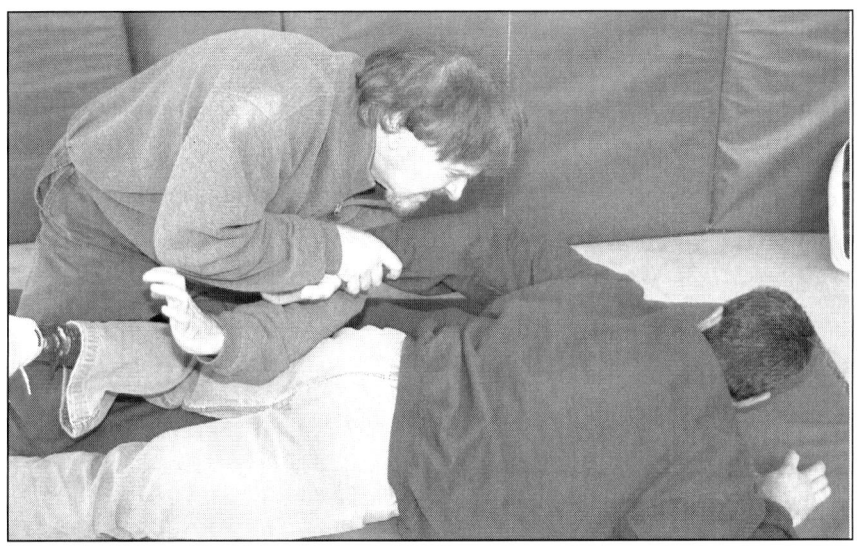

Figure 364

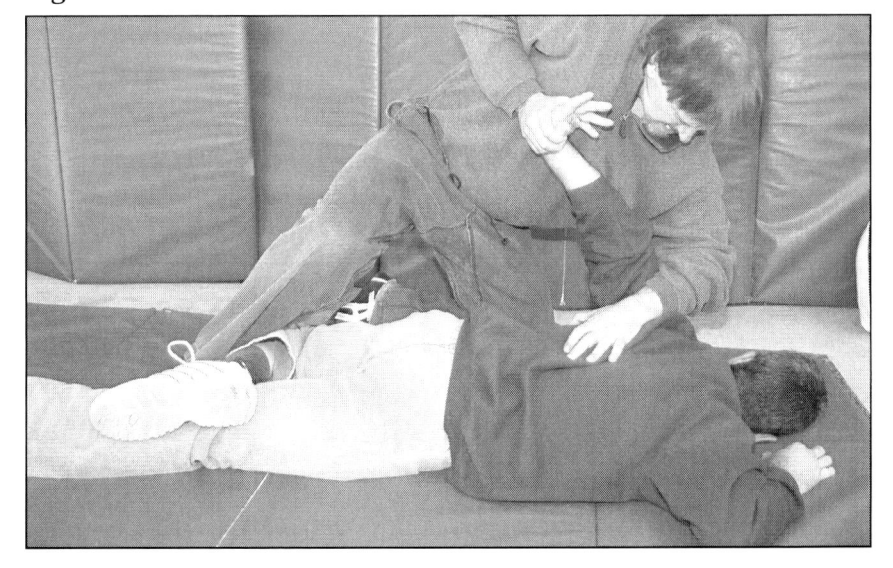

Figure 365

Inner Thigh Press

This isn't a fight stopper, but it's a good distraction device.
You and your attacker have crashed to the floor; he landed on his back and you fell between his legs.

- He grabs at your hair, shoulders, or arms in an attempt to hit you or apply a hold. (Fig. 366)
- Press your knee and as much weight as you can into his inner thigh. Wiggle and dig your knee into the meat to underscore the pain. (Fig. 367)
- When your attacker reacts, break free of his hold and counter with a blow. (Fig. 368)

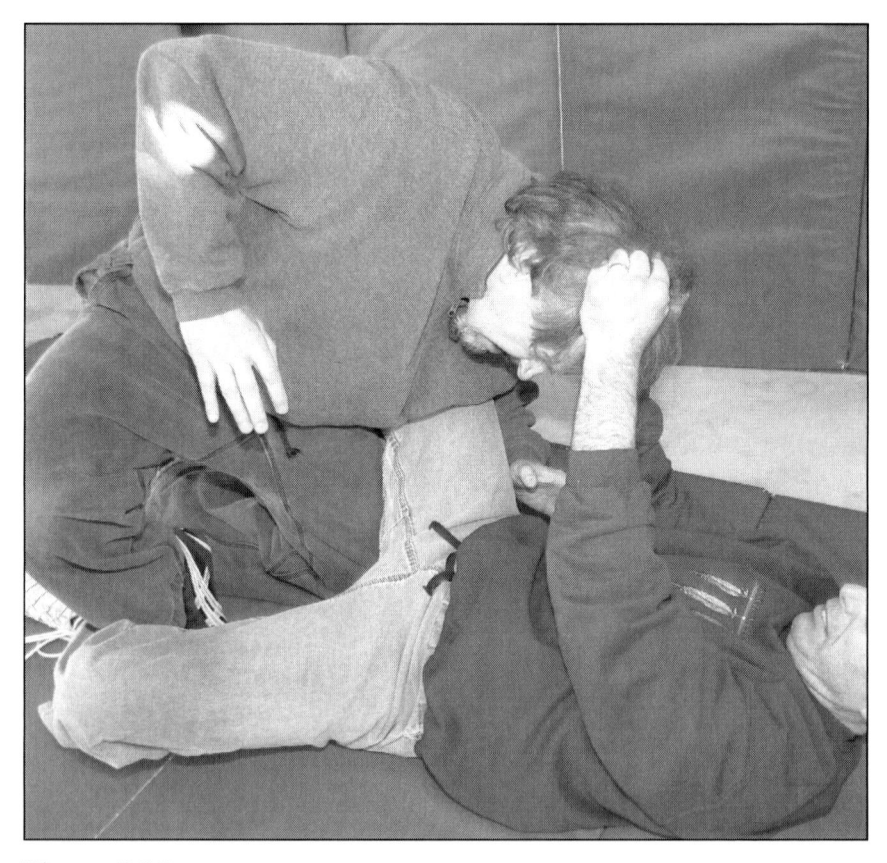

Figure 366

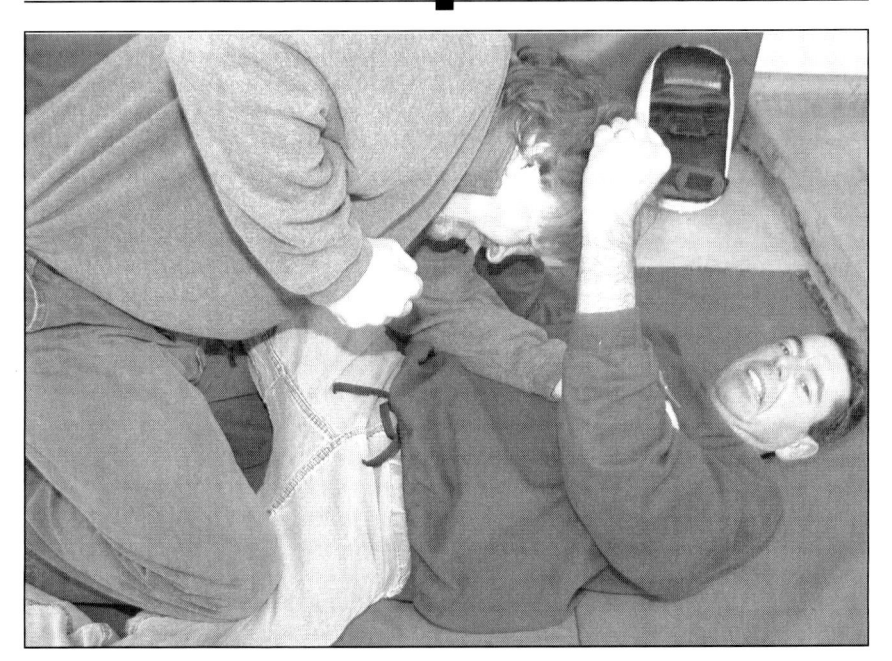

Figure 367

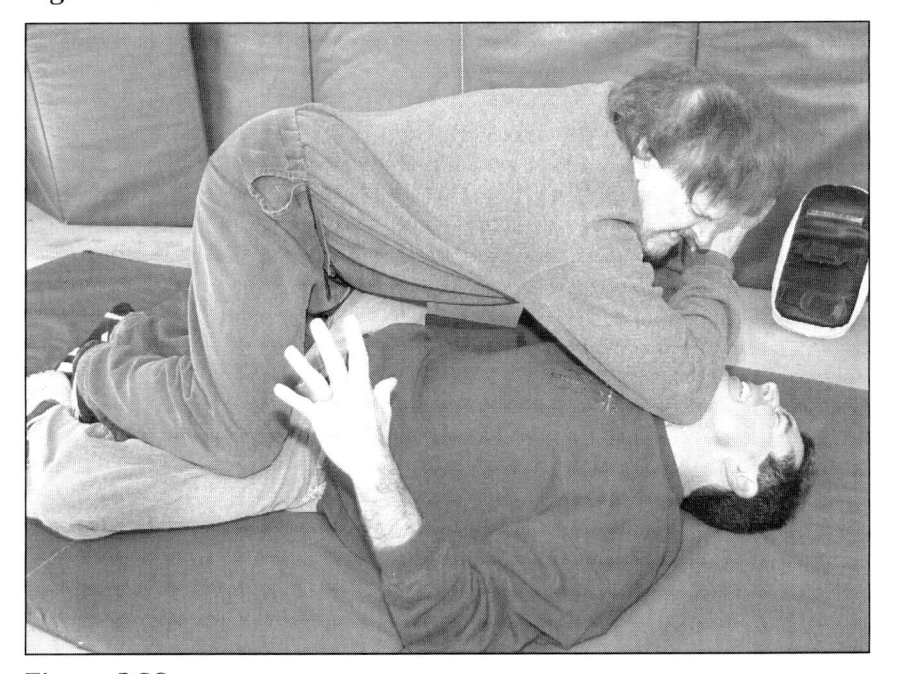

Figure 368

Variation:

- As he tries to pull you, press the point of your elbow into his inner thigh. Wiggle and dig it into his inner thigh. (Fig. 369)
- Escape or slam an elbow into his groin. (Fig. 370)

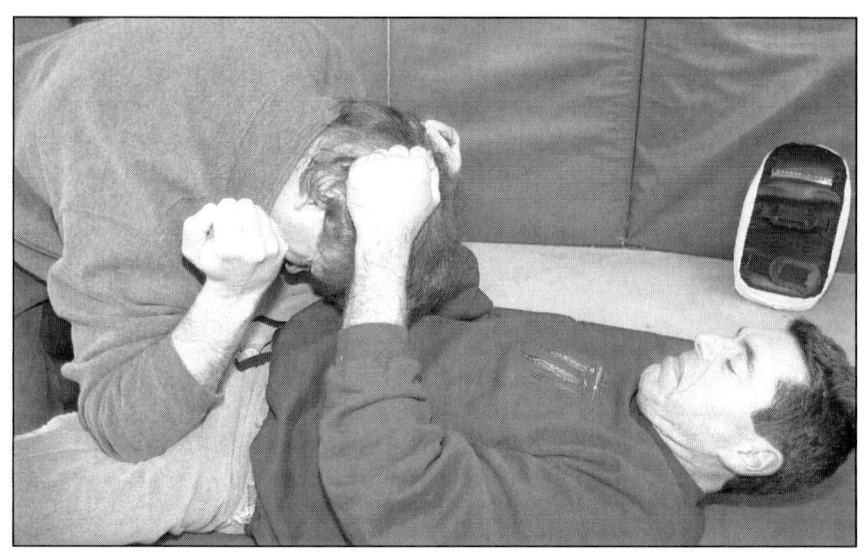

Figure 369

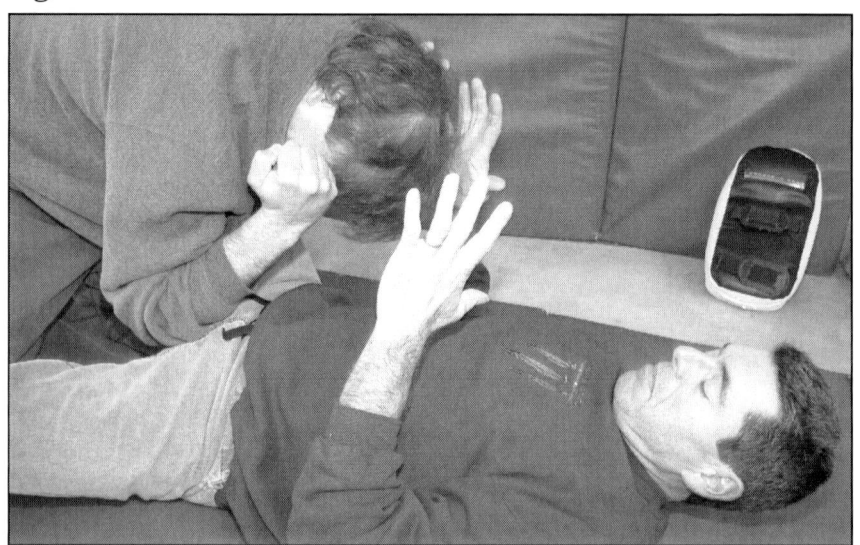

Figure 370

Legs 249

■

Calf Press with Baton or Similar Object

The following calf presses are good techniques for law enforcement or any time two people need to control a violent person. You can press one or both legs.

When his legs are flat:

- As your partner controls the attacker's upper half with an arm bar, you control the lower half with a stick or police baton. Place the object on the widest part of his calves and lean your weight on them. (Fig. 371)
- Don't have a baton? Use a 2 x 4 as shown here. (Fig. 372)

When his leg is bent:

- As your partner controls the attacker's upper half with an arm bar, you control the lower half with a stick or police baton. You have

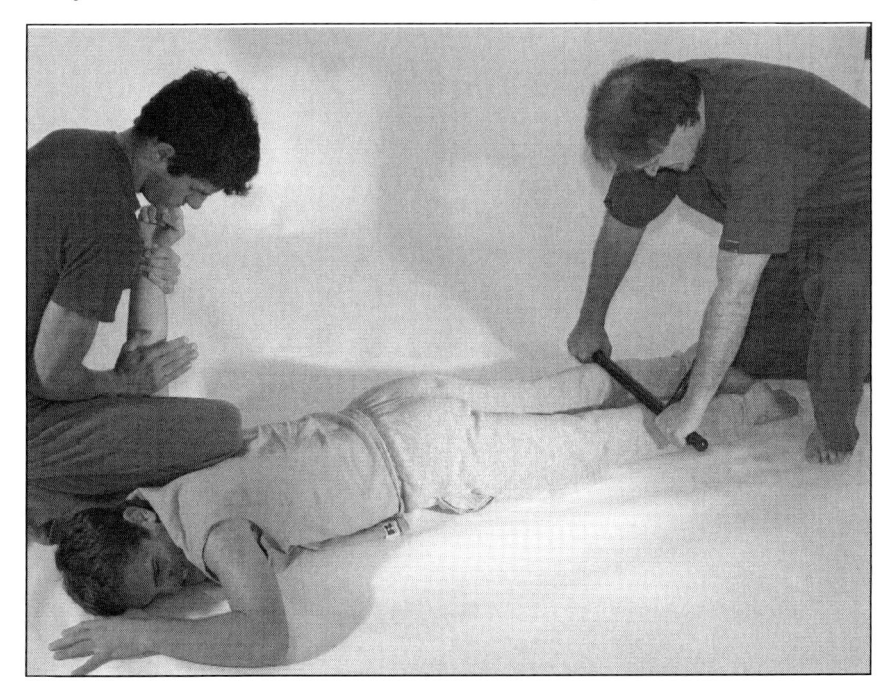

Figure 371

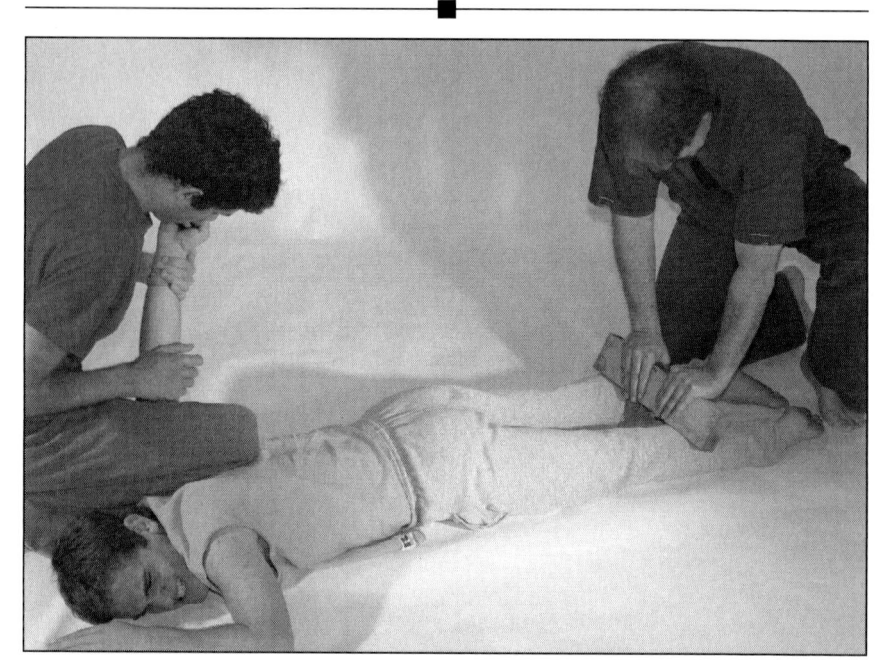

Figure 372

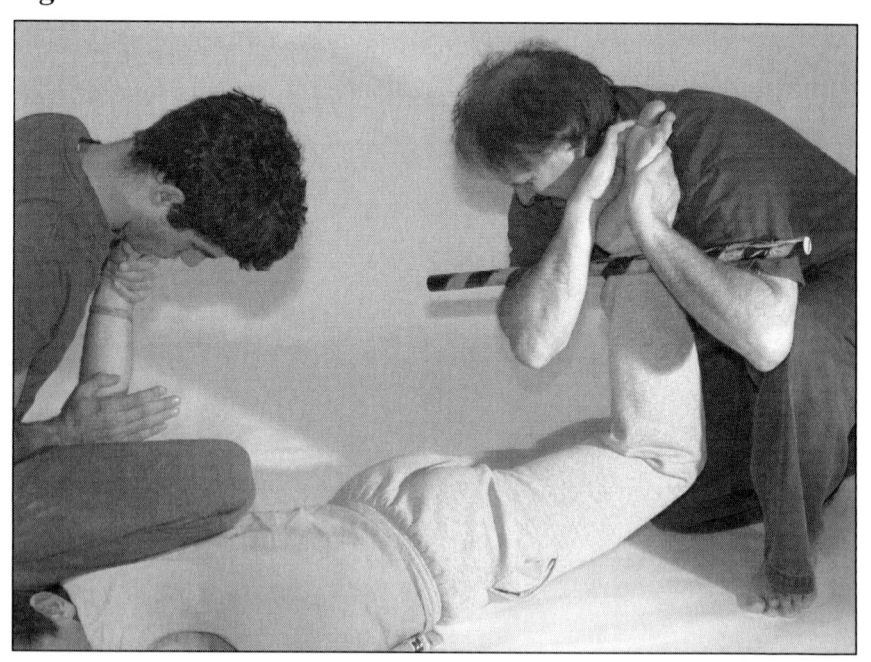

Figure 373

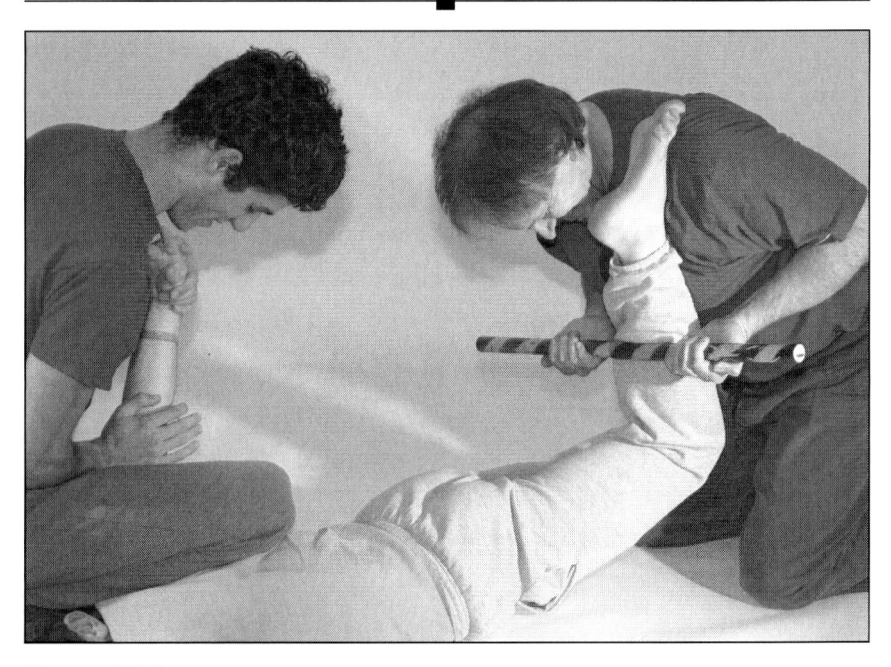

Figure 374

trapped one bent leg against your chest. Place the stick or police baton against his calf and trap the stick in the crooks of your arm. Use your hands to push his leg against the hard object. (Fig. 373)
- If your stick is too short to capture in the crooks of your arms, pull back on the ends of the stick instead. (Fig. 374)

Calf Press with Forearm When Attacker is Face Down on the Floor

This is a good alternative for the last technique when there is no stick or baton available. As your partner controls the attacker's upper half with an arm bar, you control the lower half with a naked arm press as his shin rests against your chest.

- Press your forearm into his calf muscle and pull it back with your other hand. Rotate it back and forth an inch or two in each direction to aggravate the nerves. (Fig. 375)

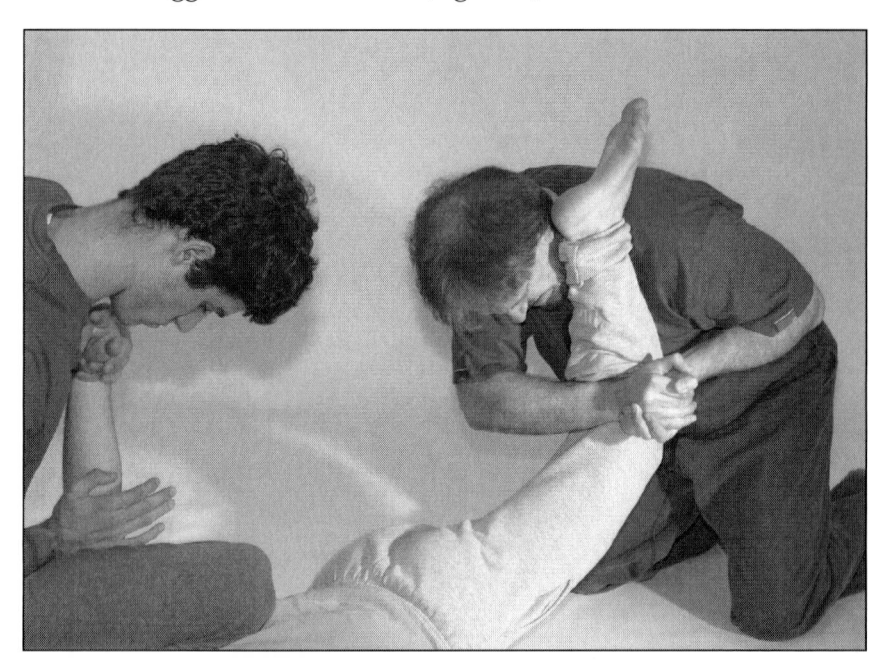

Figure 375

Legs 253

Calf Press Into a Curb

You and your partner have taken an attacker down onto his back with his legs draping over the edge of a curb. You could pull him away, but you opt to use the hard cement against him.

- As your partner applies a control hold on an arm . . . (Fig. 376)
- . . . lean on his shins to press his calf muscles into the edge of the curb. (Fig. 377)

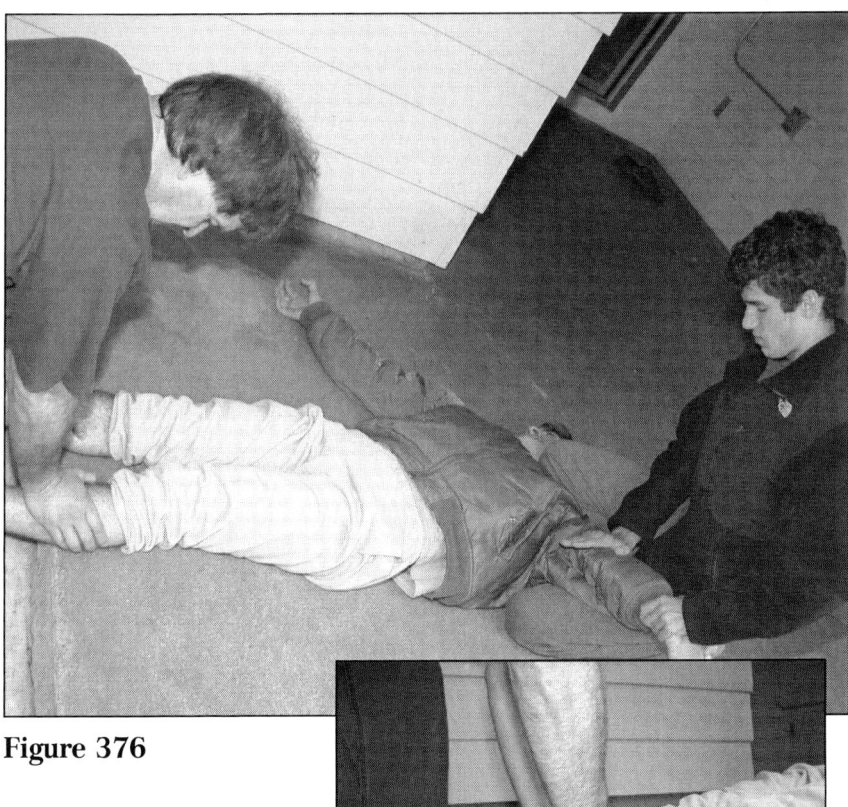

Figure 376

Figure 377

Calf Press with Elbow

This hurts like the dickens, but it's hard to apply and there are few situations in which to apply it. When you can work it in, most people react with a yelp and will do anything you say as long as you don't press.

You and your partner have taken the attacker down onto his belly.

- Before your partner can secure an armlock and you can control his lower limbs, the man begins scooting his legs to get up. (Fig. 378)
- Secure his ankle and control his other leg. Place your elbow midway between his foot and knee, between his shinbone and calf muscle, and lean your weight into a press. (Figs. 379, 380)
- The pain in the attacker's calf muscle will distract him from resisting your partner so that the arm hold can be reestablished as you transition into a leg hold. (Figs. 381, 382)

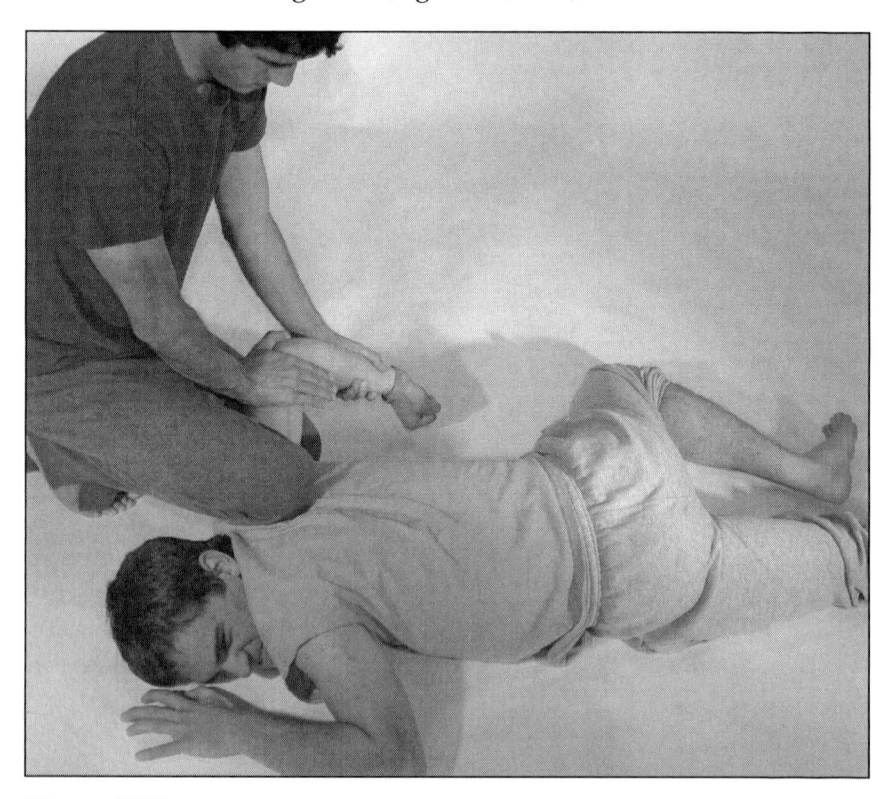

Figure 378

Legs

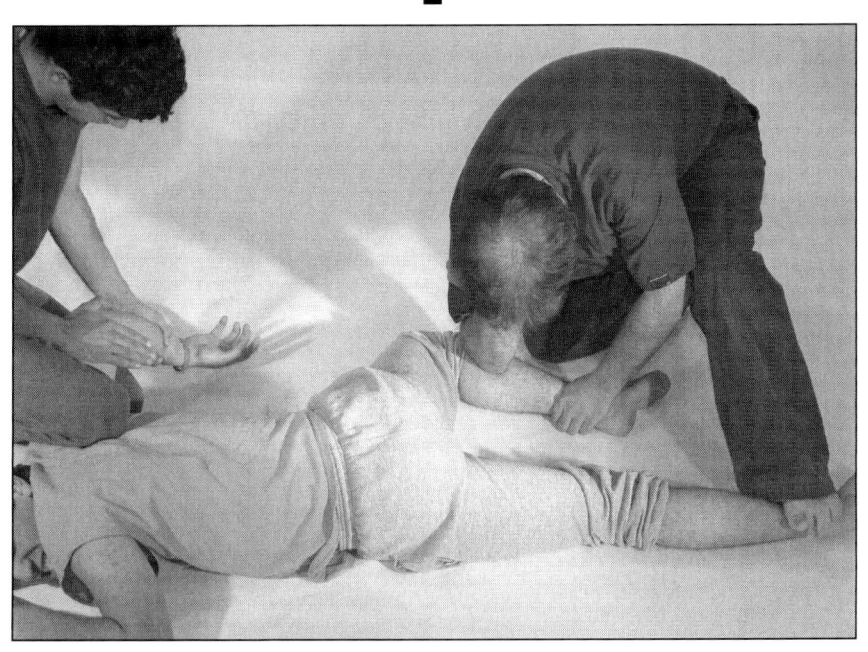

Figure 379

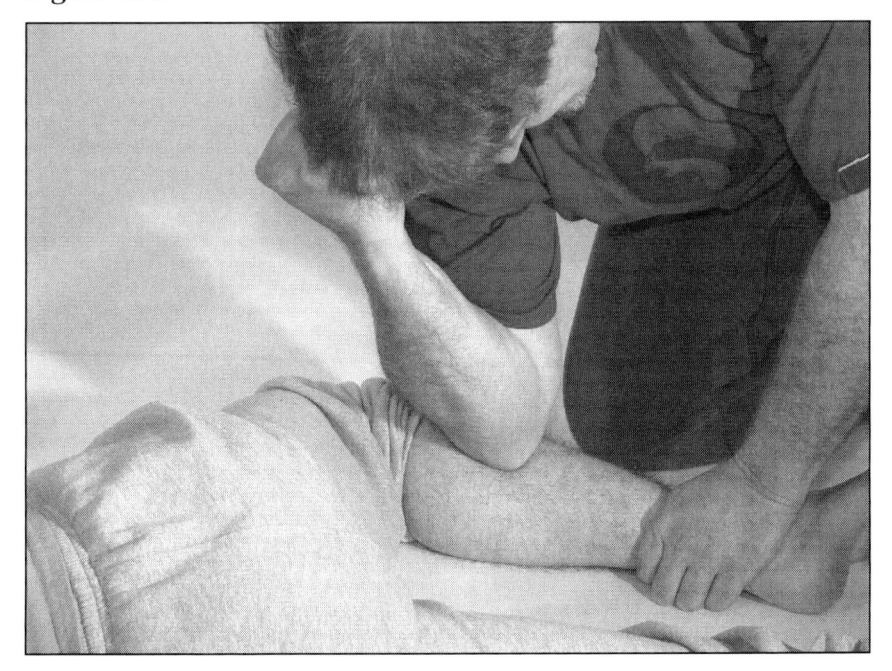

Figure 380

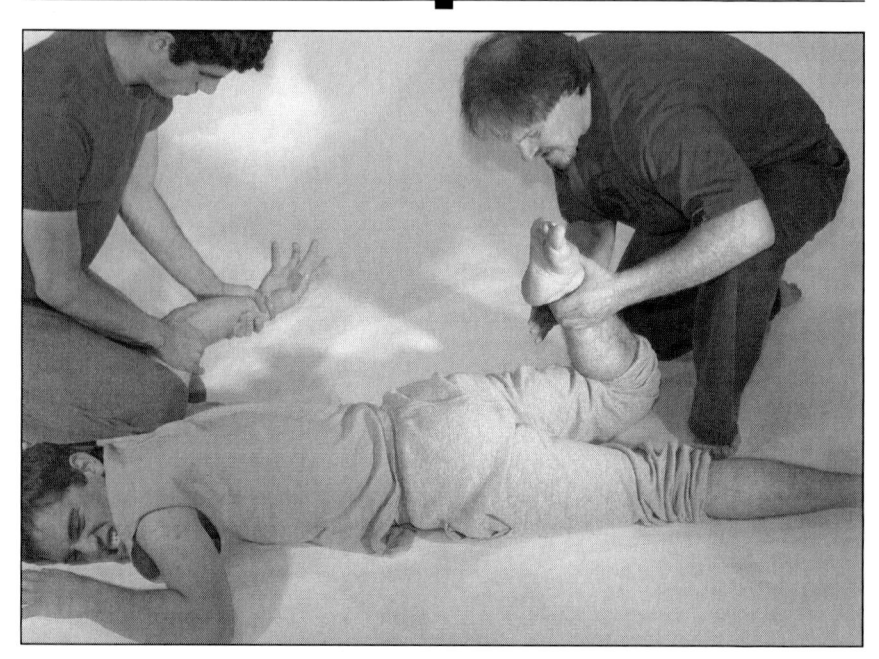

Figure 381

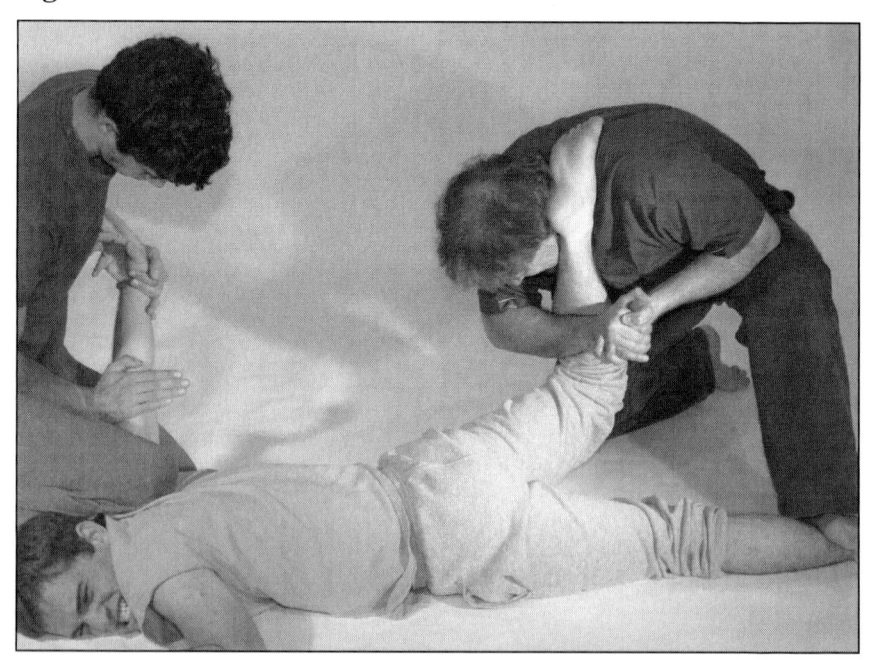

Figure 382

Legs

Calf Press with Your Leg

Since the knee has a broad, blunt surface, some attackers won't feel its press as intensely as they do your pointy elbow or a baton. Even if they don't feel any pain at all, it's still a good restraint hold.

As your partner controls the attacker's upper half, you control his lower with one of these variations of calf pain/restraint.

Variation 1:

- Apply pressure with your knee to his calf. Move your knee back and forth an inch or two in each direction to rub in the pain. (Fig. 383)

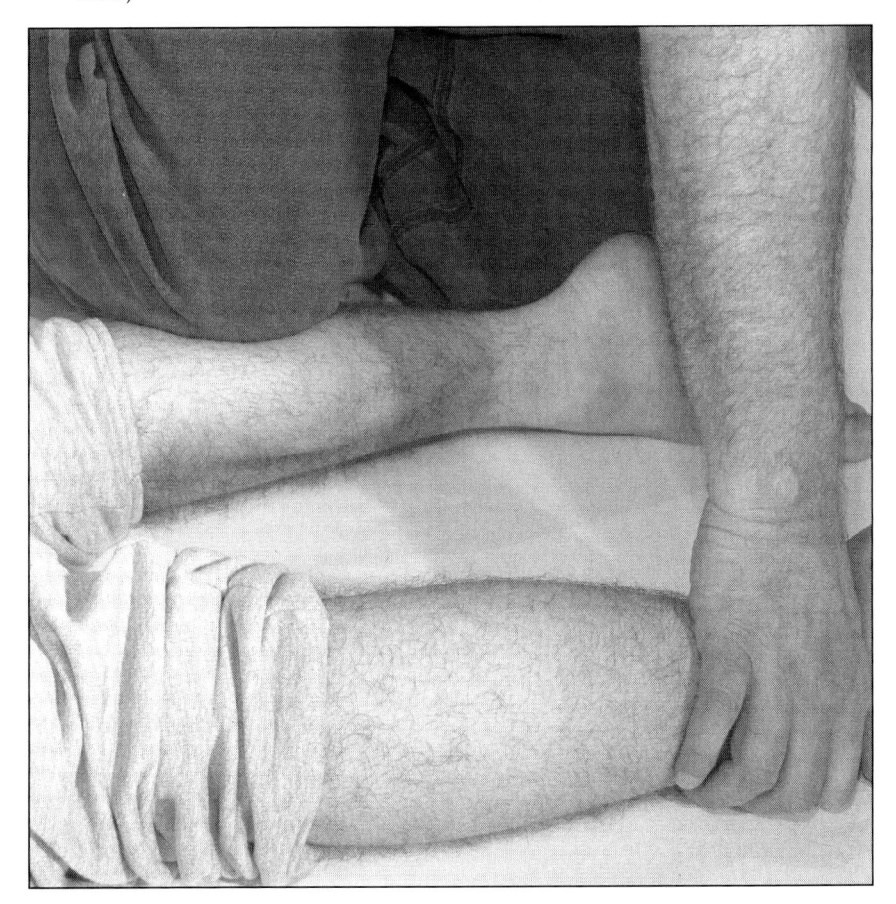

Figure 383

Variation 2:

- Place your shin, or both shins, across one or both of his calves. Press down on the widest part of his calf and then saw your shins back and forth two or three inches in both directions. (Fig. 384)

Variation 3:

- Place your shin or knee on one calf and use the point of your elbow to press into his other calf. Hold his ankle to stabilize his leg. (Fig. 385)

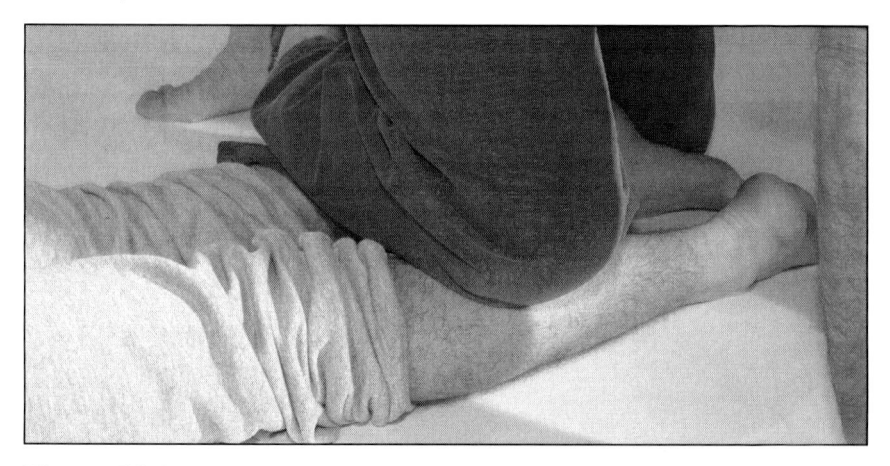

Figure 384

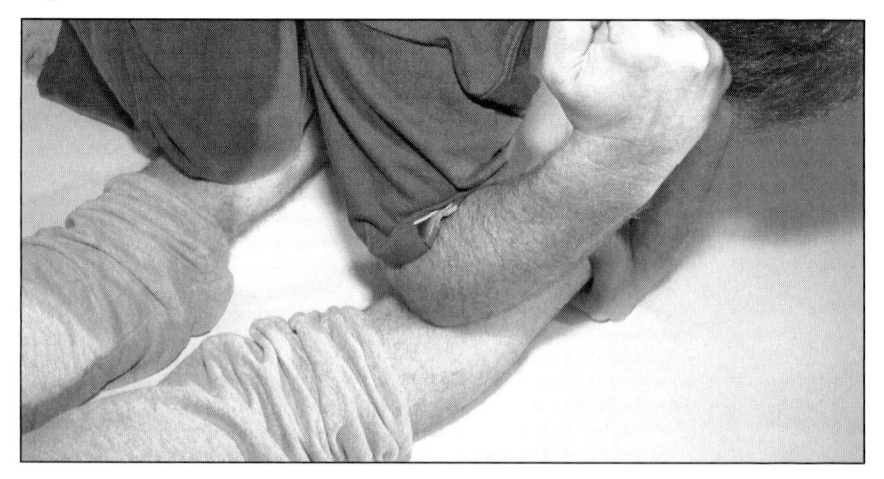

Figure 385

Shin Press with Baton or Board

This is more painful than it looks. The attacker is on his back and your partner is trying to control his upper half.

- Press a baton or board into his shins to restrain his legs. Lean your weight into it.
- Saw the object back and forth a little to dig the press into the nerves. This will distract him enough to allow your partner to apply a hold. When he stops resisting, maintain the hold on his legs to keep restraining him but reward him by reducing the pressure. Should he start to get combative, lean your weight quickly into his shins. (Fig. 386)

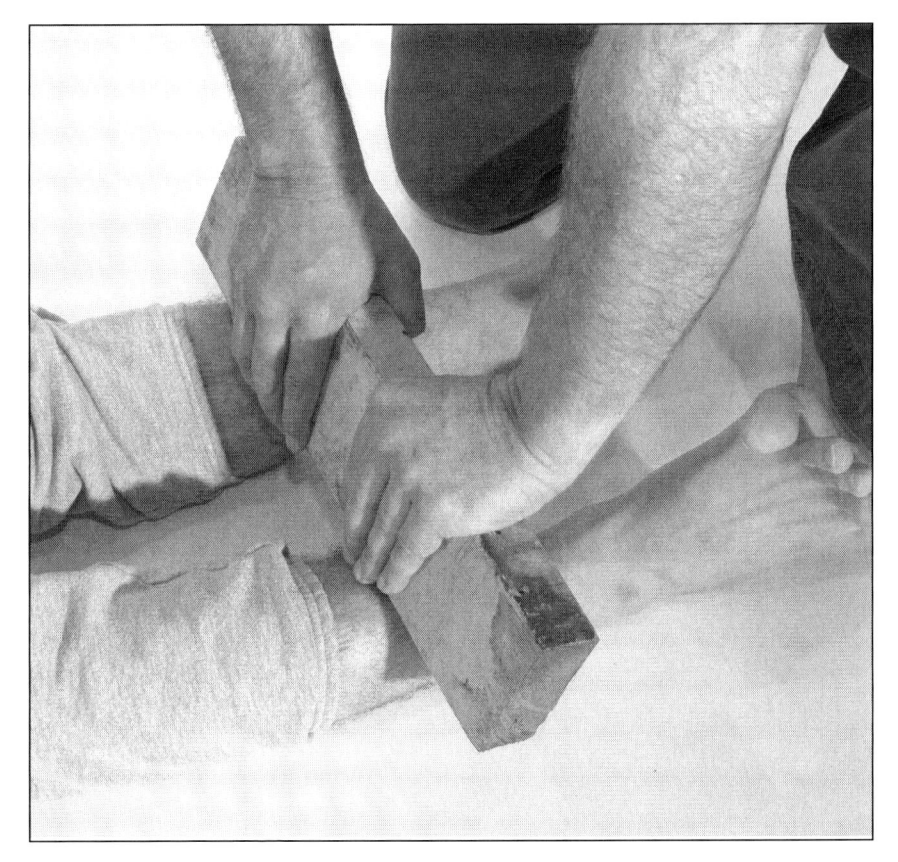

Figure 386

Shin Press into Curb

You don't need to press hard with this to cause excruciating pain and skin abrasion.

- The attacker is on his stomach with one or both legs extended over a curb or step. (Fig. 387)
- As your partner applies an arm restraint hold to control his upper body, you control his lower half by pressing one or both of his shins into the edge of the cement step. (Fig. 388)
- To add even more pain, scoot his legs back and forth in a sawing motion an inch or so in each direction. Expect bloody abrasions. (Fig. 389)

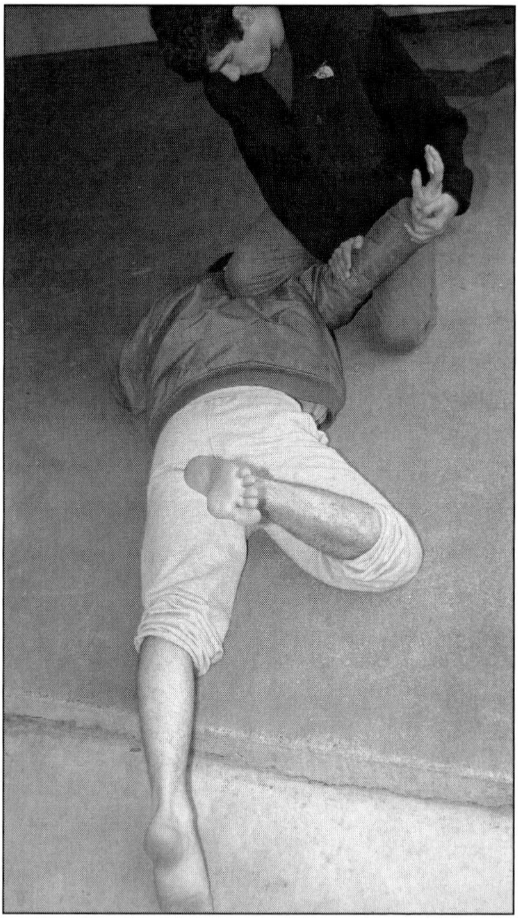

Figure 387

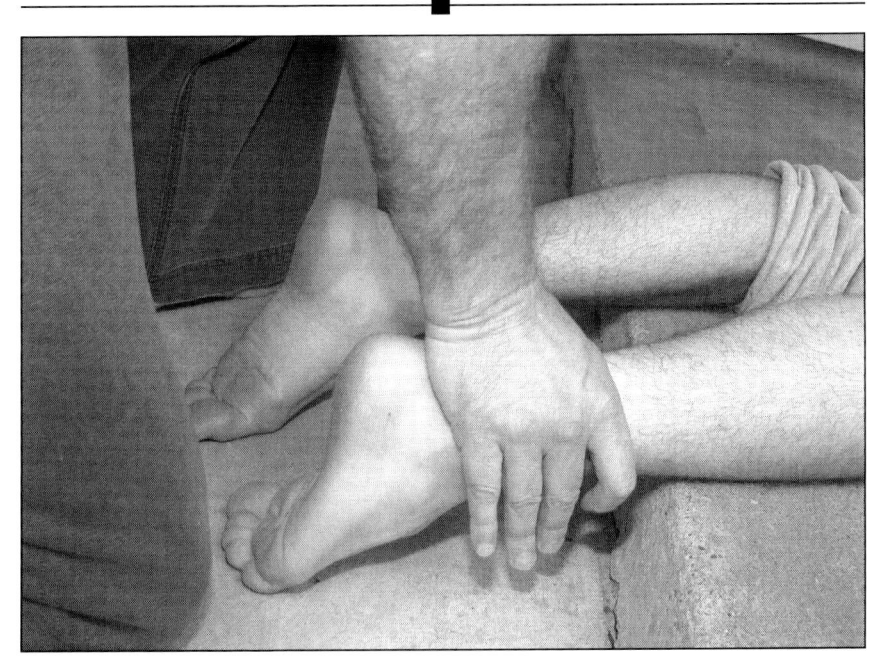

Figure 388

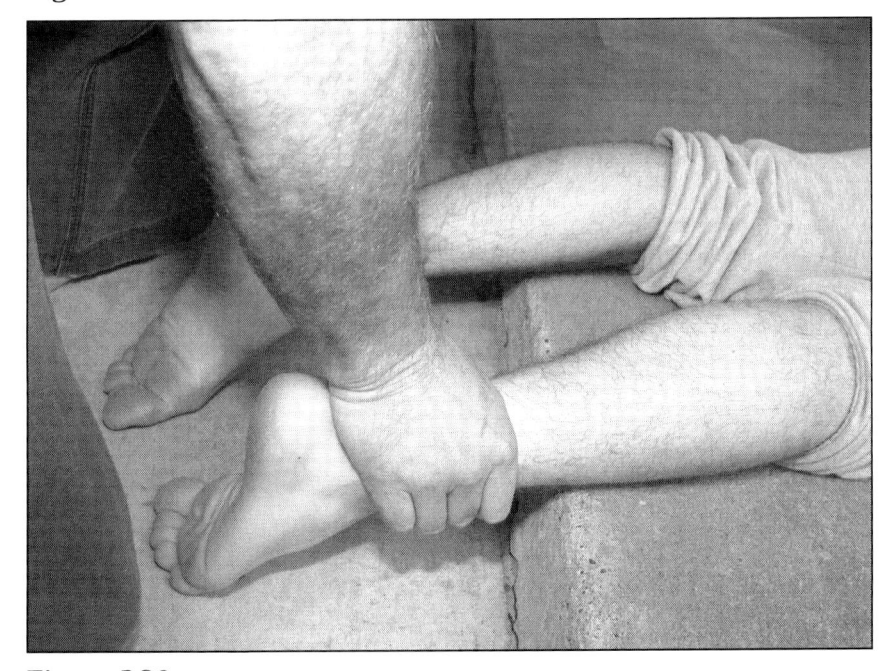

Figure 389

7
Feet

"With the thumb of your left hand, hook the most available toe and rip it outward."

Although we have all had our toes crunched agonizingly and we have all banged the tops of our feet painfully into something hard, most martial artists rarely consider them as targets. You should, though. While pressing and ripping the feet aren't as showy as drilling someone in the head with a kick, they can be distracting and debilitating. The feet are loaded with places to apply pain, from the tender toes, to the vulnerable fine bones on the top of the feet, to the highly vulnerable Achilles tendon.

Foot Press and Twist

This works great when your attacker is barefoot, it works good when he is wearing a soft athletic shoe, dress loafer, or regular shoestring shoe, and it works poorly or not at all when he is wearing heavy boots. The technique requires three elements from you: your body weight, a hard twist of your foot, and a powerful launching action off the ball of your foot. The entire move takes only a fraction of a second.

Your attacker has stepped nearly in range as he talks trash and threatens you. Your hands are up in an I-don't-want-to-fight stance.

- He jabs his fingers at you threateningly. (Fig. 390)
- Don't wait for him to attack. Stomp forward onto his foot near his ankle with as much weight as possible while still maintaining your balance, and thrust your palms against whatever is closest: his arms, chest, or shoulders. (Fig. 391)

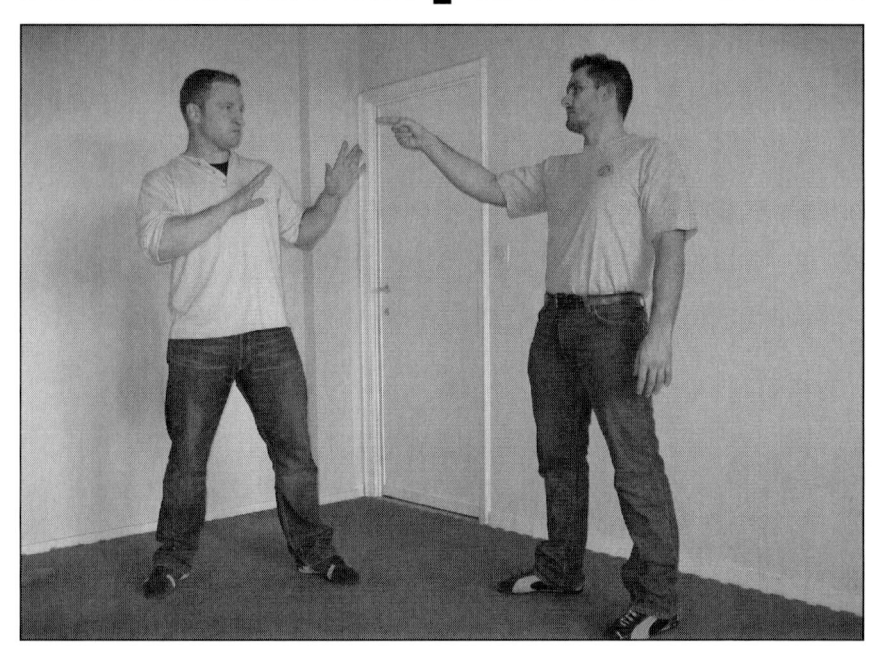

Figure 390

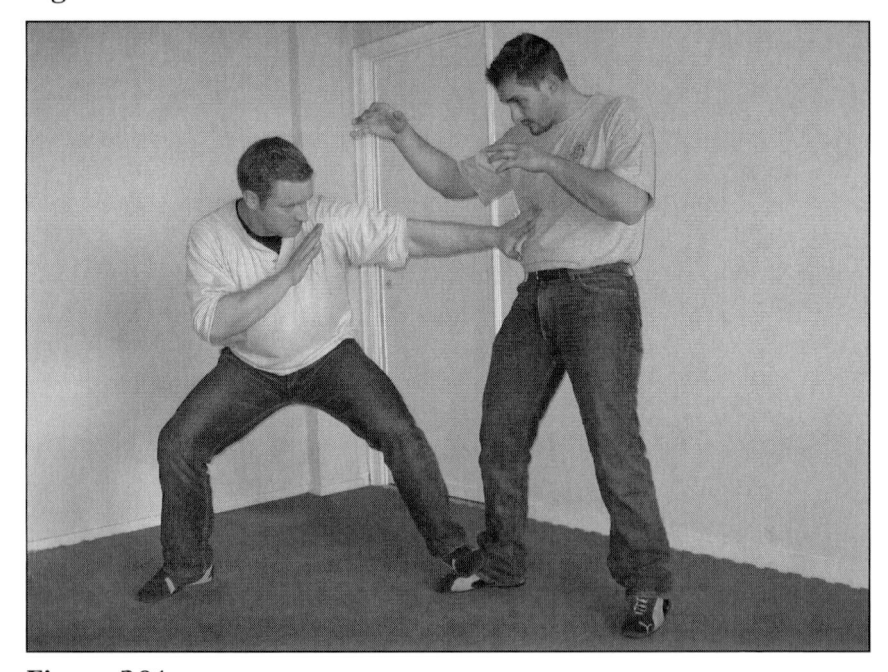

Figure 391

- Forcefully press your weight down onto his foot and twist/grind yours as you turn away from him slightly, still keeping your eyes on him. (Fig. 392)
- Push off his foot and step back a few feet, or run away. (Fig. 393)

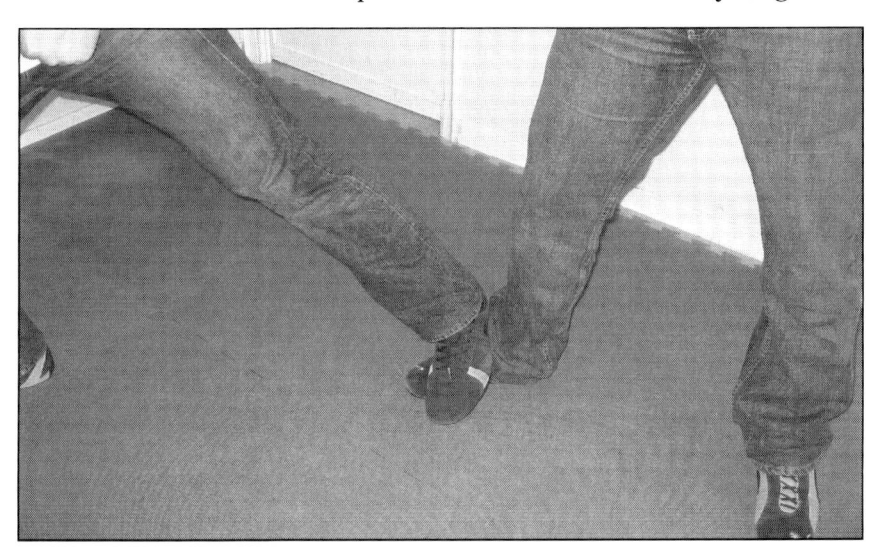

Figure 392

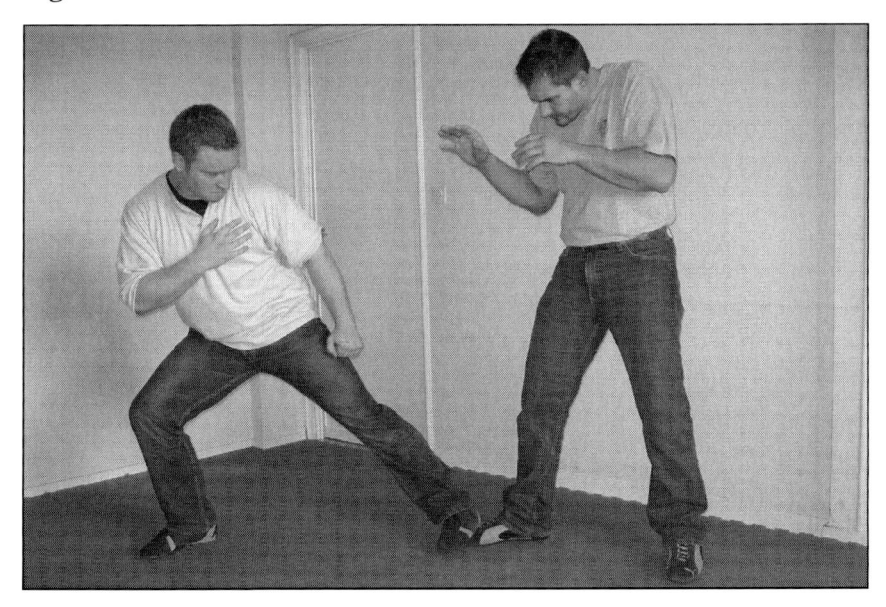

Figure 393

Variation:

- Same set up as above, but target the toes. (Fig. 394)

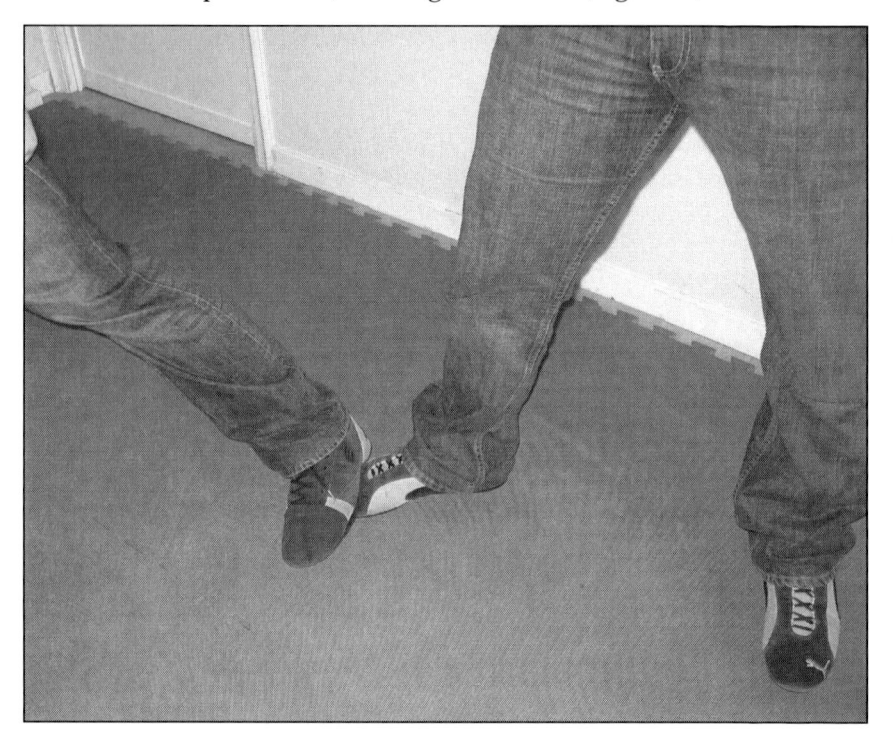

Figure 394

Knee Press

This works best against bare feet or soft athletic shoes.

You have slipped, tripped, or been knocked down onto your knees. Your attacker moves into range to finish you.

- Block his punch. (Fig. 395)
- Drop a knee down onto his foot—toes, top of foot, or instep—and press down with as much weight as you can as you drive your fist into his groin. (Fig. 396)
- Grab behind his knees and pull them toward you as your push his middle with your head. (Fig. 397)

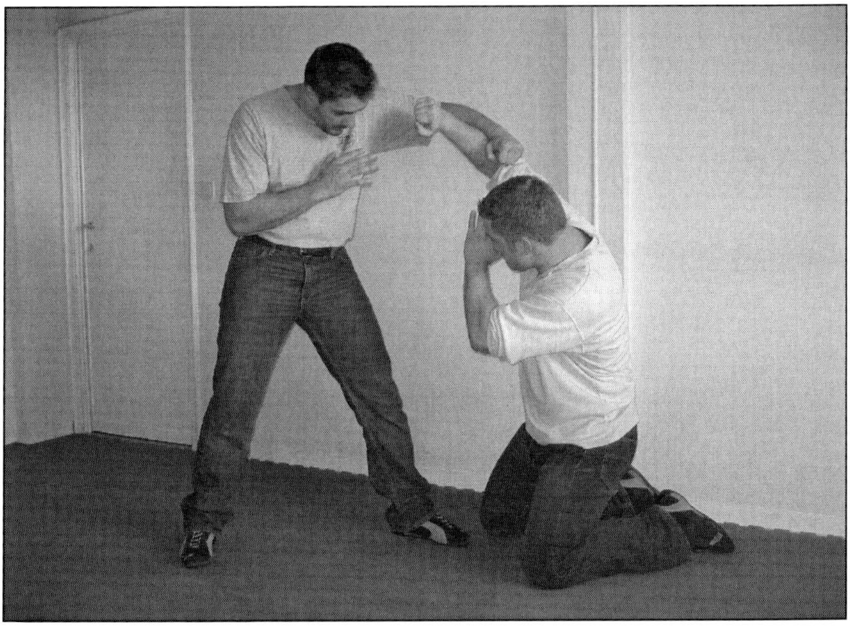

Feet 267

Figure 395

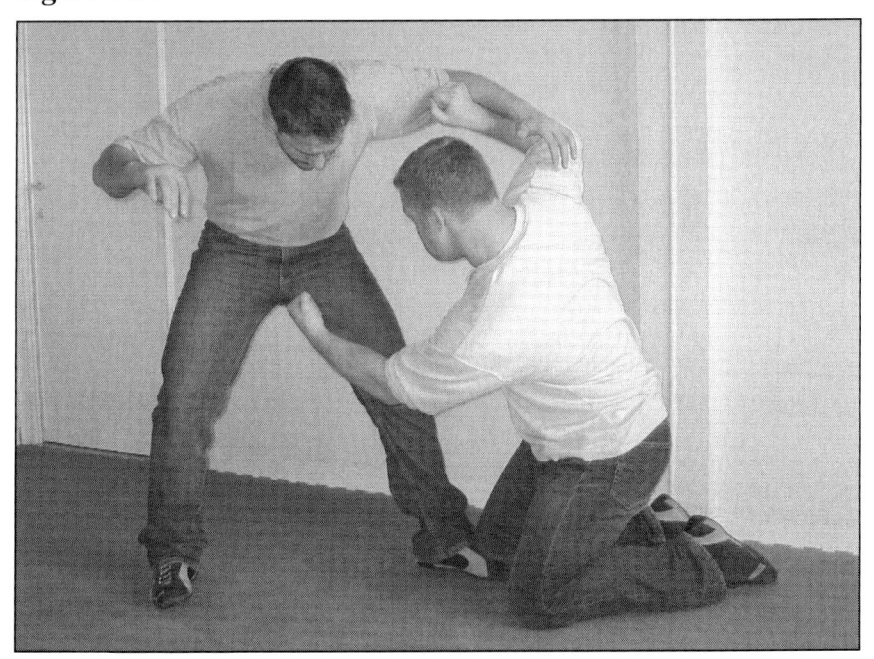

Figure 396

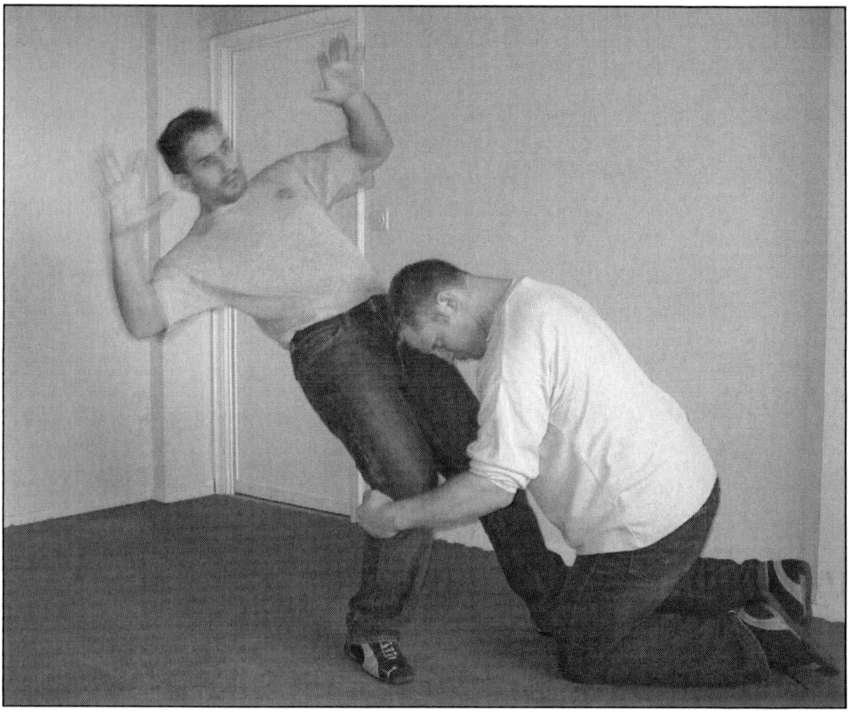

Figure 397

Toe Rip

Your attacker must be barefoot for this one. Use it on the local beach bully.

- You have caught your attacker's right kick with your right hand (though it doesn't matter which arm you use). (Fig. 398)
- Jerk his leg up a little to force him to think about his balance rather than about hitting you. (Fig. 399)
- With the thumb of your left hand, hook the most available toe and rip it outward. (Fig. 400)
- Palm him in the face with the same hand. (Fig. 401)

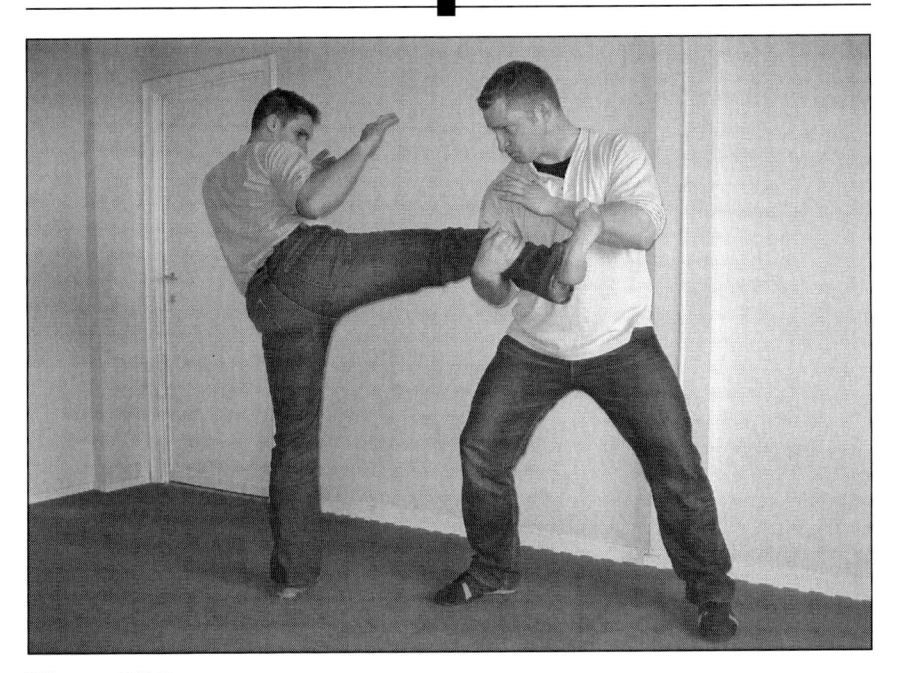

Figure 398

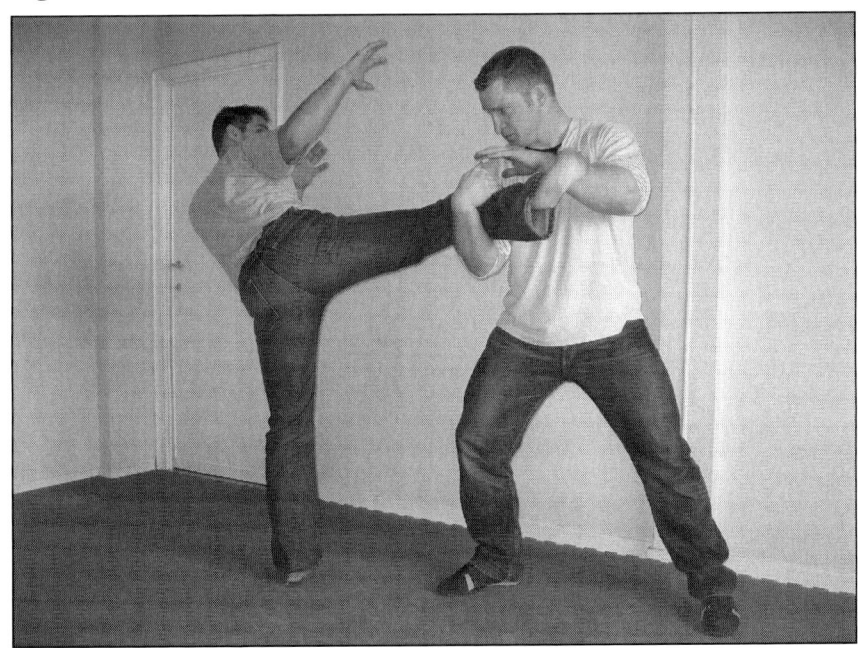

Figure 399

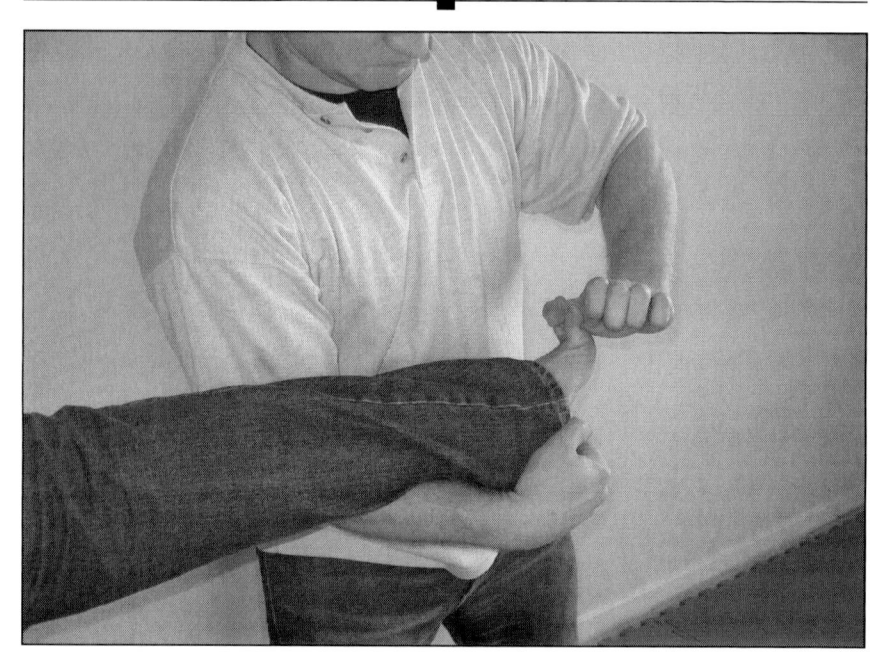

Figure 400

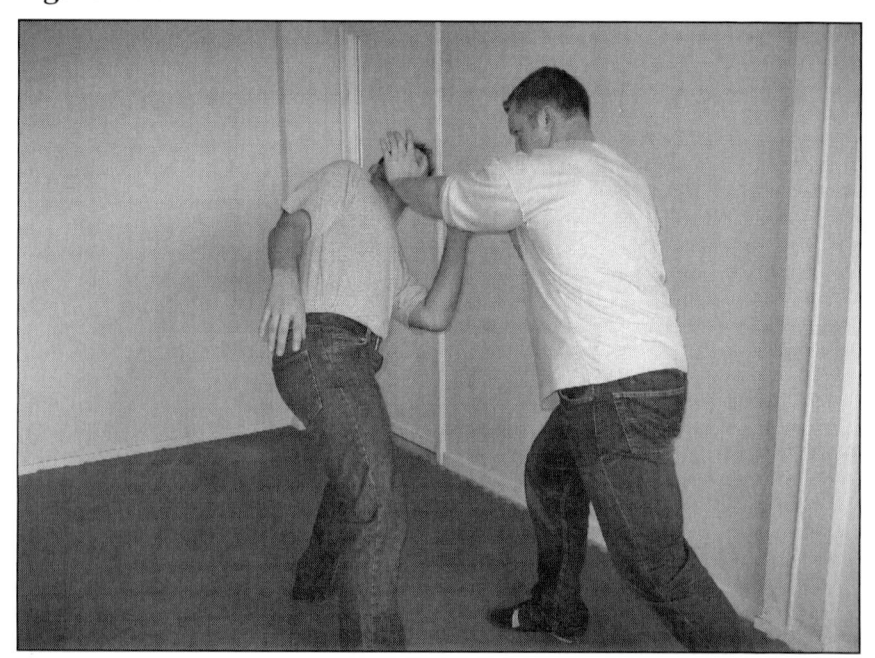

Figure 401

Feet

Achilles Press with Baton or Board

The attacker is prone and your partner is trying to control his top half.

- To restrain his legs, press a baton or board into his tender Achilles tendon. Saw it back and forth an inch or two in each direction to dig into the nerves. (Fig. 402)

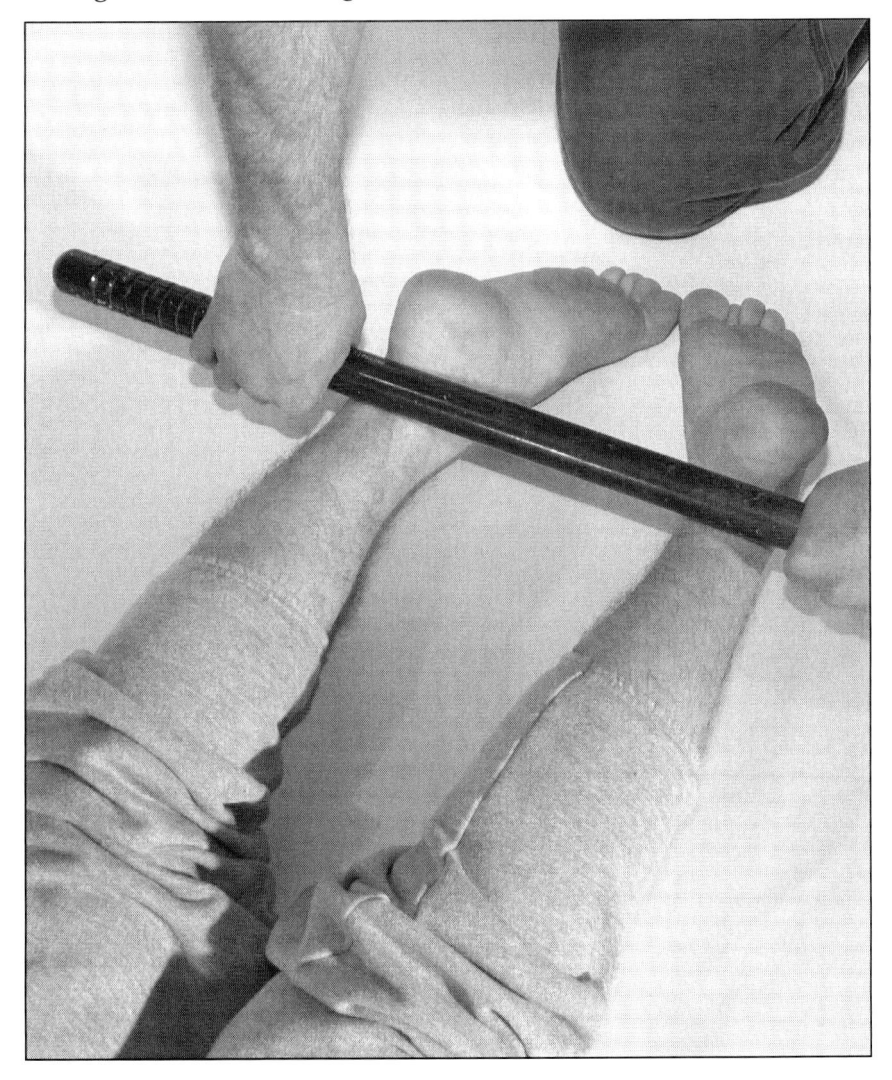

Figure 402

A Concluding Comment

Perhaps before reading this book you thought a pinch was just a pinch and a finger flick was something you did to a crumb on a tabletop. I hope you now see that a simple pinch can change the entire outcome of a fight and that a finger flick to an attacker's eye will make him long for those agony-free moments just before he decided to pick on you.

Ripping, poking, pinching, twisting, and pressing are important combat techniques that deserve an important place in your repertoire right alongside your backfists and sidekicks. Fighting successfully is about taking advantage of windows of opportunity. Sometimes a window opens wide for a big kick and sometimes it opens a crack, just enough to slip in a claw to rip at tender flesh. I encourage you to add these techniques to your repertoire and practice them often so that they are there for you when that window opens.

The goal in any fight is to survive and to go home in one piece. Whether you go home for tea or to the emergency room for bandages might very well depend on a rip, a poke, a pinch, a twist, or a press.

Train hard.

Loren W. Christensen
www.lwcbooks.com

About the Author

Loren W. Christensen is a retired police officer, Vietnam veteran, high-ranking martial artist, and prolific writer. Loren began training in the fighting arts in 1965 and over the years has earned a total of 10 black belts: seven in karate, two in jujitsu, and one in arnis. He lives in Portland, Oregon, where he writes full time and teaches martial arts.